T0195419

Lung Cancer

Editors

SARAH B. GOLDBERG
ROY S. HERBST

HEMATOLOGY/ONCOLOGY CLINICS OF NORTH AMERICA

www.hemonc.theclinics.com

Consulting Editors
GEORGE P. CANELLOS
EDWARD J. BENZ JR.

June 2023 • Volume 37 • Number 3

ELSEVIER

1600 John F. Kennedy Boulevard • Suite 1800 • Philadelphia, Pennsylvania, 19103-2899

http://www.theclinics.com

HEMATOLOGY/ONCOLOGY CLINICS OF NORTH AMERICA Volume 37, Number 3
June 2023 ISSN 0889-8588, ISBN 13: 978-0-443-18306-5

Editor: Stacy Eastman
Developmental Editor: Ann Gielou M. Posedio

Hematology/Oncology Clinics (ISSN 0889-8588) is published bimonthly by Elsevier Inc., 360 Park Avenue South, New York, NY 10010-1710. Months of issue are February, April, June, August, October, and December. Business and Editorial Offices: 1600 John F. Kennedy Blvd., Ste. 1800, Philadelphia, PA 19103−2899. Customer Service Office: 3251 Riverport Lane, Maryland Heights, MO 63043. Periodicals postage paid at New York, NY and at additional mailing offices. Subscription prices are $470.00 per year (domestic individuals), $1190.00 per year (domestic institutions), $100.00 per year (domestic students/residents), $495.00 per year (Canadian individuals), $100.00 per year (Canadian students/residents), $1232.00 per year (Canadian institutions) $563.00 per year (international individuals), $1232.00 per year (international institutions), and $255.00 per year (international students/residents). International air speed delivery is included in all *Clinics* subscription prices. All prices are subject to change without notice. **POSTMASTER:** Send address changes to *Hematology/Oncology Clinics of North America*, Elsevier Health Sciences Division, Subscription Customer Service, 3251 Riverport Lane, Maryland Heights, MO 63043. Customer Service (orders, claims, online, change of address): Elsevier Health Sciences Division, Subscription **Customer Service, 3251 Riverport Lane, Maryland Heights, MO 63043. Tel: 1-800-654-2452 (U.S. and Canada); 314-447-8871 (outside U.S. and Canada). Fax: 314-447-8029. E-mail: journalscustomerservice-usa@elsevier.com (for print support); journalsonlinesupport-usa@elsevier.com (for online support).**

Reprints. For copies of 100 or more, of articles in this publication, please contact the Commercial Reprints Department, Elsevier Inc., 360 Park Avenue South, New York, New York 10010-1710; Tel.: 212-633-3874, Fax: 212-633-3820, E-mail: reprints@elsevier.com.

Hematology/Oncology Clinics of North America is covered in *MEDLINE/PubMed (Index Medicus), EMBASE/ Excerpta Medica, and BIOSIS.*

Contributors

CONSULTING EDITORS

GEORGE P. CANELLOS, MD
William Rosenberg Professor of Medicine, Department of Medical Oncology, Dana-Farber Cancer Institute, Boston, Massachusetts, USA

EDWARD J. BENZ Jr, MD
President and CEO Emeritus, Dana-Farber Cancer Institute, Director Emeritus, Dana-Farber/Harvard Cancer Center, Richard and Susan Smith Distinguished Professor of Medicine, Professor of Pediatrics, Professor of Genetics, Harvard Medical School, Boston, Massachusetts, USA

EDITORS

SARAH B. GOLDBERG, MD, MPH
Associate Professor of Medicine (Medical Oncology), Yale School of Medicine, New Haven, Connecticut, USA

ROY S. HERBST, MD, PhD
Professor of Medicine (Medical Oncology), Yale School of Medicine, New Haven, Connecticut, USA

AUTHORS

EBAA AL-OBEIDI, MD
Division of Hematology-Oncology, University of California, Davis, Sacramento, California, USA

PATRICK BEAGEN, MD
Department of Radiation Oncology, University of California, Davis Comprehensive Cancer Center, Sacramento, California, USA

SHREYA BELLAMPALLI, BS
Medical Scientist Training Program, Mayo Clinic Alix School of Medicine, Mayo Clinic, Rochester, Minnesota, USA

JUSTIN D. BLASBERG, MD
Division of Thoracic Surgery, Yale New Haven Hospital, Yale School of Medicine, New Haven, Connecticut, USA

GEORGE N. BOTROS
Department of Radiation Oncology, Rutgers Cancer Institute of New Jersey, Rutgers Robert Wood Johnson Medical School, Rutgers University, New Brunswick, New Jersey, USA

ELLIOTT BREA, MD, PhD
Department of Medical Oncology, Dana-Farber Cancer Institute, Boston, Massachusetts, USA

ANNE CHIANG, MD, PhD
Associate Professor of Medicine (Medical Oncology), Yale School of Medicine, New Haven, Connecticut, USA

ALISSA J. COOPER, MD
Clinical Fellow in Hematology/Oncology, Massachusetts General Hospital Cancer Center, Harvard Medical School, Boston, Massachusetts, USA

SANJA DACIC, MD, PhD
Professor, Department of Pathology, Yale School of Medicine, New Haven, Connecticut, USA

MEGAN E. DALY, MD
Department of Radiation Oncology, University of California, Davis Comprehensive Cancer Center, Sacramento, California, USA

MATTHEW P. DEEK, MD
Department of Radiation Oncology, Rutgers Cancer Institute of New Jersey, Rutgers Robert Wood Johnson Medical School, Rutgers University, New Brunswick, New Jersey, USA

DAVID R. GANDARA, MD
Division of Hematology-Oncology, University of California, Davis, Sacramento, California, USA

SCOTT GETTINGER, MD
Professor of Medicine, Chief of Thoracic Oncology, Department of Internal Medicine, Yale Cancer Center, Yale School of Medicine, New Haven, Connecticut, USA

SARAH B. GOLDBERG, MD, MPH
Associate Professor of Medicine (Medical Oncology), Yale School of Medicine, New Haven, Connecticut, USA

MICHAEL J. GRANT, MD
Assistant Professor of Medicine (Medical Oncology), Yale School of Medicine, New Haven, Connecticut, USA

MISSAK HAIGENTZ, MD
Division of Thoracic Oncology, Rutgers Cancer Institute of New Jersey, Rutgers Robert Wood Johnson Medical School, Rutgers University, New Brunswick, New Jersey, USA

REBECCA S. HEIST, MD, MPH
Associate Professor of Medicine, Massachusetts General Hospital Cancer Center, Harvard Medical School, Boston, Massachusetts, USA

SALMA K. JABBOUR, MD
Department of Radiation Oncology, Rutgers Cancer Institute of New Jersey, Rutgers Robert Wood Johnson Medical School, Rutgers University, New Brunswick, New Jersey, USA

JULIA JOSEPH, MD
Yale Internal Medicine-Traditional Residency Program, Department of Internal Medicine, Yale School of Medicine, Yale University, New Haven, Connecticut, USA

JENNIFER KAPO, MD
Associate Professor, Department of General Internal Medicine, Yale School of Medicine, Yale University, New Haven, Connecticut, USA

SO YEON KIM, MD
Assistant Professor of Medicine (Medical Oncology), Yale School of Medicine, New Haven, Connecticut, USA

IAONNIS KONTOPIDIS, MD
Department of Surgery, Robert Wood Johnson University Hospital, Rutgers Robert Wood Johnson Medical School, New Brunswick, New Jersey, USA

JOHN LANGENFELD, MD
Division of Thoracic Oncology, Rutgers Cancer Institute of New Jersey, Rutgers Robert Wood Johnson Medical School, Rutgers University, New Brunswick, New Jersey, USA

MOHAMMAD H. MADANI, MD
Department of Radiology, University of California, Davis, Sacramento, California, USA

UMBERTO MALAPELLE, PhD
Department of Public Health, University of Naples Federico II, Naples, Italy

ROBERT MATERA, MD
Clinical Fellow in Hematology/Oncology, Yale New Haven Hospital, Yale School of Medicine, New Haven, Connecticut, USA

MADISON NOVOSEL, BA
Chronic Disease Epidemiology, Yale School of Public Health, Yale University, New Haven, Connecticut, USA

SARAH OH, PharmD
Department of Radiation Oncology, Rutgers Cancer Institute of New Jersey, Rutgers Robert Wood Johnson Medical School, Rutgers University, New Brunswick, New Jersey, USA

ESHAN PATEL, MD
Division of Medical Oncology, Rutgers Cancer Institute of New Jersey, New Brunswick, New Jersey, USA

MILAN PATEL
Department of Radiation Oncology, Rutgers Cancer Institute of New Jersey, Rutgers Robert Wood Johnson Medical School, Rutgers University, New Brunswick, New Jersey, USA

ELIZABETH PRSIC, MD
Assistant Professor of Medicine (Medical Oncology), Yale School of Medicine, New Haven, Connecticut, USA

JONATHAN W. RIESS, MD
Division of Hematology-Oncology, University of California, Davis, Sacramento, California, USA

CHRISTIAN ROLFO, MD, PhD, MBA
Center for Thoracic Oncology at the Tisch Cancer Institute, Icahn School of Medicine at Mount Sinai, New York, New York, USA

JULIA ROTOW, MD
Dana-Farber Cancer Institute, Boston, Massachusetts, USA

BROOKS V. UDELSMAN, MD, MHS
Division of Thoracic Surgery, Yale New Haven Hospital, Yale School of Medicine, New Haven, Connecticut, USA

GAVITT A. WOODARD, MD
Yale Cancer Center, Department of Surgery, Yale School of Medicine, New Haven, Connecticut, USA

JOHNATHAN YAO, MD
Yale Internal Medicine-Traditional Residency Program, Department of Internal Medicine, Yale School of Medicine, Yale University, New Haven, Connecticut, USA

Contents

Advances in the treatment of non-small cell lung carcinoma have resulted in improved histologic classification and the implementation of molecular testing for predictive biomarkers into the routine diagnostic workflow. Over the past decade, molecular testing has evolved from single-gene assays to high-thoroughput comprehensive next-generation sequencing. Economic barriers, suboptimal turnaround time to obtain the results, and limited tissue available for molecular assays resulted in adoption of liquid biopsies (ctDNA) into clinical practice. Multiplex immunohistochemical/immunofluorescence assays evaluating tumor microenvironment together with the AI approaches are anticipated to translate from research into clinical care.

This review article illuminates the role of liquid biopsy in the continuum of care for non-small cell lung cancer (NSCLC). We discuss its current application in advanced-stage NSCLC at the time of diagnosis and at progression. We highlight research showing that concurrent testing of blood and tissue yields faster, more informative, and cheaper answers than the standard stepwise approach. We also describe future applications for liquid biopsy including treatment response monitoring and testing for minimal residual disease. Lastly, we discuss the emerging role of liquid biopsy for screening and early detection.

Thoracic surgery for non–small cell lung cancer has evolved tremendously in the past two decades. Improvements have come on multiples fronts and include a transition to minimally invasive techniques, an incorporation of neoadjuvant treatment, and a greater utilization of sublobar resection. These advances have reduced the morbidity of thoracic surgery, while maintaining or improving long-term survival. This review highlights major advances in the surgical techniques of lung cancer and the keys to optimizing outcomes from a surgical perspective.

Video content accompanies this article at http://www.hemonc. theclinics.com.

Treatment options for medically inoperable, early-stage non-small cell lung cancer (NSCLC) include stereotactic ablative radiotherapy (SABR) and percutaneous image guided thermal ablation. SABR is delivered over 1-5 sessions of highly conformal ablative radiation with excellent tumor control. Toxicity is depending on tumor location and anatomy but is typically mild. Studies evaluating SABR in operable NSCLC are ongoing. Thermal ablation can be delivered via radiofrequency, microwave, or cryoablation, with promising results and modest toxicity. We review the data and outcomes for these approaches and discuss ongoing studies.

During the last 2 decades, the understanding of non-small cell lung cancer (NSCLC) has evolved from a purely histologic classification system to a more complex model synthesizing clinical, histologic, and molecular data. Biomarker-driven targeted therapies have been approved by the United States Food and Drug Administration for patients with metastatic NSCLC harboring specific driver alterations in EGFR, HER2, KRAS, BRAF, MET, ALK, ROS1, RET, and NTRK. Novel immuno-oncology agents have contributed to improvements in NSCLC-related survival at the population-level. However, only in recent years has this nuanced understanding of NSCLC permeated into the systemic management of patients with resectable tumors.

Consolidation immunotherapy after concurrent chemoradiation has improved five-year survival rates in unresectable, locally advanced lung cancer, but disease progression and treatment personalization remain challenges. New treatment approaches with concurrent immunotherapy and consolidative novel agents are being investigated and show promising efficacy data, but at the risk of additive toxicity. Patients with PD-L1 negative tumors, oncogenic driver mutations, intolerable toxicity, or limited performance status continue to require innovative therapies. This review summarizes historical data that galvanized new research efforts, as well as ongoing clinical trials that address the challenges of current therapeutic approaches for unresectable, locally advanced lung cancer.

Immunotherapy-based regimens are an established standard of care for the first-line treatment of driver-negative (EGFR/ALK/ROS WT) advanced non–small cell lung cancer. With multiple immune-based regimens approved in the first-line setting, clinicians are faced in practice with a variety of treatment choices. This article summarizes the most up-to-date trial data on treatments for driver-negative advanced non–small cell lung cancer, including immunotherapy monotherapy, chemoimmunotherapy, and combination immunotherapy, providing a framework for clinicians based on PD-L1 and smoking status. A multibiomarker assay that may best predict immunotherapy response remains an active area of research.

This article provides an updated review of the management of oncogene-driven non–small cell lung cancer. The use of targeted therapies for lung cancer driven by EGFR, ALK, ROS1, RET, NTRK, HER2, BRAF, MET, and KRAS are discussed, both in the first-line setting and in the setting of acquired resistance.

Small cell lung cancer (SCLC) is a rare yet aggressive lung cancer subtype with an extremely poor prognosis of around 1 year. SCLC accounts for 15% of all newly diagnosed lung cancers and is characterized by rapid growth with high potential for metastatic spread and treatment resistance. In the article the authors review some of the most notable efforts to improve outcomes, including trials of novel immunotherapy agents, novel disease targets, and multiple drug combinations.

Lung cancer carries significant mortality and morbidity. In addition to treatment advances, supportive care may provide significant benefit for patients and their caregivers. A multidisciplinary approach is critical in addressing complications of lung cancer, including disease- and treatment-related complications, oncologic emergencies, symptom management and supportive care, and addressing the psychosocial needs of affected patients.

Although lung cancer treatment has been transformed by the advent of checkpoint inhibitor immunotherapies, there remains a high unmet need for new effective therapies for patients with progressive disease. Novel treatment strategies include combination therapies with currently available programmed death ligand 1 inhibitors, targeting alternative immune checkpoints, and the use of novel immunomodulatory therapies. In addition, antibody-drug conjugates offer great promise as potent management options. As these agents are further tested in clinical trials, we anticipate that more effective therapies for patients with lung cancer are integrated into regular clinical practice.

Lung Cancer

HEMATOLOGY/ONCOLOGY CLINICS OF NORTH AMERICA

SERIES OF RELATED INTEREST

Surgical Oncology Clinics
https://www.surgonc.theclinics.com/
Advances in Oncology
https://www.advances-oncology.com/

THE CLINICS ARE AVAILABLE ONLINE!
Access your subscription at:
www.theclinics.com

Preface

Advances and Opportunities in the Management of Lung Cancer

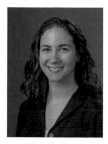 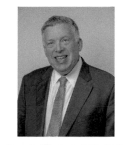

Sarah B. Goldberg, MD, MPH   Roy S. Herbst, MD, PhD
Editors

The past quarter of a century has seen tremendous advances in the diagnosis and management of lung cancer, resulting in patients living significantly longer and better than ever before. Patients with early-stage non–small cell lung cancer (NSCLC) are benefiting from innovation in surgical techniques, which results in improved outcomes and easier recovery, and those who are unable to undergo resection are benefiting from progress in radiation therapy technology, such as stereotactic body radiotherapy. We have known for many years that neoadjuvant and adjuvant therapy for resectable NSCLC can improve the change of cure; however, relapse is unfortunately common with standard chemotherapy alone. We have now witnessed the remarkable improvement in patient outcomes when adding immunotherapy or targeted therapy into the management of early-stage and locally advanced NSCLC, resulting in the incorporation of these therapies into the management of patients. With this progress comes many questions about how to choose the most appropriate strategy for patients, and more work remains to fully understand the best sequence for any given scenario.

Progress in managing metastatic NSCLC has arguably been the most remarkable advance in recent years, stemming from our enhanced understanding of the biology of lung cancer at a molecular and immunologic level. There is no other malignancy that demonstrates the power of precision medicine more than lung cancer: we now can successfully target many different alterations that dramatically impact our ability to successfully treat this disease. Knowing how to assess for these alterations has become paramount in the field, and the emergence of liquid biopsies in addition to next-generation sequencing of the tumor has revolutionized the way in which we can identify targetable alterations in lung cancer. Small cell lung cancer continues to be a devastating malignancy, but new therapies are now emerging that offer promise in this difficult disease. Despite this incredible progress in treating lung cancer,

Hematol Oncol Clin N Am 37 (2023) xi–xii
https://doi.org/10.1016/j.hoc.2023.03.001
0889-8588/23/© 2023 Published by Elsevier Inc.

hemonc.theclinics.com

supportive care remains as important as ever before, and fortunately, our understanding of how to optimally provide it has improved over the years. We have come so far from the one-size-fits-all management strategies of the past, and it is only with further exploration of the molecular underpinnings of lung cancer, the development of predictive biomarkers, and the ability for all patients to access cutting-edge therapies that we will fully realize the power of precision medicine in lung cancer.

Sarah B. Goldberg, MD, MPH
Yale School of Medicine
333 Cedar Street, FMP130
New Haven, CT 06510, USA

Roy S. Herbst, MD, PhD
Yale School of Medicine
333 Cedar Street, WWW221
New Haven, CT 06510, USA

E-mail addresses:
sarah.goldberg@yale.edu (S.B. Goldberg)
roy.herbst@yale.edu (R.S. Herbst)

State of the Art of Pathologic and Molecular Testing

Sanja Dacic, MD, PhD

KEYWORDS

- Lung cancer • Molecular testing • PD-L1 • NGS-AI

KEY POINTS

- Testing for predictive biomarkers of response to targeted therapies and immunotherapies is standard of care in patients with lung cancer.
- Next-generation sequencing deoxyribonucleic acid/ribonucleic acid (DNA/RNA) comprehensive assays are the preferred testing approach rather than single-gene assays.
- Low output multiplex immunohistochemistry/immunofluorescence assays assessing biomarkers in the tumor microenvironment will be adopted into clinical practice.
- The artificial intelligence (AI) algorithms are valuable tools that enhance pathologists' role in biomarker testing.

INTRODUCTION

Rapidly evolving targeted and immunotherapies in non-small cell lung carcinoma (NSCLC) have resulted in an enormous pressure to develop and implement laboratory assays that will rapidly and accurately identify predictive biomarkers of responses.[1-4] Molecular testing over the past decade has evolved from low-throughput assays (fluorescence in situ hybridization [FISH], immunohistochemistry [IHC], single or limited panel polymerase chain reaction [PCR]) to high-throughput comprehensive next-generation sequencing (NGS) (**Table 1**).[5] Molecular testing plays a key role in the management of patients with advanced lung cancer and therefore should be implemented into routine diagnostic workflow.[1] Despite the clinical need for detection of actionable targets and predictors of response, the rate of molecular testing in lung cancer remains suboptimal mainly due to economical obstacles and limited access to new technologies.[6,7] The selection of appropriate molecular assay is essential for optimal detection of established standard of care as well as emerging biomarkers.[8] Therefore, it is important to understand the limitations of available assays, which may be gene or molecular alteration-specific.[8-10]

Department of Pathology, Yale School of Medicine, 200 South Frontage Road, EP2-631, New Haven, CT 06510, USA
E-mail address: sanja.dacic@yale.edu

Hematol Oncol Clin N Am 37 (2023) 463–473
https://doi.org/10.1016/j.hoc.2023.02.001
0889-8588/23/© 2023 Elsevier Inc. All rights reserved.

Table 1
Standard biomarker testing for NSCLC

Predictive Biomarker	Clinical Assay			
	IHC	FISH	PCR	NGS
Targeted therapies				
Gene mutations				
EGFR			+	+
KRAS				+
BRAF				+
MET	(+)	(+)		+
ERBB2/HER2				+
Gene fusions				
ALK	+	+		+
ROS1	+	+		+
RET		+	+	+
NTRK	+	+	+	+
Immunotherapy				
PD-L1	+			
TMB				+

A frequently encountered issue is that the quantity of tumor tissue available for molecular analysis after the initial diagnostic work up is inadequate.[11] ctDNA ("liquid biopsy") has emerged as an alternative minimally invasive, usually faster, approach.[12–15] This approach has become clinically more important with the development of high-sensitivity technologies and includes both single-gene PCR-based assays and multigene NGS assays.

Choosing between testing workflow and the assay itself can be influenced by laboratory expertise in running different commercial or laboratory developed tests, test performance, expected turnaround time, or reimbursements.

This review focus on the current and emerging testing approaches for predictive biomarkers in lung cancer.

DISCUSSION
Pathology Diagnosis and Ancillary Testing

Histologic classification of lung carcinoma significantly evolved in the past two decades mostly because of the significant progress in understanding genetics and the development of molecular-targeted therapies. These advances have led to the implementation of immunohistochemistry as a diagnostic tool which allows pathologists to precisely subclassify lung carcinomas. The principles of diagnostic work remain the same, starting with morphology, followed by immunohistochemistry, and then molecular testing. Depending on the carcinoma subtype, further molecular testing may be needed to identify targetable molecular alterations (**Fig. 1**). From a diagnostic standpoint, morphology can be sufficient, but if immunohistochemistry is needed for subtyping, the current recommendation is to use a single adenocarcinoma marker (eg, transcription termination factor 1 [TTF-1]) and a single squamous marker (eg, p40).[16,17] If morphology suggests neuroendocrine differentiation, neuroendocrine marker (eg, synaptophysin) should be performed.

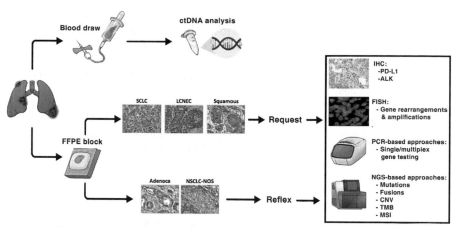

Fig. 1. Implementation of tissue-based and liquid biopsy molecular testing into diagnostic workflow of NSCLC. For adenocarcinoma and NSCLC NOS reflex testing initiated by pathologist at the time of initial diagnosis in preferred. For other histologic subtypes depending on clinical characteristics, molecular testing should be performed at the request of oncologists. Liquid biopsy can be performed as a complementary or alternative approach to tissue-based molecular profiling. FFPE, formalin fixed formalin embedded tissue; LCNEC, large cell neuroendocrine carcinoma; NOS, not otherwise specified; SCLC, small cell lung carcinoma.

The small biopsy or cytology specimens are the only sample in over 70% of patients with lung cancer who are not surgical candidates. To secure adequate tissue for diagnosis and molecular testing, rapid on-site evaluation at the time of diagnostic sampling procedure may be implemented, although practices vary between institutions.[11,18] Tissue conservation protocols such as upfront cutting of unstained slides should also be considered.[11]

There is no standardized approach to what represents adequate tissue because of the broad spectrum of molecular assays used in the clinical practice, which may have different tissue requirements. Recently, European Expert Group recommended that for tissue samples, at least five endobronchial/transbronchial forceps biopsies are obtained, whereas additional five forceps biopsies or two cryo-biopsies could be considered. For cytology specimens, the same group recommended at least four endobronchial ultrasound/endoscopic needle aspiration passes per target needle and at least two percutaneous core needle biopsies (18- to 20-gauge needle) or three to six core needle biopsies.[19]

Tissue-Based Assays

Immunohistochemistry
Molecular-targeted therapies. Immunohistochemistry is a standard assay used in all pathology laboratories and can be performed on limited tumor samples which may not be suitable for complex molecular assays. The major application of immunohistochemistry is for fusion gene testing and PD-L1.[20,21] The US Food and Drug Administration (FDA)-approved VENTANA ALK (D5F3) CDx IHC assay as a primary therapy-determining test for ALK kinase inhibitors. Based on the published evidence, properly validated IHC assays show great concordance with FDA-approved FISH assays with 97% sensitivity and 99% specificity and more recently with NGS platforms.[22–25] Studies also showed that IHC-positive ALK protein expression correlates with response to ALK inhibitors even in *ALK* FISH-negative cases.[26] In contrast, ROS1 and NTRK-IHC positive tumors should be confirmed by another

molecular method such as FISH or NGS because of nonspecific expressions that could be difficult to interpret and may lead to false positive results.[27,28] For rearranged during transfection (*RET*) fusions, IHC is not recommended because false positive and negative results have been reported.[29] IHC assays for fusion gene testing are mostly used as a screening tool or complementary to NGS or FISH testing, particularly on limited small samples.

The use of mutation-specific antibodies is not recommended as negative staining does not exclude the presence of actionable mutations.[1] For example, epidermal growth factor receptor (EGFR) mutation-specific antibodies show cross-reactivity and suboptimal detection particularly of exon 19 deletions.[30]

More recently developed BRAF V600E mutation-specific antibodies show better specificity and may be considered as a screening option for V600E mutations. However, in NSCLC, non-V600E mutations are more common, and therefore, the use of BRAF V600E IHC is of limited value.[31,32]

Many commercially available antibodies directed against various MET epitopes are available; however, they are not predictive of efficacy of MET inhibitors, and therefore, their use is not recommended.[33] Similarly, HER2 IHC is not entirely predictive of response and therefore is not recommended for routine clinical use.[34]

Immunotherapy

PD-L1 According to the NCCN guidelines, all advanced NSCLC should be reflex tested with a PD-L1 IHC assay. One of the main issues is that five different PD-L1 IHC assays with various regulatory approval status have been recommended as predictive biomarkers of response to specific PD1/PD-L1 inhibitors (**Table 2**). From practical and economical standpoints, pathology laboratories cannot afford to implement all approved or available PD-L1 assays into clinical practice. The main challenge for pathology laboratories is a choice of assay. Several studies showed that the PD-L1 clones Dako 22-8, Dako 22C3, and Ventana SP263 are analytically interchangeable.[35–38] Laboratory developed tests (LDTs) are commonly developed, and it was demonstrated that adequately validated assay can use different antibodies on different staining platforms.[39] Recent study showed that LDT for particular clone should be used for the same indication as FDA-approved assay.[40] In contrast, French harmonization study showed that only half of the LDTs demonstrated sufficient concordance with the reference assays.[39] However, it has to be mentioned that not

Table 2
PD-L1 immunohistochemical assays for lung cancer

PD-L1 Assay	Scoring Criteria	Drug	Regulatory Status
22C3 Dako pharmDx	TPS ≥50% for 1st line ≥1% for 2nd line	Pembrolizumab (Keytruda)	Companion
28–8 Dako pharmDx	TPS ≥1% non-squamous NSCLC	Nivolumab (Opdivo)	Complementary
SP263	TPS ≥1%	Durvalumab (Imfinzi)	Complementary
SP142	TC ≥ 50% IC ≥ 10%	Atezolizumab (Tecentriq)	Complementary
73–10 pharmDx	TC ≥ 1%	Avelumab (Bavencio)	-

Abbreviations: IC, immune cells; TC, tumor cells; TPS, tumor proportion score.

all of the LDTs used in the study were subjected to a rigorous validation against approved assay. Pathologists showed good concordance in the interpretation of the tumor cell scoring, whereas low concordance was observed for inflammatory cells.[35] PD-L1 scoring is another area where AI using digital platforms can be potentially useful. Some algorithms are already available and show consistency between pathologists and AI models.[41,42] Discrepancies are usually observed in cases with weak staining and when immune cells are admixed with tumor cells.

Next-generation sequencing

Large NGS panels implemented into diagnostic workflow of tumor samples from patients with advanced lung cancer are the most efficient way to test for both standard-of-care and desirable actionable driver mutations and gene fusions. There are several NGS approaches including targeted NGS, whole-exome sequencing (WES) and whole-genome sequencing (WGS).[9,43] Targeted NGS assays provide high depth of sequencing and high sensitivity in detection of alterations of typically 100–500 cancer-relevant genes included in the panel. WES and WGS have a lower depth of sequencing, but a better ability to discover novel mutations and structural variants. However, they require more DNA/RNA input, longer sequencing time, and more

Table 3
Summary of common comprehensive next-generation sequencing assays

Assay	Nucleic Acid Input	Target Enrichment Method	Number of Genes/ Targets
Oncomine Comprehensive Assay v3	DNA, RNA	Amplicon-based	161 genes; 87 hotspot regions, 43 focal copy number variation (CNV) gains, 48 full CDS for del mutations, 51 fusion drivers
Oncomine Comprehensive Assay Plus	DNA, RNA	Amplicon-based	333 genes with focal CNV gains/loss, 227 full CDS, 49 fusion drivers
QIAseq Pan-cancer Multimodal Panel	DNA, RNA	Amplicon-based (simultaneous DNA/ RNA enrichment)	523 genes, 56 fusion, 26 microsatellite instability (MSI) loci
AmpliSeq for Illumina Comprehensive Panel v3	DNA, RNA	Amplicon-based	161 genes, 86 hotspot regions, 48 full-length genes, copy number genes, inter- and intragenic gene fusions
AmpliSeq for Illumina Comprehensive Cancer Panel	DNA	Amplicon-based	Full exon coverage of 409 genes
TruSight Oncology 500	DNA, RNA	Hybrid-based	523 targeted biomarkers, 523 Single nucleotide variation (SNVs) and indels, 60 focal amplifications, 55 fusions

complex bioinformatics support that leads to a longer TAT to generate reports. Therefore, their use in clinical practice is currently limited. The panel size is also essential for the assessment of tumor mutation burden (TMB).[44,45] Commercially available NGS assays, as summarized in **Table 3**, have different capabilities in detection of single-nucleotide variants, small insertions/deletions, copy number variances, and gene fusions.[8,46] For the optimal use of available NGS platforms, a minimal understanding of the assay characteristics is necessary and includes knowledge about gene targets included in the panel, enrichment approaches, and whether the panel is designed to analyze DNA, RNA, or both. This is necessary to adequately interpret the results and include the available information in the treatment-decision algorithm. The gene coverage is different between the panels, and therefore, the discordant results may be obtained. The target-enrichment approaches (amplicon-based vs hybrid capture) play a major role in the ability of the assay to detect certain alterations.[8,9,43] For example, *MET* exon 14 skipping shows a large spectrum of alterations that are not identified by comprehensive NGS panels if those are not specifically designed to detect those alterations.[10] It has been shown that amplicon-based targeted DNA NGS panels such as TruSight Tumor26 or Ion AmpliSeq Cancer Hotspot panel would not be able to detect *MET* exon 14 alterations in more than about 60% of cases, particularly fusions of exons 13 and 15 that are best detected by RNA-based testing. Required DNA/RNA input also varies between different platforms. Factors such as fixation and storage of paraffin blocks may impact the quantity and quality of extracted DNA/RNA from a sample that based on tumor cellularity is deemed to be optimal. DNA-based panels have been more prevalent in the clinical practice than RNA panels, but limitations are well-known.[47] Therefore, DNA/RNA hybrid panels are becoming increasingly popular. Another proposed workflow would be sequential targeted RNA sequencing, if DNA sequencing assays appear driver negative.

Liquid Biopsy

Liquid biopsy is increasingly important diagnostic tool in the management of patients with lung cancer.[12,13] It is based on the detection of circulating cancer cell markers such as cell free DNA (cfDNA) or circulating tumor DNA (ctDNA), predominantly in plasma although other fluid types such as CSF are also being explored.[48] The main advantages of liquid biopsies over tissue-based molecular profiling are that it requires less invasive procedures for the patient and provides rapid results. Liquid biopsies show a high concordance (>90%) with tissue-based assays for common genes such as EGFR.[14] The analytical sensitivity is variable, and the identified actionable alterations can be used for treatment decisions, whereas negative results should be confirmed by tissue-based testing.[12,13] There are several assays that are used for liquid biopsies including real-time PCR, digital droplet polymerase chain reaction (ddPCR), and NGS. Similar to tissue-based testing, clinically validated NGS platforms rather than single-gene PCR assays are strongly recommended. Technically, there has been a major improvement in the plasma-based NGS assays over the past several years that has resulted in FDA approval of two different assays (Guadrant360 CDx and FoundationOne Liquid CDx) for ctDNA analysis and subsequently growing clinical implementation.

The most common dilemma for the treating physician is which sample to test first-tissue or plasma. International Association for the Study of Lung Cancer (IASLC) evidence-based recommendations provide a guideline on when to order which test and how to interpret the results.[12] Plasma ctDNA is considered to be complementary to tissue-based tests in patients with newly diagnosed advanced NSCLC and can be ordered at the same time as tissue-based assays. "Plasma first" is preferred in patients who developed acquired resistance after tyrosine kinase inhibitor (TKI) therapy in oncogene-driven NSCLC.[12] Repeat tissue biopsy should be considered if liquid biopsy is noninformative. ctDNA is also the preferred method for real-time monitoring of response to therapy. The role of liquid biopsy in detection of early-stage disease is challenging because the low level of ctDNA shedding from the tumor causes low sensitivity.[12,49] However, ctDNA detected after complete surgical resection minimally residual disease (MRD) may be helpful in identifying patients with high risk for recurrence.[49,50] The role of liquid biopsy in non-oncogene-addicted NSCLC is less defined, although several studies showed the predictive value of TMB analyzed in blood.[51,52] Similar to tissue-based assays, it is essential for treating physicians to be aware of the liquid biopsy assay performance characteristics, limitations, and the significance of the results.

Emerging Assays

The clinical practice has been highly impacted by the current "second generation" of NGS despite its known shortcomings such as sequence gaps and PCR artifacts among others.[9] The third-generation sequencing technologies also known as single-molecule sequencing addressed those limitations. There are two main technologies that represent the third-generation sequencing—Pacific Bioscience single-molecule real-time and Oxford Nanopores.[53] The main advantages of the third-generation sequencing is shorter sample preparation and sequencing run time, longer sequencing reads, and reduced sequencing errors due to PCR amplification. However, these techniques still have high error rate.[9] Another interesting approach is a single-cell sequencing that has been shown to be very helpful in studying intratumoral heterogeneity and tumor evolution.[54,55]

Recently developed multiplex immunohistochemistry and multiplex immunofluorescence assays can be used to help quantify immune cell subsets and their spatial arrangements between different tumor compartments.[56] A meta-analysis comparing tumor mutational burden, gene expression profiling for interferon-gamma gene signatures, PD-L1 IHC, and multiplex immunohistochemistry and immunofluorescence approaches showed that the multiplex approaches were better predictors of objective response to anti-PD-(L)1 therapies.[57] The multiplexing approaches can analyze 2 to 50 markers expressed on a single-cell level. Multiple platforms exist for techniques, including standard immunfluorescence (IF) scopes which can support 4 to 5 plex assays, and multispectral technologies (Vectra 3.0/Polaris), which can support 6- to 8-plex assays.[2] The higher-order plex approaches include multiplex ion beam imaging, by time of flight, imaging mass cytometry, and digital spatial profiling, among others. The main disadvantage of these assays is that they are technically challenging, time-consuming, and require digital imaging support and analysis.[2] Most of these approaches are discovery tools and limited for use in research only; however, some relatively limited multiplex approaches may be implemented in the clinical practice sooner.[2]

Recently, image-based models for the detection on lung carcinoma driver mutations or gene fusions directly from routine H&E scanned slides using the deep learning algorithms have been developed.[58–60]

SUMMARY

Molecular testing for predictive biomarkers of response to targeted therapies, immunotherapies or combination therapies should be implemented into routine diagnostic workup of advanced lung carcinomas. Comprehensive NGS panels rather than single-gene tests should be standard of care. NGS testing of tissue and liquid biopsies should be complementary, with liquid biopsies providing faster results. Treating physicians to provide excellent clinical care to the patients with lung cancer should be aware of advantages and limitations of clinically available comprehensive assays.

CLINICS CARE POINTS

- All patients with unresectable non-small cell lung carcinoma (NSCLC) require testing for predictive biomarkers at the time of diagnosis.
- Comprehensive next-generation sequencing (NGS) DNA/RNA assays provide characterization of the standard and emerging targetable alterations.
- NGS assays are different in terms of sample requirements, gene coverage, enrichment approaches, and whether the panel is designed to analyze DNA, RNA, or both.
- Plasma ctDNA (liquid biopsy) is considered complementary to tissue-based tests in patients with newly diagnosed advanced NSCLC.
- Repeat tissue biopsy should be considered if liquid biopsy is noninformative.
- "Plasma first" is preferred in patients who developed acquired resistance after TKI therapy in oncogene-driven NSCLC and also for the real-time monitoring of response to therapy.

REFERENCES

1. Lindeman NI, Cagle PT, Aisner DL, et al. Updated molecular testing guideline for the selection of lung cancer patients for treatment with targeted tyrosine kinase inhibitors: guideline from the college of american pathologists, the international association for the study of lung cancer, and the association for molecular pathology. J Mol Diagn 2018;20(2):129–59.
2. Taube JM, Akturk G, Angelo M, et al. The society for immunotherapy of cancer statement on best practices for multiplex immunohistochemistry (IHC) and immunofluorescence (IF) staining and validation. J Immunother Cancer 2020;8(1): e000155.
3. Pentheroudakis G, Committee EG. Recent eUpdate to the ESMO clinical practice guidelines on early and locally advanced non-small-cell lung cancer (NSCLC). Ann Oncol 2020;31(9):1265–6.
4. Ettinger DS, Wood DE, Aisner DL, et al. Non-small cell lung cancer, version 3.2022, NCCN clinical practice guidelines in oncology. J Natl Compr Canc Netw 2022;20(5):497–530.
5. Kerr KM, Bibeau F, Thunnissen E, et al. The evolving landscape of biomarker testing for non-small cell lung cancer in Europe. Lung Cancer 2021;154:161–75.
6. Pennell NA, Arcila ME, Gandara DR, et al. Biomarker testing for patients with advanced non-small cell lung cancer: real-world issues and tough choices. Am Soc Clin Oncol Educ Book 2019;39:531–42.
7. Smeltzer MP, Wynes MW, Lantuejoul S, et al. The international association for the study of lung cancer global survey on molecular testing in lung cancer. J Thorac Oncol 2020;15(9):1434–48.
8. Ionescu DN, Stockley TL, Banerji S, et al. Consensus recommendations to optimize testing for new targetable alterations in non-small cell lung cancer. Curr Oncol 2022;29(7):4981–97.
9. Zhong Y, Xu F, Wu J, et al. Application of next generation sequencing in laboratory medicine. Ann Lab Med 2021;41(1):25–43.
10. Poirot B, Doucet L, Benhenda S, et al. MET Exon 14 Alterations and new resistance mutations to tyrosine kinase inhibitors: risk of inadequate detection with current amplicon-based NGS panels. J Thorac Oncol 2017;12(10):1582–7.

11. Penault-Llorca F, Kerr KM, Garrido P, et al. Expert opinion on NSCLC small specimen biomarker testing - Part 1: tissue collection and management. Virchows Arch 2022;481(3):335–50.
12. Rolfo C, Mack PC, Scagliotti GV, et al. Liquid biopsy for advanced non-small cell lung cancer (NSCLC): a statement paper from the IASLC. J Thorac Oncol 2018; 13(9):1248–68.
13. Aggarwal C, Rolfo CD, Oxnard GR, et al. Strategies for the successful implementation of plasma-based NSCLC genotyping in clinical practice. Nat Rev Clin Oncol 2021;18(1):56–62.
14. Odegaard JI, Vincent JJ, Mortimer S, et al. Validation of a plasma-based comprehensive cancer genotyping assay utilizing orthogonal tissue- and plasma-based methodologies. Clin Cancer Res 2018;24(15):3539–49.
15. Gerber T, Taschner-Mandl S, Saloberger-Sindhoringer L, et al. Assessment of pre-analytical sample handling conditions for comprehensive liquid biopsy analysis. J Mol Diagn 2020;22(8):1070–86.
16. Nicholson AG, Tsao MS, Beasley MB, et al. The 2021 WHO classification of lung tumors: impact of advances since 2015. J Thorac Oncol 2022;17(3):362–87.
17. Yatabe Y, Dacic S, Borczuk AC, et al. Best practices recommendations for diagnostic immunohistochemistry in lung cancer. J Thorac Oncol 2019;14(3): 377–407.
18. Roy-Chowdhuri S., Dacic S., Ghofrani M., et al., Collection and handling of thoracic small biopsy and cytology specimens for ancillary studies: guideline from the college of american pathologists in collaboration with the american college of chest physicians, association for molecular pathology, american society of cytopathology, american thoracic society, pulmonary pathology society, papanicolaou society of cytopathology, society of interventional radiology, and society of thoracic radiology, Arch Pathol Lab Med, 2020;144(8):933–958.
19. Dietel M, Bubendorf L, Dingemans AM, et al. Diagnostic procedures for non-small-cell lung cancer (NSCLC): recommendations of the European Expert Group. Thorax 2016;71(2):177–84.
20. Hung YP, Sholl LM. Diagnostic and predictive immunohistochemistry for non-small cell lung carcinomas. Adv Anat Pathol 2018;25(6):374–86.
21. Mino-Kenudson M. Immunohistochemistry for predictive biomarkers in non-small cell lung cancer. Transl Lung Cancer Res 2017;6(5):570–87.
22. Jurmeister P, Lenze D, Berg E, et al. Parallel screening for ALK, MET and ROS1 alterations in non-small cell lung cancer with implications for daily routine testing. Lung Cancer 2015;87(2):122–9.
23. Minca EC, Portier BP, Wang Z, et al. ALK status testing in non-small cell lung carcinoma: correlation between ultrasensitive IHC and FISH. J Mol Diagn 2013; 15(3):341–6.
24. Blackhall FH, Peters S, Bubendorf L, et al. Prevalence and clinical outcomes for patients with ALK-positive resected stage I to III adenocarcinoma: results from the European Thoracic Oncology Platform Lungscape Project. J Clin Oncol 2014;32(25):2780–7.
25. Peled N, Palmer G, Hirsch FR, et al. Next-generation sequencing identifies and immunohistochemistry confirms a novel crizotinib-sensitive ALK rearrangement in a patient with metastatic non-small-cell lung cancer. J Thorac Oncol 2012; 7(9):e14–6.
26. Sun JM, Choi YL, Won JK, et al. A dramatic response to crizotinib in a non-small-cell lung cancer patient with IHC-positive and FISH-negative ALK. J Thorac Oncol 2012;7(12):e36–8.

27. Gatalica Z, Xiu J, Swensen J, et al. Molecular characterization of cancers with NTRK gene fusions. Mod Pathol 2019;32(1):147–53.

28. Solomon JP, Linkov I, Rosado A, et al. NTRK fusion detection across multiple assays and 33,997 cases: diagnostic implications and pitfalls. Mod Pathol 2020; 33(1):38–46.

29. Yang SR, Aypar U, Rosen EY, et al. A performance comparison of commonly used assays to detect RET fusions. Clin Cancer Res 2021;27(5):1316–28.

30. Brevet M, Arcila M, Ladanyi M. Assessment of EGFR mutation status in lung adenocarcinoma by immunohistochemistry using antibodies specific to the two major forms of mutant EGFR. J Mol Diagn 2010;12(2):169–76.

31. Ilie M, Long E, Hofman V, et al. Diagnostic value of immunohistochemistry for the detection of the BRAFV600E mutation in primary lung adenocarcinoma Caucasian patients. Ann Oncol 2013;24(3):742–8.

32. Seto K, Haneda M, Masago K, et al. Negative reactions of BRAF mutation-specific immunohistochemistry to non-V600E mutations of BRAF. Pathol Int 2020;70(5):253–61.

33. Jorgensen JT, Mollerup J. Companion diagnostics and predictive biomarkers for MET-targeted therapy in NSCLC. Cancers 2022;14(9):2150–61.

34. Ren S, Wang J, Ying J, et al. Consensus for HER2 alterations testing in non-small-cell lung cancer. ESMO Open 2022;7(1):100395.

35. Hirsch FR, McElhinny A, Stanforth D, et al. PD-L1 immunohistochemistry assays for lung cancer: results from phase 1 of the blueprint PD-L1 IHC assay comparison project. J Thorac Oncol 2017;12(2):208–22.

36. Tsao MS, Kerr KM, Kockx M, et al. PD-L1 immunohistochemistry comparability study in real-life clinical samples: results of blueprint phase 2 project. J Thorac Oncol 2018;13(9):1302–11.

37. Ratcliffe MJ, Sharpe A, Midha A, et al. Agreement between Programmed cell death ligand-1 diagnostic assays across multiple protein expression cutoffs in non-small cell lung cancer. Clin Cancer Res 2017;23(14):3585–91.

38. Rimm DL, Han G, Taube JM, et al. A prospective, multi-institutional, pathologist-based assessment of 4 immunohistochemistry assays for PD-L1 expression in non-small cell lung cancer. JAMA Oncol 2017;3(8):1051–8.

39. Adam J, Le Stang N, Rouquette I, et al. Multicenter harmonization study for PD-L1 IHC testing in non-small-cell lung cancer. Ann Oncol 2018;29(4):953–8.

40. Torlakovic E, Lim HJ, Adam J, et al. "Interchangeability" of PD-L1 immunohistochemistry assays: a meta-analysis of diagnostic accuracy. Mod Pathol 2020; 33(1):4–17.

41. Cheng G, Zhang F, Xing Y, et al. Artificial intelligence-assisted score analysis for predicting the expression of the immunotherapy biomarker PD-L1 in lung cancer. Front Immunol 2022;13:893198.

42. Wu J, Liu C, Liu X, et al. Artificial intelligence-assisted system for precision diagnosis of PD-L1 expression in non-small cell lung cancer. Mod Pathol 2022;35(3): 403–11.

43. Gagan J, Van Allen EM. Next-generation sequencing to guide cancer therapy. Genome Med 2015;7(1):80.

44. Merino DM, McShane LM, Fabrizio D, et al. Establishing guidelines to harmonize tumor mutational burden (TMB): in silico assessment of variation in TMB quantification across diagnostic platforms: phase I of the Friends of Cancer Research TMB Harmonization Project. J Immunother Cancer 2020;8(1):e000147.

45. Vega DM, Yee LM, McShane LM, et al. Aligning tumor mutational burden (TMB) quantification across diagnostic platforms: phase II of the Friends of Cancer Research TMB Harmonization Project. Ann Oncol 2021;32(12):1626–36.
46. Kazdal D, Hofman V, Christopoulos P, et al. Fusion-positive non-small cell lung carcinoma: Biological principles, clinical practice, and diagnostic implications. Genes Chromosomes Cancer 2022;61(5):244–60.
47. Benayed R, Offin M, Mullaney K, et al. High Yield of RNA sequencing for targetable kinase fusions in lung adenocarcinomas with no mitogenic driver alteration detected by DNA sequencing and low tumor mutation burden. Clin Cancer Res 2019;25(15):4712–22.
48. Bale TA, Yang SR, Solomon JP, et al. Clinical experience of cerebrospinal fluid-based liquid biopsy demonstrates superiority of cell-free DNA over cell pellet genomic DNA for molecular profiling. J Mol Diagn 2021;23(6):742–52.
49. Chaudhuri AA, Chabon JJ, Lovejoy AF, et al. Early detection of molecular residual disease in localized lung cancer by circulating tumor DNA profiling. Cancer Discov 2017;7(12):1394–403.
50. Moding EJ, Liu Y, Nabet BY, et al. Circulating tumor DNA dynamics predict benefit from consolidation immunotherapy in locally advanced non-small cell lung cancer. Nat Cancer 2020;1(2):176–83.
51. Gandara DR, Paul SM, Kowanetz M, et al. Blood-based tumor mutational burden as a predictor of clinical benefit in non-small-cell lung cancer patients treated with atezolizumab. Nat Med 2018;24(9):1441–8.
52. Herbst RS, Giaccone G, de Marinis F, et al. Atezolizumab for First-Line Treatment of PD-L1-Selected Patients with NSCLC. N Engl J Med 2020;383(14):1328–39.
53. Midha MK, Wu M, Chiu KP. Long-read sequencing in deciphering human genetics to a greater depth. Hum Genet 2019;138(11–12):1201–15.
54. Bowes AL, Tarabichi M, Pillay N, et al. Leveraging single-cell sequencing to unravel intratumour heterogeneity and tumour evolution in human cancers. J Pathol 2022;257(4):466–78.
55. Duckworth AD, Gherardini PF, Sykorova M, et al. Multiplexed profiling of RNA and protein expression signatures in individual cells using flow or mass cytometry. Nat Protoc 2019;14(3):901–20.
56. Moutafi M, Martinez-Morilla S, Divakar P, et al. Discovery of biomarkers of resistance to immune checkpoint blockade in NSCLC using high-plex digital spatial profiling. J Thorac Oncol 2022;17(8):991–1001.
57. Lu S, Stein JE, Rimm DL, et al. Comparison of biomarker modalities for predicting response to PD-1/PD-L1 checkpoint blockade: a systematic review and meta-analysis. JAMA Oncol 2019;5(8):1195–204.
58. Ninatti G, Kirienko M, Neri E, et al. Imaging-based prediction of molecular therapy targets in NSCLC by radiogenomics and AI approaches: a systematic review. Diagnostics 2020;10(6):359–82.
59. Mayer C, Ofek E, Fridrich DE, et al. Direct identification of ALK and ROS1 fusions in non-small cell lung cancer from hematoxylin and eosin-stained slides using deep learning algorithms. Mod Pathol 2022;35:1882–7.
60. Tan X, Li Y, Wang S, et al. Predicting EGFR mutation, ALK rearrangement, and uncommon EGFR mutation in NSCLC patients by driverless artificial intelligence: a cohort study. Respir Res 2022;23(1):132.

Convergence of Precision Oncology and Liquid Biopsy in Non-Small Cell Lung Cancer

Ebaa Al-Obeidi, MD[a],*, Jonathan W. Riess, MD[a],
Umberto Malapelle, PhD[b], Christian Rolfo, MD, PhD, MBA[c],
David R. Gandara, MD[a]

KEYWORDS

- Liquid biopsy • Circulating tumor DNA (ctDNA) • Next-generation sequencing (NGS)
- Minimal residual disease (MRD) • Tumor mutational burden (TMB)
- Non-small cell lung cancer (NSCLC)

KEY POINTS

- Studies have shown that oncogene drivers observed in plasma are clinically actionable and responsive to targeted therapies, even at low levels of detection.
- There is growing evidence that concurrent testing of blood and tissue yields faster, more informative, and less expensive diagnostic information than the standard stepwise approach.
- In advanced-stage non-small cell lung cancer (NSCLC), liquid biopsy plays an important role in selection of therapy, identifying recurrence, determining mechanisms of resistance, and monitoring response to therapy.
- In early-stage NSCLC, there is research into the application of liquid biopsy for minimal residual disease detection after local treatment as well as screening and early diagnosis.

INTRODUCTION

Precision medicine, also known as personalized medical care, is a concept easily embraced by physicians and patients alike. In brief, considering the genomic complexities revealed by the human genome project and other such efforts, each patient should be viewed as unique, and management should be tailored to that individual. Despite initial enthusiasm for this approach, some have raised concerns regarding

[a] Division of Hematology-Oncology, University of California, Davis, 4501 X Street, Suite 3016, Sacramento, CA 95817, USA; [b] Department of Public Health, University of Naples Federico II, Via Sergio Pansini 5, 80131, Naples, Italy; [c] Center for Thoracic Oncology at the Tisch Cancer Institute, Icahn School of Medicine at Mount Sinai, One Gustave Levy Place, Box 1079, New York, NY 10029, USA
* Corresponding author.
E-mail address: ealobeidi@ucdavis.edu
Twitter: @UmbertoMalapel1 (U.M.); @ChristianRolfo (C.R.); @drgandara (D.R.G.)

Hematol Oncol Clin N Am 37 (2023) 475–487
https://doi.org/10.1016/j.hoc.2023.02.005
0889-8588/23/© 2023 Elsevier Inc. All rights reserved.

hemonc.theclinics.com

its shortcoming and skepticism about lack of progress in medicine overall.[1,2] However, as applied to oncology, and especially non-small cell lung cancer (NSCLC), the concept of precision oncology is, by every measure, clearly fulfilling its promise. NSCLC is uniquely suited to personalized care strategies because of both its genomic and immunologic characteristics. Genomically, recent studies have shown that NSCLC is complex and highly variable from one individual to the next, with a multitude of potential oncogenes known to drive tumor growth and proliferation.[3–5] Current guidelines recommend that a total of nine oncogene drivers should be assessed in the initial diagnostic evaluation of patients with advanced-stage disease, particularly applicable to adenocarcinomas.[6–9] From a practical viewpoint, in 2022 this goal is best accomplished by the use of broad-based genomic profiling via next-generation sequencing (NGS),[10] providing the ability to simultaneously test for all relevant abnormalities. In a similar fashion, NSCLC is quantitatively and qualitatively well-suited for a precision oncology strategy, being quantitatively a cancer with one of the highest tumor mutational burdens (TMBs) and qualitatively an ideal candidate for checkpoint immunotherapy in a large subset of patients, based on a high proportion of C > A transversion mutations characteristic of tobacco carcinogenesis and neo-antigenicity.[11] Recently, the advent of liquid biopsy has provided the opportunity to accelerate or optimize precision oncology strategies and to broaden its scope in areas such as screening for early detection and determination of minimal residual disease (MRD) following surgical resection.[12,13] Here, we discuss this growing convergence of precision oncology and liquid biopsy in NSCLC.

LIQUID BIOPSY THROUGHOUT THE CONTINUUM OF CARE IN NON-SMALL CELL LUNG CANCER

The term liquid biopsy encompasses a variety of fluid sources, technologies, and products (Fig. 1).[14,15] Within the context of this review, we refer specifically to plasma as the source, NGS as the technology and largely circulating tumor (ct) DNA as the product of liquid biopsy assays. Liquid biopsy is emerging as an

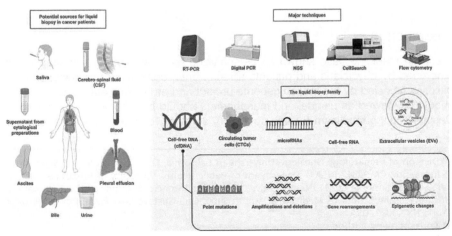

Fig. 1. Liquid biopsy as a path to precision oncology. Liquid biopsy sources, techniques, components, and specific products assessed by plasma ctDNA assays. (*Figure from* Malapelle U, Pisapia P, Addeo A, et al. Liquid biopsy from research to clinical practice: focus on non-small cell lung cancer. Expert Rev Mol Diagn. 2021;21(11):1165–1178. https://doi.org/10.1080/14737159.2021.1985468.)

investigational strategy or as a standard approach across the continuum of care of NSCLC,[16] as shown in **Fig. 2**. NGS in plasma offers several potential advantages over tissue biopsy: (1) Provides a global perspective by reflecting shed tumor DNA or other tumor-related components in plasma from all tumor sites; (2) Abrogates the issue of tumor heterogeneity; (3) Relatively non-invasive and can be repeated serially to monitor tumor response & progression; (4) High acceptance rate by patients[17]; (5) Can determine mechanisms of acquired resistance in plasma before radiographic detection; (6) Can define the presence of MRD after surgical resection of early-stage NSCLC; and (7) Can be incorporated into screening in pre-diagnostic settings.[7] It is notable that in contrast to tumor tissue analysis, liquid biopsy is unique in its ability to be applied in screening and MRD detection. Recent technologic advances have shown that commercially available plasma ctDNA assays, referred to as broad genomic profiling, have both the sensitivity and specificity necessary for a breadth of clinical applications.[18–21] In an analysis of over 21,000 patients with advanced-stage cancer, 85% had detectable ctDNA in plasma, including 87% of patients with NSCLC. Importantly, the median variant allele frequency (VAF) was only 0.41%, range 0.03% to 97.6%.[22] Even at low levels of detection, subsequent studies have shown that oncogene drivers observed in plasma are clinically actionable and responsive to targeted therapies. In one such trial, PENN2, response rate to targeted therapies was independent of VAF, confirming the actionability of positive findings in baseline liquid biopsy.[23]

LIQUID BIOPSY IN ADVANCED-STAGE NON-SMALL CELL LUNG CANCER: ESTABLISHING NEW STANDARDS OF CARE AT INITIAL DIAGNOSIS AND AT PROGRESSIVE DISEASE IN ONCOGENE-DRIVEN DISEASE

Convergence of precision oncology and liquid biopsy is undoubtedly best exemplified in the setting of stage IV NSCLC. NGS analysis of ctDNA is now guideline-recommended as a potential alternative to tumor tissue analysis in the molecular

Liquid biopsy Across the Cancer Care Continuum in Individual Patients (Precision Oncology)

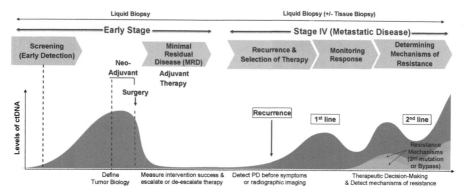

Fig. 2. Different uses of ctDNA analysis over the course of the cancer care continuum. Liquid biopsy can be implemented at various points during the care of an individual patient as illustrated in this figure. (*Data from* Wan JCM, Massie C, Garcia-Corbacho J, et al. Liquid biopsies come of age: towards implementation of circulating tumour DNA. Nat Rev Cancer 2017 174. 2017;17(4):223–238. https://doi.org/10.1038/nrc.2017.7.)

testing algorithm at the time of initial diagnosis of advanced-stage NSCLC, as reported in a recent update of the IASLC consensus statement on liquid biopsy.[16] As shown in **Fig. 3** for newly diagnosed advanced stage NSCLC, in addition to the classic algorithm of using plasma ctDNA to perform initial molecular testing when tissue is inadequate or unrevealing and the well-established role in the detection of mechanisms of resistance at the time of progressive disease (PD) in oncogene-driven cancers, there is growing evidence that a concurrent plasma-tissue approach is complementary, more informative, faster and even more cost-efficient than the classic sequential tissue-first algorithm.[24–26] For example, in the NILE study, patients with newly diagnosed non-squamous metastatic NSCLC, undergoing physician discretion standard of care (SOC) tissue genotyping were prospectively also evaluated by plasma ctDNA testing using a validated and clinically available assay.[25] With tissue-based SOC testing only 18% had complete genotyping for all guideline-recommended biomarkers. If plasma ctDNA was the first test done, 87% had a guideline-recommended biomarker identified versus 67% with SOC tissue testing ($p < 0.0001$). Furthermore, ctDNA testing had a faster turnaround time, with a median of 9 days versus 15 days for SOC tissue testing, $p < 0.0001$.

At the time of PD in an advanced stage oncogene-driven NSCLC, practicing oncologists generally have two options for new systemic therapy: (1) empiric selection of next-generation targeted therapy or chemotherapy with or without immunotherapy, or (2) a precision medicine approach of re-biopsy or liquid biopsy to determine potential mechanisms of resistance and subsequent therapy (**Fig. 4**).[27,28] A classic example of the precision medicine approach is the identification of the epidermal growth factor receptor (EGFR) resistance mutation T790M at the time of PD following first- to second-generation tyrosine kinase inhibitors (TKIs). Multiple studies have shown that plasma ctDNA is equivalent to tissue re-biopsy in this setting in terms of

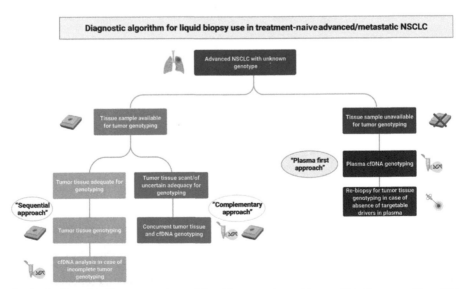

Fig. 3. Outline for the sequencing of liquid versus tissue biopsy. This figure outlines the different approaches ("plasma first" versus "tissue first" versus "concurrent" approach) to obtaining genomic information for patients with newly diagnosed advanced stage NSCLC. Created with BioRender.com.

Progressive Disease (PD) after 1ˢᵗ line TKI Therapy in Oncogene-driven Advanced NSCLC (e.g. EGFR or ALK)

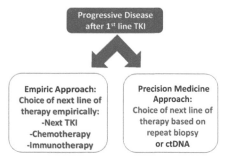

Fig. 4. Approaches to progressive disease. At the time of progressive disease in NSCLC, two pathways exist to select subsequent therapy: the empiric approach versus the precision medicine approach. (*Data from* Melosky B, Popat S, Gandara DR. An Evolving Algorithm to Select and Sequence Therapies in EGFR Mutation-positive NSCLC: A Strategic Approach. Clin Lung Cancer. 2018;19(1):42–50. https://doi.org/10.1016/J.CLLC.2017.05.019.)

actionability.[29–31] In the ALK space, a more recent report by Shaw and colleagues[32] suggested that a precision medicine approach was more effective than an empiric approach in identifying patients who benefit from lorlatinib following failure on earlier generation ALK inhibitors. Using plasma ctDNA, the investigators showed that those patients with cancers in which a resistance mutation was identified had a response rate of 62% and median PFS of 7.3 months, versus those in which no resistance mutation was identified where the response rate was 32% and median PFS was 5.3 months (**Fig. 5**). Clearly, a precision medicine approach appears worth pursuing in this scenario.

LIQUID BIOPSY IN TREATMENT RESPONSE MONITORING

Multiple potential applications for liquid biopsy in therapeutic monitoring are under investigation. Evidence is emerging that liquid biopsy monitoring can detect early evidence of treatment response by reduction in total ctDNA or by reduction in VAF of selected genomic parameters. Conversely, monitoring may serve as an early indicator of PD or assist in differentiating true PD versus so-called pseudo-progression. For example, in true PD the plasma ctDNA would be higher than at baseline while in pseudo-progression the VAFs would be lower or, at worst, stable. Within the setting of advanced-stage NSCLC, preliminary reports suggest that monitoring is accurate in predicting subsequent PD and that it can do so much earlier than radiographic or clinical parameters.

Moreover, liquid biopsy, primarily using plasma ctDNA, has been shown in multiple studies to be prognostic of subsequent therapeutic outcomes: complete or partial clearance of ctDNA is associated with improved tumor response, progression-free survival (PFS), and overall survival (OS).[33,34] In a recent report of clinical trial S1403 by Mack and colleagues[35] in the setting of EGFR-mutated NSCLC receiving targeted therapy, patients with clearance of ctDNA had marked improvements in survival in comparison to those who did not: median PFS of 15.1 months versus 2.8 months (hazard ratio, HR 0.24 [95% CI 0.13 to 0.44]), and median OS of 27.2 versus 15 months (HR 0.30 [95% CI 0.14 to 0.66]). Despite the reproducibility of such studies, the question remains about the actionability of such findings. At present,

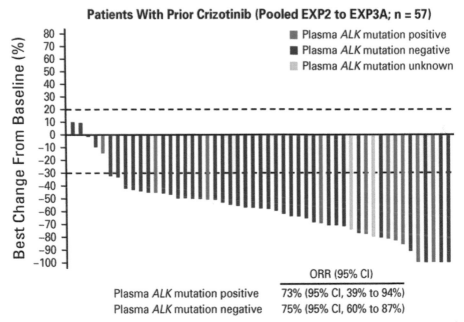

Fig. 5. Lorlatinib activity in patients with ALK + NSCLC who have failed previous second-generation ALK inhibitors. Patients previously treated with ALK inhibitors who had ALK mutations detected by plasma ctDNA had significantly higher response rates to lorlatinib in the second-line setting compared with mutation-negative patients. (*Figure from* Shaw AT, Solomon BJ, Besse B, et al. ALK Resistance Mutations and Efficacy of Lorlatinib in Advanced Anaplastic Lymphoma Kinase-Positive Non-Small-Cell Lung Cancer. J Clin Oncol. 2019;37(16):1370–1379. https://doi.org/10.1200/JCO.18.02236.)

there are no data in NSCLC indicating that changing therapy early based on ctDNA levels is associated with improved clinical outcomes. However, trials designed to address this question of "biomarker switch therapy" are ongoing, as reflected in a randomized trial of osimertinib in EGFR-mutated NSCLC (**Fig. 6**).[36] In this trial, patients with a reduction in ctDNA continue osimertinib alone, whereas those with no reduction or increase in ctDNA are randomized to continued osimertinib monotherapy versus osimertinib plus platinum chemotherapy. Positive results from trials such as this will be required before this approach can be accepted as a reasonable SOC. Recent reports also suggest the potential to use plasma monitoring for early determination of efficacy from checkpoint immunotherapy or chemotherapy, as shown in the study of Zou and colleagues[37] using a "plasma-informed" ctDNA assay. Further studies will be required to determine the clinical validity of incorporating these findings into clinical practice.

LIQUID BIOPSY IN DETECTION OF MINIMAL RESIDUAL DISEASE

Owing to its low invasiveness and repeatability, liquid biopsy lends itself well to MRD detection after surgery, for the purpose of selecting therapeutic regimens such as adjuvant chemotherapy, targeted therapy, or immunotherapy.[38] Tumor-derived analytes in the blood include ctDNA, ctRNA, circulating tumor cells (CTCs), and extracellular vesicles (EVs).[39] Liquid biopsy, in particular ultra-sensitive techniques such as digital polymerase chain reaction (dPCR) and NGS, are reported to provide evidence

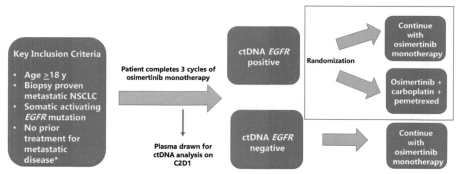

Fig. 6. Clinical trial NCT04410796 evaluating "biomarker switch therapy." A phase 2 trial (NCT04410796) is looking to advance the utility of liquid biopsy by evaluating how best to manage persistent EGFR mutant ctDNA in plasma after initiation of osimertinib treatment. Patients with metastatic EGFR-mutant NSCLC will receive first-line osimertinib therapy. Participants with persistent ctDNA detected in plasma samples will then be randomized to receive either osimertinib alone or addition of chemotherapy. The primary endpoint is progression free survival.

of tumor relapse much sooner than standard radiological tools, potentially enabling an early change in therapy.[40–42] In NSCLC, De Kock and colleagues[43] were able to detect mutations in plasma with an allelic frequency as low as 0.25% by using a droplet digital PCR (ddPCR) pentaplex assay, enabling the identification of the EGFR T790M resistance mutation in all tested patients who experienced PD after TKI administration. Similar results have been obtained by using ultra-deep NGS approaches. In the experience by Chaudhuri and colleagues,[44] the presence of ctDNA at any post-treatment time point was shown to be predictive of lower PFS than patients with undetectable ctDNA. To date, retrospective ctDNA analyses have shown variable results after adjuvant or neoadjuvant chemo-immunotherapy.[45] In the adjuvant setting, whereas MRD analysis of plasma from the IMpower 010 atezolizumab study using a tissue-informed assay was associated with improved patient outcomes in both MRD positive and negative patients, there was a continuous pattern of relapse in both groups (**Fig. 7**). Thus, results could not be used to omit therapy. Nevertheless, prospective trials using different MRD assays are currently under investigation in two clinical trials of adjuvant durvalumab (MERMAID-1 and -2).[46,47] Therapeutic decision-making based on MRD detection may be limited in clinical applicability by two factors. First, the limited number of circulating analytes requires the adoption of ultra-sensitive approaches, leading to the risk of generating false-positive results. Thus, it is crucial to have careful validation and rigorous error-proofing methods to reduce the chance of assay-based false-positive signals.[14] Second, dependent on the technique used, mutations induced by clonal hematopoiesis may cloud interpretation.[48–50] Beyond ctDNA, CTCs are of interest in monitoring the evolution of the tumor under treatment pressure.[51] CTCs offer another avenue for MRD-based therapies. As an example, Wu and colleagues[52] measured a significant reduction of CTCs after surgical excision and a higher level in patients subsequently experiencing PD.

Finally, the inclusion of methylation status or other epigenetic markers together with mutation status may prove enlightening and is under investigation. In this setting, the Guardant Reveal assay has shown promising preliminary results and is now in Phase III adjuvant therapy trials of treatment acceleration or omission in a cohort of colorectal cancer patients after surgical resection.[53,54]

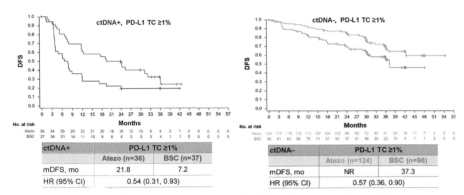

Fig. 7. Exploratory analysis of disease-free survival (DFS) outcomes by ctDNA status in patients enrolled in IMPower010. The exploratory analysis showed that ctDNA positivity post-operatively was a poor prognostic factor as it corresponded with lower DFS across all stages. Atezolizumab after adjuvant chemotherapy showed DFS benefit in both ctDNA-positive and ctDNA-negative patients. (*Adapted from* C. Zhou, M. Das Thakur, M.K. Srivastava, W. Zou, H. Xu, M. Ballinger, E. Felip, H. Wakelee, N.K. Altorki, M. Reck, R. Liersch, A. Kryzhanivska, M. Harada, H. Tanaka, J. Hamm, S. McCune, V. McNally, E. Bennett, B. Gitlitz, S. Novello, 2O IMpower010: Biomarkers of disease-free survival (DFS) in a phase III study of atezolizumab (atezo) vs best supportive care (BSC) after adjuvant chemotherapy in stage IB-IIIA NSCLC, Annals of Oncology, 32, Supplement 7, 2021, Page S1374, https://doi.org/10.1016/j.annonc.2021.10.018.)

EMERGING ROLE OF LIQUID BIOPSY IN SCREENING AND EARLY DETECTION

Liquid biopsy is also undergoing evaluation in lung cancer screening and early detection.[14,55] False positive results[56] and the low abundance of somatic molecular alterations in patients with early-stage cancer remain concerns.[57,58] However, the CancerSEEK assay, consisting of a wide integrating DNA/protein panel able to detect eight of the most recurrent mutations in the early stages of adult solid tumors, has shown interesting results in patients with cancer, albeit with higher sensitivity and specificity in advanced stage compared with early-stage patients. To this end, clinical trials are ongoing to evaluate applicability. For example, the Circulating Cell-free Genome Atlas (NCT02889978) is assessing the combination of ctDNA and methylation profile analysis with a machine learning approach to identify patients with cancer in the early stages.[59] Large-scale epigenetic modification assays using fragmentomics wherein the ctDNA fragment size is evaluated as a means to detect tumor cell "molecular fingerprints" are also under evaluation.[60] A scoring system known as DNA evaluation of fragments for early interception (DELFI) has been developed to increase sensitivity. In a study of healthy individuals and patients with a clinical suspicion of lung cancer, there was a high degree of discrimination between the noncancer group who had a DELFI score 0.16 to 0.21 as compared with the cancer group who had a DELFI score 0.35 to 0.99 (score varied according to tumor stage).[61] In addition, results suggest that clinical outcome is strongly associated with modifications in the fragmentome profile.[61] Beyond cancer screening and early detection, there is also a new field of investigation known as cancer interception.[62] This is related to the possibility of identifying biological hallmarks and altered pathways that increase individual cancer risk in healthy people.[63,64] In this scenario, miRNAs are of interest. The role of specific miRNA signatures has been shown to have the predictive potential for cancer development in high-risk healthy individuals.[65,66] In another study, a combination of ctDNA and ctRNA analysis has been used for the evaluation of high-risk healthy individuals.[67] Lastly, Sequist and colleagues have developed and validated a CTC-based chip as a tool for lung cancer interception.[68–70]

SUMMARY

This review article illuminates the role of liquid biopsy in the continuum of care for NSCLC. We discuss its current application in advanced-stage NSCLC at the time of diagnosis and at progression. We highlight research showing that concurrent testing of blood and tissue yields faster, more informative, and cheaper answers than the standard stepwise approach. We also describe future applications for liquid biopsy including treatment response monitoring and testing for MRD. Lastly, we discuss the emerging role of liquid biopsy for screening and early detection.

CLINICS CARE POINTS

- Studies have shown that oncogene drivers observed in plasma are clinically actionable and responsive to targeted therapies, even at low levels of detection.
- There is growing evidence that concurrent testing of blood and tissue yields faster, more informative, and less-expensive diagnostic information than the standard stepwise approach.
- In advanced-stage non-small cell lung cancer (NSCLC), liquid biopsy plays an important role in selection of therapy, identifying recurrence, determining mechanisms of resistance, and monitoring response to therapy.
- In early-stage NSCLC, there is research into the application of liquid biopsy for minimal residual disease detection after local treatment as well as screening and early diagnosis.

DISCLOSURE

E. Al-Obeidi has nothing to disclose. J. W. Riess discloses consulting/advisory board fees from Blueprint, Beigene, Daiichi Sankyo, EMD Serano, Janssen, Regeneron, Turning Point, Bristol Myers Squibb, Jazz Pharmaceuticals, Novartis, Roche/Genentech, Boehringer Ingelheim, Biodesix, Sanofi; research funding to institution from Merck, AstraZeneca, Spectrum, and Revolution Medicines. U. Malapelle has received personal fees (as a consultant and/or speaker bureau) from Boehringer Ingelheim, Roche, MSD, Amgen, Thermo Fisher Scientifics, Eli Lilly, Diaceutics, Diatech, GSK, Janssen, Merck and AstraZeneca, unrelated to the current work. C. Rolfo discloses consulting fees from Novartis, Boston Pharmaceuticals, EMD Serono, Pfizer, Mirati, Eisai, Daiichi Sankyo, Sanofi Genzyme-Regeneron, Blueprint, and Bayer U.C. LLC; fees for non-CME/CE services from Astra Zeneca, Roche, Guardant Health, MSD, COR2ED, Physicians Education Resource LLC, and Intellisphere LLC; ownership interest in Novartis. D.R. Gandara discloses institutional research grants from Amgen, AstraZeneca, Genentech, and Merck; consultant/advisory board for Adagene, AstraZeneca, Roche-Genentech, Guardant, IO Biotech, Oncocyte, OncoHost, Lilly, Merck, Novartis.

REFERENCES

1. Bayer R, Galea S. Public health in the precision-medicine ERA. Beyond Bioeth Towar a New Biopolitics 2018;267–70. https://doi.org/10.1056/NEJMP1506241.

2. Joyner MJ, Paneth N. Promises, promises, and precision medicine. J Clin Investig 2019;129. https://doi.org/10.1172/JCI126119.

3. Imielinski M, Berger AH, Hammerman PS, et al. Mapping the hallmarks of lung adenocarcinoma with massively parallel sequencing. Cell 2012;150(6):1107–20.

4. Park KH, Choi JY, Lim AR, et al. Genomic landscape and clinical utility in korean advanced pan-cancer patients from prospective clinical sequencing: K-MASTER program. Cancer Discov 2022;12(4):938–48.

5. Jordan EJ, Kim HR, Arcila ME, et al. Prospective comprehensive molecular characterization of lung adenocarcinomas for efficient patient matching to approved and emerging therapies. Cancer Discov 2017;7(6):596–609.

6. Lindeman NI, Cagle PT, Aisner DL, et al. Updated molecular testing guideline for the selection of lung cancer patients for treatment with targeted tyrosine kinase inhibitors: guideline from the college of american pathologists, the international association for the study of lung cancer, and the association for molecular pathology. J Thorac Oncol 2018;13(3):323–58.

7. Aggarwal C, Rolfo CD, Oxnard GR, et al. Strategies for the successful implementation of plasma-based NSCLC genotyping in clinical practice. Nat Rev Clin Oncol 2020;18(1):56–62.

8. Mosele F, Remon J, Mateo J, et al. Recommendations for the use of next-generation sequencing (NGS) for patients with metastatic cancers: a report from the ESMO Precision Medicine Working Group. Ann Oncol 2020;31(11):1491–505.

9. Ettinger DS, Wood DE, Aisner DL, et al. Non–small cell lung cancer, version 3.2022, NCCN clinical practice guidelines in oncology. J Natl Compr Cancer Netw 2022;20(5):497–530.

10. Pennell N.A., Mutebi A., Zhou Z.-Y., et al., Economic impact of next-generation sequencing versus single-gene testing to detect genomic alterations in metastatic non–small-cell lung cancer using a decision analytic model. JCO Precis Oncol, 2019;(3):1-9. https://doi.org/10.1200/PO.18.00356.

11. Rizvi NA, Hellmann MD, Snyder A, et al. Mutational landscape determines sensitivity to PD-1 blockade in non-small cell lung cancer. Science 2015;348(6230):124–8.

12. Rolfo C, Russo A. Liquid biopsy for early stage lung cancer moves ever closer. Nat Rev Clin Oncol 2020;17(9):523–4.

13. Wang B, Pei J, Wang S, et al. Prognostic potential of circulating tumor DNA detection at different time periods in resectable non-small cell lung cancer: Evidence from a meta-analysis. Crit Rev Oncol Hematol 2022;177:103771.

14. Malapelle U, Pisapia P, Pepe F, et al. The evolving role of liquid biopsy in lung cancer. Lung Cancer 2022;172:53–64.

15. Wan JCM, Massie C, Garcia-Corbacho J, et al. Liquid biopsies come of age: towards implementation of circulating tumour DNA. Nat Rev Cancer 2017;17(4):223–38.

16. Rolfo C, Mack P, Scagliotti GV, et al. Liquid Biopsy for Advanced NSCLC: a consensus statement from the international association for the study of lung cancer. J Thorac Oncol 2021;16(10):1647–62.

17. Lee MJ, Hueniken K, Kuehne N, et al. Cancer patient-reported preferences and knowledge for liquid biopsies and blood biomarkers at a comprehensive cancer center. Cancer Manag Res 2020. https://doi.org/10.2147/CMAR.S235777.

18. Schrock AB, Welsh A, Chung JH, et al. Hybrid capture-based genomic profiling of circulating tumor DNA from patients with advanced non-small cell lung cancer. J Thorac Oncol 2019;14(2):255–64.

19. Odegaard JI, Vincent JJ, Mortimer S, et al. Validation of a plasma-based comprehensive cancer genotyping assay utilizing orthogonal tissue- and plasma-based methodologies. Clin Cancer Res 2018;24(15):3539–49.

20. Sabari JK, Offin M, Stephens D, et al. A prospective study of circulating tumor DNA to guide matched targeted therapy in lung cancers. JNCI J Natl Cancer Inst 2019;111(6):575–83.

21. Remon J, Lacroix L, Jovelet C, et al. Real-world utility of an amplicon-based next-generation sequencing liquid biopsy for broad molecular profiling in patients with advanced non-small-cell lung cancer. JCO Precis Oncol 2019;3(3):1–14.

22. Zill OA, Banks KC, Fairclough SR, et al. The landscape of actionable genomic alterations in cell-free circulating tumor DNA from 21,807 advanced cancer patients. Clin Cancer Res 2018;24(15):3528–38.

23. Aggarwal C, Thompson JC, Black TA, et al. Clinical implications of plasma-based genotyping with the delivery of personalized therapy in metastatic non-small cell lung cancer. JAMA Oncol 2019;5(2):173–80.

24. Cui W, Milner-Watts C, McVeigh TP, et al. A pilot of Blood-First diagnostic cell free DNA (cfDNA) next generation sequencing (NGS) in patients with suspected advanced lung cancer. Lung Cancer 2022;165:34–42.

25. Leighl NB, Page RD, Raymond VM, et al. Clinical utility of comprehensive cell-free DNA Analysis to identify genomic biomarkers in patients with newly diagnosed metastatic non-small cell lung cancer. Clin Cancer Res 2019;25(15):4691–700.

26. Englmeier F, Bleckmann A, Brückl W, et al. Clinical benefit and cost-effectiveness analysis of liquid biopsy application in patients with advanced non-small cell lung cancer (NSCLC): a modelling approach. J Cancer Res Clin Oncol 2022;1–17. https://doi.org/10.1007/S00432-022-04034-W/FIGURES/7.

27. Aldea M, Andre F, Marabelle A, et al. Overcoming resistance to tumor-targeted and immune-targeted therapies. Cancer Discov 2021;11(4):874–99.

28. Cooper AJ, Sequist LV, Lin JJ. Third-generation EGFR and ALK inhibitors: mechanisms of resistance and management. Nat Rev Clin Oncol 2022;19(8):499–514.

29. Oxnard GR, Paweletz CP, Kuang Y, et al. Noninvasive detection of response and resistance in EGFR-mutant lung cancer using quantitative next-generation genotyping of cell-free plasma DNA. Clin Cancer Res 2014;20(6):1698–705.

30. Oxnard GR, Thress KS, Alden RS, et al. Association between plasma genotyping and outcomes of treatment with osimertinib (AZD9291) in advanced non-small-cell lung cancer. J Clin Oncol 2016;34(28):3375–82.

31. Jenkins S, Yang JCH, Ramalingam SS, et al. Plasma ctDNA Analysis for Detection of the EGFR T790M Mutation in Patients with Advanced Non-Small Cell Lung Cancer. J Thorac Oncol 2017;12(7):1061–70.

32. Shaw AT, Solomon BJ, Besse B, et al. ALK resistance mutations and efficacy of lorlatinib in advanced anaplastic lymphoma kinase-positive non-small-cell lung cancer. J Clin Oncol 2019;37(16):1370–9.

33. Zhang Q, Luo J, Wu S, et al. Prognostic and predictive impact of circulating tumor DNA in Patients with advanced cancers treated with immune checkpoint blockade. Cancer Discov 2020;10(12):1842.

34. García-Pardo M, Makarem M, Li JJN, et al. Integrating circulating-free DNA (cfDNA) analysis into clinical practice: opportunities and challenges. Br J Cancer 2022;127(4):592–602.

35. Mack PC, Miao J, Redman MW, et al. Circulating tumor DNA (ctDNA) kinetics predict progression-free and overall survival in EGFR TKI-treated patients with EGFR-mutant NSCLC (SWOG S1403). Clin Cancer Res 2022;OF1–9. https://doi.org/10.1158/1078-0432.CCR-22-0741.

36. Osimertinib Alone or With Chemotherapy for EGFR-Mutant Lung Cancers - Full Text View - ClinicalTrials.gov. Available at: https://clinicaltrials.gov/ct2/show/NCT04410796. Accessed August 25, 2022.

37. Zou W., Yaung S.J., Fuhlbrück F., et al., ctDNA Predicts Overall Survival in Patients With NSCLC Treated With PD-L1 Blockade or With Chemotherapy, JCO Precis Oncol, 5, 2021, 827-838.

38. Russo A, De Miguel Perez D, Gunasekaran M, et al. Liquid biopsy tracking of lung tumor evolutions over time. Expert Rev Mol Diagn 2019;19(12):1099–108.

39. Luskin MR, Murakami MA, Manalis SR, et al. Targeting minimal residual disease: a path to cure? Nat Rev Cancer 2018;18(4):255–63.

40. Goddard ET, Bozic I, Riddell SR, et al. Dormant tumour cells, their niches and the influence of immunity. Nat Cell Biol 2018;20(11):1240–9.

41. Crowley E, Di Nicolantonio F, Loupakis F, et al. Liquid biopsy: monitoring cancer-genetics in the blood. Nat Rev Clin Oncol 2013;10(8):472–84.

42. Schwarzenbach H, Hoon DSB, Pantel K. Cell-free nucleic acids as biomarkers in cancer patients. Nat Rev Cancer 2011;11(6):426–37.

43. de Kock R, van den Borne B, Youssef-El Soud M, et al. Therapy Monitoring of EGFR-Positive Non-Small-Cell Lung Cancer Patients Using ddPCR Multiplex Assays. J Mol Diagn 2021;23(4):495–505.

44. Chaudhuri AA, Chabon JJ, Lovejoy AF, et al. Early Detection of Molecular Residual Disease in Localized Lung Cancer by Circulating Tumor DNA Profiling. Cancer Discov 2017;7(12):1394–403.

45. Reuss JE, Anagnostou V, Cottrell TR, et al. Neoadjuvant nivolumab plus ipilimumab in resectable non-small cell lung cancer. J Immunother cancer 2020;8(2). https://doi.org/10.1136/JITC-2020-001282.

46. Peters S, Spigel D, Ahn M, et al. P03.03 MERMAID-1: a phase III study of adjuvant durvalumab plus chemotherapy in resected NSCLC patients with MRD+ post-surgery. J Thorac Oncol 2021;16(3):S258–9.

47. MERMAID-2: Phase 3 study of durvalumab in patients with resected, Stage II-III NSCLC who become MRD+ after curative-intent therapy | OncologyPRO. Available at: https://oncologypro.esmo.org/meeting-resources/european-lung-cancer-congress-2021/mermaid-2-phase-3-study-of-durvalumab-in-patients-with-resected-stage-ii-iii-nsclc-who-become-mrd-after-curative-intent-therapy. Accessed August 25, 2022.

48. Chabon JJ, Hamilton EG, Kurtz DM, et al. Integrating genomic features for non-invasive early lung cancer detection. Nature 2020;580(7802):245–51.

49. Leal A, van Grieken NCT, Palsgrove DN, et al. White blood cell and cell-free DNA analyses for detection of residual disease in gastric cancer. Nat Commun 2020;11(1). https://doi.org/10.1038/S41467-020-14310-3.

50. Marass F, Stephens D, Ptashkin R, et al. Fragment size analysis may distinguish clonal hematopoiesis from tumor-derived mutations in cell-free DNA. Clin Chem 2020;66(4):616–8.

51. Tognela A, Spring KJ, Becker T, et al. Predictive and prognostic value of circulating tumor cell detection in lung cancer: a clinician's perspective. Crit Rev Oncol Hematol 2015;93(2):90–102.

52. Wu CY, Lee CL, Wu CF, et al. Circulating tumor cells as a tool of minimal residual disease can predict lung cancer recurrence: a longitudinal, prospective trial. Diagnostics 2020;10(3).

53. Parikh AR, van Seventer EE, Siravegna G, et al. Minimal residual disease detection using a plasma-only circulating tumor DNA assay in patients with colorectal cancer. Clin Cancer Res 2021;27(20):OF1–9.

54. Chen X, Dong Z, Hubbell E, et al. Prognostic significance of blood-based multi-cancer detection in plasma cell-free DNA. Clin Cancer Res 2021;27(15):4221–9.
55. Bozic I, Reiter JG, Allen B, et al. Evolutionary dynamics of cancer in response to targeted combination therapy. Elife 2013;2(2). https://doi.org/10.7554/ELIFE.00747.
56. Cree IA, Uttley L, Buckley Woods H, et al. The evidence base for circulating tumour DNA blood-based biomarkers for the early detection of cancer: a systematic mapping review. BMC Cancer 2017;17(1). https://doi.org/10.1186/S12885-017-3693-7.
57. Scimia M, Du J, Pepe F, et al. Evaluation of a novel liquid biopsy-based Colo-Scape assay for mutational analysis of colorectal neoplasia and triage of FIT+ patients: a pilot study. J Clin Pathol 2018;71(12):1123–6.
58. Cohen JD, Javed AA, Thoburn C, et al. Combined circulating tumor DNA and protein biomarker-based liquid biopsy for the earlier detection of pancreatic cancers. Proc Natl Acad Sci U S A 2017;114(38):10202–7.
59. Liu MC, Oxnard GR, Klein EA, et al. Sensitive and specific multi-cancer detection and localization using methylation signatures in cell-free DNA. Ann Oncol Off J Eur Soc Med Oncol 2020;31(6):745–59.
60. Shen SY, Singhania R, Fehringer G, et al. Sensitive tumour detection and classification using plasma cell-free DNA methylomes. Nature 2018;563(7732):579–83.
61. Mathios D, Johansen JS, Cristiano S, et al. Detection and characterization of lung cancer using cell-free DNA fragmentomes. Nat Commun 2021;12(1):1–14.
62. Beane J, Campbell JD, Lel J, et al. Genomic approaches to accelerate cancer interception. Lancet Oncol 2017;18(8):e494–502.
63. Serrano MJ, Garrido-Navas MC, Mochon JJD, et al. Precision prevention and cancer interception: the new challenges of liquid biopsy. Cancer Discov 2020; 10(11):1635–44.
64. Malapelle U, Pisapia P, Addeo A, et al. Liquid biopsy from research to clinical practice: focus on non-small cell lung cancer. Expert Rev Mol Diagn 2021; 21(11):1165–78.
65. Sozzi G, Boeri M, Rossi M, et al. Clinical utility of a plasma-based miRNA signature classifier within computed tomography lung cancer screening: a correlative MILD trial study. J Clin Oncol 2014;32(8):768–73.
66. Montani F, Marzi MJ, Dezi F, et al. miR-Test: a blood test for lung cancer early detection. J Natl Cancer Inst 2015;107(6). https://doi.org/10.1093/JNCI/DJV063.
67. Beane JE, Mazzilli SA, Campbell JD, et al. Molecular subtyping reveals immune alterations associated with progression of bronchial premalignant lesions. Nat Commun 2019;10(1). https://doi.org/10.1038/S41467-019-09834-2.
68. Sequist LV, Nagrath S, Toner M, et al. The CTC-chip: an exciting new tool to detect circulating tumor cells in lung cancer patients. J Thorac Oncol 2009;4(3):281–3.
69. Melosky B, Popat S, Gandara DR. An evolving algorithm to select and sequence therapies in EGFR mutation-positive NSCLC: a strategic approach. Clin Lung Cancer 2018;19(1):42–50.
70. Zhou C, Thakur M Das, Srivastava MK, et al. IMpower010: biomarkers of disease-free survival (DFS) in a Phase 3 study of atezolizumab (atezo) vs best supportive care (BSC) after adjuvant chemo... | OncologyPRO. ESMO Immuno-Oncology Congress 2021, Abstract 2O. Available at: https://oncologypro.esmo.org/meeting-resources/esmo-immuno-oncology-congress/impower010-biomarkers-of-disease-free-survival-dfs-in-a-phase-3-study-of-atezolizumab-atezo-vs-best-supportive-care-bsc-after-adjuvant-chemo. Accessed September 20, 2022.

Advances in Surgical Techniques for Lung Cancer

Brooks V. Udelsman, MD, MHS[a,b], Justin D. Blasberg, MD[a,b,*]

KEYWORDS

- Thoracic surgery • Non–small cell lung cancer
- Video-assisted thoracoscopic surgery • Robotic-assisted thoracoscopic surgery
- Neoadjuvant therapy • Navigational bronchoscopy

KEY POINTS

- Minimally invasive thoracoscopic surgery reduces perioperative morbidity while maintaining long-term survival.
- Parenchymal-sparing segmentectomy can offer the same oncologic benefits as lobectomy in highly selected patients with small (<2 cm) peripheral tumors.
- Increased thresholds for intervention and parenchymal-sparing techniques can reduce morbidity and avoid unnecessary procedures in patients with ground-glass opacities.

BACKGROUND

The goals of thoracic surgery for non–small cell lung cancer (NSCLC) are to achieve an R0 resection, perform an adequate nodal staging, and reduce any associated morbidity. Although these goals have been present since the first oncologic resections were performed nearly 100 years ago, the techniques by which they are achieved have evolved tremendously in the past 3 decades. Improvements have come on multiple fronts and include a transition to minimally invasive approaches, an incorporation of neoadjuvant treatment, and a greater utilization of sublobar resection. These advances have reduced the morbidity of thoracic surgery, while preserving or improving long-term survival. This review highlights the major advances in the surgical management of NSCLC and the keys to optimizing outcomes from a surgical perspective.

CURRENT OPERATIVE TECHNIQUES

The first description of a successful oncologic resection for lung cancer with a survival greater than 1 year was by Drs Evarts Graham and J.J. Singer in 1933.[1] In their original

[a] Division of Thoracic Surgery, Yale-New Haven Hospital, New Haven, CT, USA; [b] Yale University School of Medicine, New Haven, CT, USA
* Corresponding author. 330 Cedar Street, Boardman 204N, PO Box 208039, New Haven, CT 06510.
E-mail address: justin.blasberg@yale.edu

Hematol Oncol Clin N Am 37 (2023) 489–497
https://doi.org/10.1016/j.hoc.2023.02.006
0889-8588/23/© 2023 Elsevier Inc. All rights reserved.

report, a left pneumonectomy was performed through a generous thoracotomy along with removal of the third through ninth rib from the spine to the anterior axillary line.[1] In the intervening decades, advances have been made to reduce the incision size, reduce morbidity, and improve safety. A modern open thoracotomy is typically performed with a posterior-lateral incision in the fifth intercostal space. A rib may be purposefully cut or "shingled" to allow for better access to the chest, but unless there is direct tumor invasion of the chest wall no ribs are resected. The serratus anterior and latissimus dorsi muscle may be preserved in a "muscle-sparing" technique in which they are retracted and spread between their fibers.[2] Using muscle-sparing techniques in combination with intercostal nerve blocks, discharge home on postoperative day 1 has been reported, all be it in highly selected patients.[3] Although these "open" techniques require a larger incision, they do allow the surgeon nearly unrestricted access to the lung and can facilitate identification of subtle lesions through digital palpation.

In the past 25 years the expansion of fiber-optic technology has allowed for surgery to be performed through small incisions with visualization provided by a camera or thoracoscope. Video-assisted thoracoscopic surgery (VATS) was adopted in the 1990s and steadily gained popularity in the 2000s.[4,5] In this technique a camera is inserted into the chest through a 5-mm incision; 3 or 4 additional incisions are made with the largest being up to 4 to 5 cm, which is necessary for extraction of the specimen. Although digital palpation of the lung is more challenging compared with open techniques, it is still possible to palpate almost all the parenchymal surface to identify and remove a nodule of interest. As a result, this technique is commonly used for surgical biopsy of a suspicious nodule or parenchymal process.

Numerous retrospective studies have compared VATS with traditional thoracotomy. These studies have consistently demonstrated a reduction in perioperative complications and hospital length of stay.[6–10] Several adjusted and propensity-matched analyses have demonstrated at least equivalent long-term survival.[8,9,11,12] However, the nodal dissection of N1 and N2 nodes can be more challenging using a VATS approach, and reduction in nodal harvest and upstaging has been observed in several large database series.[7,8,10,13] The impact of nodal evaluation on long-term survival also remains a controversial point given equivalent long-term survival in most large series.

In addition to VATS, robotic-assisted thoracoscopic surgery (RATS) has emerged as a minimally invasive approach. This technology primarily uses the da Vinci surgical system (Intuitive Surgical, Sunnyvale, CA, USA), although new platforms are in development. The first published reports on RATS were from the early 2000s, and since that time the technology has been rapidly adopted.[14–16] The popularity of a RATS approach is partly explained by the shorter learning curve necessary to obtain competency and mastery of the technique. As opposed to VATS lobectomy in which an estimated 50 cases are required for competency, the learning curve for RATS is an estimated 22 lobectomies.[17–19] The advantages of robotics are founded in the platform using a hybrid of both open and VATS approaches: instruments that move and perform functions similar to a human hand through an open incision, however, miniaturized and through keyhole incisions to achieve the patient-specific benefits of VATS.

Direct comparison of RATS and VATS has demonstrated minimal differences. In multiple studies, perioperative morbidity is equivalent.[20–22] There is a slight advantage to RATS in nodal harvest, but so far this has not been associated with an increase in nodal upstaging or survival.[20,24] RATS may be associated with increased cost, but this can be partially explained by the upfront costs associated with early adoption.[25,26] Although a minimally invasive approach is preferred over open thoracotomy, there is no clear advantage of one minimally invasive approach over the other (**Table 1**).

Table 1 Approaches to surgical resection of lung cancer			
Approach	**First Adoption**	**Advantages**	**Disadvantages**
Thoracotomy	1930s	• Direct palpation of lung • Direct visualization of the lung surface	• Increased postoperative pain • Increased length of stay
VATS	1990s	• Reduced postoperative morbidity • Reduced length of stay • Digital palpation of most of the lung surface	• Visualization dependent on quality of thoracoscope • Longer learning curve • More difficult nodal dissection
RATS	2000s	• Reduced postoperative morbidity • Reduce length of stay • High-definition thoracoscope • Reduced learning curve	• No access for digital palpation • Lack of hepatic feedback • Increased cost

SURGERY IN THE SETTING OF NEOADJUVANT THERAPY

Chemoradiotherapy and more recently chemotherapy plus immunotherapy is the preferred treatment in patients who present with locally advanced, stage IIIa/IIIb disease or larger central node-negative tumors in which neoadjuvant therapy may improve resectability.[27–30] Compared with upfront surgery, operative resection after neoadjuvant has shown a clear benefit in this patient population.[31,32] Surgery after neoadjuvant treatment can be challenging due to treatment-related changes, which can make operative resection more difficult and increase the risk of bronchial stump breakdown. Despite this risk several studies have demonstrated the safety of surgery after immunotherapy.[33] Yang and colleagues[34] showed no difference in perioperative mortality or morbidity in a cohort of patients receiving chemotherapy as well as ipilimumab compared with historical controls. Likewise, Bott and colleagues[35] demonstrated the safety of neoadjuvant treatment with nivolumab followed by surgical resection. Such results served as the foundation for larger neoadjuvant trials, including Checkmate 816, in which combination neoadjuvant nivolumab plus chemotherapy was associated with longer event-free survival and higher rate of complete pathologic response compared with chemotherapy alone.[36] Although these trials cast a wide net regarding patients for inclusion, these results are more provocative for patients with locoregional disease and a greater than 1% expression of Programmed death-ligand 1 (PD-L1). Additional studies using larger cohorts and greater follow-up will be needed to determine the true benefit of immunotherapy in the neoadjuvant setting.

Equally important is the role of salvage surgery in patients with locally advanced disease that either recurs or demonstrates only a partial response to treatment. In these patients with locoregional failure, surgery can offer a potential benefit.[37] The benefits of salvage surgery vary widely in the literature with a 3-year survival ranging from 20% to 78%.[38,39] Complication rates in patients undergoing salvage surgery tend to be higher, and there is a frequent need for pneumonectomy or bilobectomy.[40] In a meta-analysis comparing long-term survival there is a clear advantage to surgical resection in patients when a pneumonectomy can be avoided.[41] There is also significant heterogeneity with patients who have early recurrence and death as well as long-term survivors (>5 years).[42] Predicting which patients may benefit from salvage surgery remains an area of continued investigation.

SEGMENTECTOMY AND SUBLOBAR RESECTION FOR EARLY-STAGE NON–SMALL CELL LUNG CANCER

Surgical resection for NSCLC can be accomplished through 3 methods: lobectomy, segmentectomy, or wedge resection. Lobectomy mandates the formal resection of the associated bronchus, pulmonary artery, and pulmonary vein to the specified lobe. Segmentectomy mandates the resection of the segmental bronchus and at least 1 of the associated vascular structures (typically the segmental pulmonary artery).[43] In both cases the associated nodal basin is taken with the specimen. In contrast, a wedge resection simply requires the resection of tumor and associated parenchyma without regard to the underlying anatomic structures. The nature of this operation restricts the opportunity to fully resect local lymph nodes and draining lymphatic pathways in a similar fashion to anatomic resection.

In 1995 the North American Lung Cancer Study Group published the results of a randomized clinical trial comparing lobectomy to limited resection (wedge resection or segmentectomy) for early-stage NSCLC (T1N0). The results of that trial demonstrated an unequivocal disadvantage to limited resection, with a 30% increase in death rate and a 50% increase in observed death with cancer rate.[44] However, accrual for the study occurred between 1982 and 1988 before the widespread adoption of computed tomography (CT) and PET. In addition, a significant proportion of patients in the sublobar resection group were treated with wedge resection.

Given the significant improvements in staging that have occurred with the rise of CT and PET-CT, 2 additional trials were performed to reassess the benefits of limited resection. The first, JCOG0802, compared lobectomy with segmentectomy for small (≤2 cm) clinical stage Ia tumors with a consolidation-to-tumor ratio (CTR) greater than 0.5.[45] The results showed a modest but statistically significant 5-year survival advantage to segmentectomy over lobectomy (94.3% vs 91.1%). Similarly, the CALGB/Alliance 140503 demonstrated noninferiority of sublobar (wedge or segmentectomy) resection in node-negative NSCLC less than 2 cm in diameter.[46] Although the impact of these recently reported studies remains uncertain, there is evidence supporting the use of anatomic segmentectomy in carefully selected small early-stage tumors with slow growth kinetics and low risk of nodal spread.

SURGICAL MANAGEMENT OF GROUND-GLASS OPACITIES

As a result of improvement and widespread adoption of CT scans, small subsolid nodules are commonly encountered.[47] Unlike sold nodules, ground-glass opacities (GGOs) are defined as hazy lung opacities with preservation of bronchial and vascular markings.[48,49] In the setting of pneumonia, interstitial lung disease, or other inflammation they can represent benign disease. However, persistent or growing GGOs, especially those that develop a solid component, may represent an early-stage adenocarcinoma.

Determining the threshold for intervention for GGOs is an ongoing challenge to the field. In up to 30% of individuals, GGOs are multifocal and overly aggressive intervention at one site (eg, lobectomy) can result in unnecessary morbidity or limited treatment options for additional sites.[50] Conversely, these tumors can eventually metastasize to lymph nodes and other organs and if surgery is delayed the opportunity for cure may be lost. Fortunately, 5-year survival is greater than 90% in most series, and for this reason the threshold for intervention has gradually increased over the past 2 decades.[51] Features on serial imaging warranting surgical intervention include maximal size greater than 3 cm, new solid area or growth of prior solid area by greater than or equal to 2 mm on mediastinal windows, or growth by greater than or equal to 25% in a single year (total or solid area).[52] Likewise, the extent of resection for GGOs has gradually decreased. Most recently, the Japan Clinical Oncology Group and the West Japan Oncology Group demonstrated a 5-year relapse-free survival of 99.7% for peripheral GGOs with a CTR less than 0.25 treated with wide wedge resection or segmentectomy.[53] Based on these results sublobar resection seems to be efficacious along with systematic sampling of N1 and N2 nodes for this particular subgroup.[47]

Perhaps the greatest challenge for the thoracic surgeon in the operating room is the difficulty encountered in palpating these lesions. Unlike solid nodules, which can readily be identified, GGOs can often elude digital palpation.[54] In a RATS approach this is even more challenging because only the gentle brushing of the robotic instruments provides clues to the exact location of the GGO. For this reason fiducial markers or injectable agents are often placed by interventional radiology before surgery.[55,56] These agents include radiotracers, metal clips, and lipiodol. These agents can be used in combination with a thoracotomy, VATS, or RATS approach and are associated with 95% to 98% success rate in most series.[57–62]

NAVIGATIONAL BRONCHOSCOPY

The evolution of robotics in surgical practice also includes opportunities for nodule localization and biopsy. Although initially difficult to use and only a small improvement from traditional bronchoscopic options such as endobronchial ultrasonography,[63] the newest generation of robotic navigation platforms allow for access to more peripheral targets or nodules at challenging angles to the airway. In this format, the camera is mounted to a robotic arm, the control and movement of a robotic bronchoscope is precise and robotically driven, and angles for biopsy can be achieved without deflection in the airway to improve diagnostic yield. In a recently reported multicenter study including more than 50 patients enrolled from 5 centers, the diagnostic yield was greater than 90%.[64] This is an operator-dependent technology and best performed at centers of excellence with expertise and volume, which are both likely associated with successful sampling. Future iterations of robotic navigation harmonized with ablative technologies could have therapeutic applications for subgroups of high-risk patients or nodules not amenable to radiation or peripheral ablation.

SUMMARY

Thoracic surgery has made major strides in the past 3 decades. The advent of minimally invasive techniques has allowed for a significant reduction in perioperative complications and postoperative pain. Going forward, the field will be challenged to integrate neoadjuvant treatment while maintaining these hard-fought improvements in perioperative morbidity. Equally important, disparities in treatment need to be addressed. Despite clear advantages to minimal invasive techniques, open thoracotomy is still performed in more than 40% of patients with stage I NSCLC.[65] As in many other areas of medicine, poorer patients and those living in rural areas tend to have reduced access to optimal care.[66] For the full advantages of recent advancements to be realized equity of care needs to become a priority.

DISCLOSURES

The authors have no financial disclosures to report.

FUNDING

No outside funding was used in the completion of this work.

AUTHOR CONTRIBUTIONS

B.V. Udelsman: conception, analysis, interpretation of data, and drafting of article.
J.D. Blasberg: conception, analysis, interpretation of data, and drafting of article.

REFERENCES

1. Graham EA, Singer JJ. Successful removal of an entire lung for carcinoma of the bronchus. J Am Med Assoc 1933;101(18):1371–4.
2. Tovar EA, Roethe RA, Weissig MD, et al. Muscle-sparing minithoracotomy with intercostal nerve cryoanalgesia: an improved method for major lung resections. Am Surg 1998;64(11):1109–15.
3. Tovar EA, Roethe RA, Weissig MD, et al. One-day admission for lung lobectomy: an incidental result of a clinical pathway. Ann Thorac Surg 1998;65(3):803–6.
4. Abbas AE. Surgical management of lung cancer: history, evolution, and modern advances. Curr Oncol Rep 2018;20(12):98.
5. Cheng X, Onaitis MW, D'amico TA, et al. Minimally invasive thoracic surgery 3.0: lessons learned from the history of lung cancer surgery. Ann Surg 2018; 267(1):37–8.
6. Scott WJ, Allen MS, Darling G, et al. Video-assisted thoracic surgery versus open lobectomy for lung cancer: a secondary analysis of data from the American College of Surgeons Oncology Group Z0030 randomized clinical trial. J Thorac Cardiovasc Surg 2010;139(4):976–81 [discussion: 981-3].
7. Nwogu CE, Groman A, Fahey D, et al. Number of lymph nodes and metastatic lymph node ratio are associated with survival in lung cancer. Ann Thorac Surg 2012;93(5):1614–9 [discussion: 1619-20].
8. Licht PB, Jørgensen OD, Ladegaard L, et al. A national study of nodal upstaging after thoracoscopic versus open lobectomy for clinical stage I lung cancer. Ann Thorac Surg 2013;96(3):943–9 [discussion: 949-50].
9. Flores RM, Park BJ, Dycoco J, et al. Lobectomy by video-assisted thoracic surgery (VATS) versus thoracotomy for lung cancer. J Thorac Cardiovasc Surg 2009;138(1):11–8.
10. Boffa DJ, Kosinski AS, Paul S, et al. Lymph node evaluation by open or video-assisted approaches in 11,500 anatomic lung cancer resections. Ann Thorac Surg 2012;94(2):347–53 [discussion: 353].
11. Nwogu CE, D'Cunha J, Pang H, et al. VATS lobectomy has better perioperative outcomes than open lobectomy: CALGB 31001, an ancillary analysis of CALGB 140202 (Alliance). Ann Thorac Surg 2015;99(2):399–405.
12. Al-Ameri M, Bergman P, Franco-Cereceda A, et al. Video-assisted thoracoscopic versus open thoracotomy lobectomy: a Swedish nationwide cohort study. J Thorac Dis 2018;10(6):3499–506.
13. Denlinger CE, Fernandez F, Meyers BF, et al. Lymph node evaluation in video-assisted thoracoscopic lobectomy versus lobectomy by thoracotomy. Ann Thorac Surg 2010;89(6):1730–5 [discussion: 1736].
14. Bodner J, Wykypiel H, Wetscher G, et al. First experiences with the da Vincie operating robot in thoracic surgery. Eur J Cardio Thorac Surg 2004;25:844–51.

15. Park BJ, Flores RM, Rusch VW. Robotic assistance for video-assisted thoracic surgical lobectomy: technique and initial results. J Thorac Cardiovasc Surg 2006;131(1):54–9.
16. Subramanian MP, Liu J, Chapman WC Jr, et al. Utilization trends, outcomes, and cost in minimally invasive lobectomy. Ann Thorac Surg 2019;108(6):1648–55.
17. Arnold BN, Thomas DC, Bhatnagar V, et al. Defining the learning curve in robot-assisted thoracoscopic lobectomy. Surgery 2019;165(2):450–4.
18. McKenna RJ Jr. Complications and learning curves for video-assisted thoracic surgery lobectomy. Thorac Surg Clin 2008;18(3):275–80.
19. Petersen RH, Hansen HJ. Learning curve associated with VATS lobectomy. Ann Cardiothorac Surg 2012;1(1):47–50.
20. Louie BE, Wilson JL, Kim S, et al. Comparison of video-assisted thoracoscopic surgery and robotic approaches for clinical stage I and stage II non-small cell lung cancer using the society of thoracic surgeons database. Ann Thorac Surg 2016;102(3):917–24.
21. Haruki T, Kubouchi Y, Takagi Y, et al. Comparison of medium-term survival outcomes between robot-assisted thoracoscopic surgery and video-assisted thoracoscopic surgery in treating primary lung cancer. Gen Thorac Cardiovasc Surg 2020;68(9):984–92.
22. Ma J, Li X, Zhao S, et al. Robot-assisted thoracic surgery versus video-assisted thoracic surgery for lung lobectomy or segmentectomy in patients with non-small cell lung cancer: a meta-analysis. BMC Cancer 2021;21(1):498.
23. Udelsman BV, Chang DC, Boffa DJ, et al. Association of Lymph node sampling and clinical volume in lobectomy for non-small cell lung cancer. Ann Thorac Surg 2022. https://doi.org/10.1016/j.athoracsur.2022.05.051.
24. Merritt RE, Abdel-Rasoul M, D'Souza DM, et al. Lymph node upstaging for robotic, thoracoscopic, and open lobectomy for stage T2-3N0 lung cancer. Ann Thorac Surg 2022. https://doi.org/10.1016/j.athoracsur.2022.05.041.
25. Swanson SJ, Miller DL, McKenna RJ Jr, et al. Comparing robot-assisted thoracic surgical lobectomy with conventional video-assisted thoracic surgical lobectomy and wedge resection: Results from a multihospital database (Premier). J Thorac Cardiovasc Surg 2014;47(3):929–37.
26. Nasir BS, Bryant AS, Minnich DJ, et al. Performing robotic lobectomy and segmentectomy: cost, profitability, and outcomes. Ann Thorac Surg 2014;98(1):203–8 [discussion: 208-9].
27. Bradley JD, Paulus R, Komaki R, et al. Standard-dose versus high-dose conformal radiotherapy with concurrent and consolidation carboplatin plus paclitaxel with or without cetuximab for patients with stage IIIA or IIIB non-small-cell lung cancer (RTOG 0617): a randomised, two-by-two factorial phase 3 study. Lancet Oncol 2015;16(2):187–99.
28. Aupérin A, Le Péchoux C, Rolland E, et al. Meta-analysis of concomitant versus sequential radiochemotherapy in locally advanced non-small-cell lung cancer. J Clin Oncol 2010;28(13):2181–90.
29. Antonia SJ, Villegas A, Daniel D, et al. Overall survival with durvalumab after chemoradiotherapy in stage III NSCLC. N Engl J Med 2018;379(24):2342–50.
30. Jabbour SK, Berman AT, Decker RH, et al. Phase 1 trial of pembrolizumab administered concurrently with chemoradiotherapy for locally advanced non-small cell lung cancer: a nonrandomized controlled trial. JAMA Oncol 2020;6(6):848–55.
31. Rosell R, Gómez-Codina J, Camps C, et al. A randomized trial comparing preoperative chemotherapy plus surgery with surgery alone in patients with non-small-cell lung cancer. N Engl J Med 1994;330(3):153–8.

32. Roth JA, Fossella F, Komaki R, et al. A randomized trial comparing perioperative chemotherapy and surgery with surgery alone in resectable stage IIIA non-small-cell lung cancer. J Natl Cancer Inst 1994;86(9):673–80.

33. Jia X-H, Xu H, Geng L-Y, et al. Efficacy and safety of neoadjuvant immunotherapy in resectable nonsmall cell lung cancer: A meta-analysis. Lung Cancer 2020;147:143–53.

34. Yang C-FJ, McSherry F, Mayne NR, et al. Surgical outcomes after neoadjuvant chemotherapy and ipilimumab for non-small cell lung cancer. Ann Thorac Surg 2018;105(3):924–9.

35. Bott MJ, Yang SC, Park BJ, et al. Initial results of pulmonary resection after neoadjuvant nivolumab in patients with resectable non-small cell lung cancer. J Thorac Cardiovasc Surg 2019;158(1):269–76.

36. Forde PM, Spicer J, Lu S, et al. Neoadjuvant nivolumab plus chemotherapy in resectable lung cancer. N Engl J Med 2022;386(21):1973–85.

37. Dickhoff C, Dahele M, Paul MA, et al. Salvage surgery for locoregional recurrence or persistent tumor after high dose chemoradiotherapy for locally advanced non-small cell lung cancer. Lung Cancer 2016;94:108–13.

38. Casiraghi M, Maisonneuve P, Piperno G, et al. Salvage Surgery after definitive chemoradiotherapy for non-small cell lung cancer. Semin Thorac Cardiovasc Surg 2017;29(2):233–41.

39. Shimada Y, Suzuki K, Okada M, et al. Feasibility and efficacy of salvage lung resection after definitive chemoradiation therapy for Stage III non-small-cell lung cancer. Interact Cardiovasc Thorac Surg 2016;23(6):895–901.

40. Dickhoff C, Otten RHJ, Heymans MW, et al. Salvage surgery for recurrent or persistent tumour after radical (chemo)radiotherapy for locally advanced non-small cell lung cancer: a systematic review. Ther Adv Med Oncol 2018;10. 1758835918804150.

41. Swaminath A, Vella ET, Ramchandar K, et al. Surgery after chemoradiotherapy in patients with stage III (N2 or N3, excluding T4) non-small-cell lung cancer: a systematic review. Curr Oncol 2019;26(3):e398–404.

42. Schreiner W, Dudek W, Lettmaier S, et al. Long-term survival after salvage surgery for local failure after definitive chemoradiation therapy for locally advanced non-small cell lung cancer. Thorac Cardiovasc Surg 2018;66(2):135–41.

43. Weiss KD, Deeb AL, Wee JO, et al. When a segmentectomy is not a segmentectomy: quality assurance audit and evaluation of required elements for an anatomic segmentectomy. J Thorac Cardiovasc Surg 2022. https://doi.org/10. 1016/j.jtcvs.2022.08.042.

44. Ginsberg RJ, Rubinstein LV. Randomized trial of lobectomy versus limited resection for T1 N0 non-small cell lung cancer. Lung Cancer Study Group. Ann Thorac Surg 1995;60(3):615–22 [discussion: 622-3].

45. Saji H, Okada M, Tsuboi M, et al. Segmentectomy versus lobectomy in small-sized peripheral non-small-cell lung cancer (JCOG0802/WJOG4607L): a multicentre, open-label, phase 3, randomised, controlled, non-inferiority trial. Lancet 2022;399(10335):1607–17.

46. Altorki NK, Wang X, Kozono D, et al. PL03.06 lobar or sub-lobar resection for peripheral clinical stage IA = 2 cm non-small cell lung cancer (NSCLC): results from an international randomized phase III trial (CALGB 140503 [Alliance]). J Thorac Oncol 2022;17(9, Supplement):S1–2.

47. Detterbeck FC, Homer RJ. Approach to the ground-glass nodule. Clin Chest Med 2011;32(4):799–810.

48. Müller NL. Differential diagnosis of chronic diffuse infiltrative lung disease on high-resolution computed tomography. Semin Roentgenol 1991;26(2):132–42.
49. Zhang Y, Fu F, Chen H. Management of ground-glass opacities in the lung cancer spectrum. Ann Thorac Surg 2020;110(6):1796–804.
50. Kim TJ, Goo JM, Lee KW, et al. Clinical, pathological and thin-section CT features of persistent multiple ground-glass opacity nodules: comparison with solitary ground-glass opacity nodule. Lung Cancer 2009;64(2):171–8.
51. Suzuki K. Whack-a-mole strategy for multifocal ground glass opacities of the lung. J Thorac Dis 2017;9(Suppl 3):S201–7.
52. Detterbeck FC. Achieving clarity about lung cancer and opacities. Chest 2017; 151(2):252–4.
53. Suzuki K, Watanabe S-I, Wakabayashi M, et al. A single-arm study of sublobar resection for ground-glass opacity dominant peripheral lung cancer. J Thorac Cardiovasc Surg 2022;163(1):289–301.e2.
54. Suzuki K, Nagai K, Yoshida J, et al. Video-assisted thoracoscopic surgery for small indeterminate pulmonary nodules: indications for preoperative marking. Chest 1999;115(2):563–8.
55. Yang SC, Oh where. oh where can that little nodule be? J Thorac Cardiovasc Surg 2015;149(1):33–4.
56. Predina JD, Fedor D, Newton AD, et al. Intraoperative molecular imaging: the surgical oncologist's north star. Ann Surg 2017;266(6):e42–4.
57. Fan L, Yang H, Yu L, et al. Multicenter, prospective, observational study of a novel technique for preoperative pulmonary nodule localization. J Thorac Cardiovasc Surg 2020;160(2):532–9.e2.
58. Tyng CJ, Baranauskas MVB, Bitencourt AGV, et al. Preoperative computed tomography-guided localization of ground-glass opacities with metallic clip. Ann Thorac Surg 2013;96(3):1087–9.
59. Park CH, Han K, Hur J, et al. Comparative effectiveness and safety of preoperative lung localization for pulmonary nodules: a systematic review and meta-analysis. Chest 2017;151(2):316–28.
60. Park CH, Lee SM, Lee JW, et al. Hook-wire localization versus lipiodol localization for patients with pulmonary lesions having ground-glass opacity. J Thorac Cardiovasc Surg 2020;159(4):1571–9.e2.
61. Grogan EL, Jones DR, Kozower BD, et al. Identification of small lung nodules: technique of radiotracer-guided thoracoscopic biopsy. Ann Thorac Surg 2008; 85(2):S772–7.
62. Stiles BM, Altes TA, Jones DR, et al. Clinical experience with radiotracer-guided thoracoscopic biopsy of small, indeterminate lung nodules. Ann Thorac Surg 2006;82(4):1191–6 [discussion: 1196-7].
63. Oki M, Saka H, Ando M, et al. Ultrathin bronchoscopy with multimodal devices for peripheral pulmonary lesions. a randomized trial. Am J Respir Crit Care Med 2015;192(4):468–76.
64. Chen AC, Pastis NJ Jr, Mahajan AK, et al. Robotic bronchoscopy for peripheral pulmonary lesions: a multicenter pilot and feasibility study (BENEFIT). Chest 2021;159(2):845–52.
65. Medbery RL, Fernandez FG, Kosinski AS, et al. Costs associated with lobectomy for lung cancer: an analysis merging STS and medicare data. Ann Thorac Surg 2021;111(6):1781–90.
66. Stitzenberg KB, Shah PC, Snyder JA, et al. Disparities in access to video-assisted thoracic surgical lobectomy for treatment of early-stage lung cancer. J Laparoendosc Adv Surg Tech 2012;22(8):753–7.

Nonsurgical Therapy for Early-Stage Lung Cancer

Megan E. Daly, MD[a],*, Patrick Beagen, MD[a], Mohammad H. Madani, MD[b]

KEYWORDS

- Non-small cell lung cancer • SABR • SBRT • Thermal ablation

KEY POINTS

- Non-surgical treatment approaches for early stage, medically inoperable NSCLC now offer the potential of cure to patients who historically had limited treatment options.
- Stereotactic ablative radiotherapy (SABR) is the delivery of highly conformal, high dose per fraction radiation to the tumor and results in high rates of primary tumor control.
- Toxicity following SABR is largely dependent on tumor location, adjacent anatomy, and dose to critical structures.
- Percutaneous imaging guided thermal ablation provides an additional non-surgical treatment approach for inoperable NSCLC with promising outcomes and low toxicity.

 Video content accompanies this article at http://www.hemonc.theclinics.com.

INTRODUCTION

The standard treatment for early-stage non-small cell lung cancer (NSCLC) has historically been surgical, through either lobectomy or sublobar resection. However, many patients with early-stage NSCLC are medically inoperable, with cardiac, pulmonary, or other comorbidities that preclude safe surgical resection, and other patients decline surgery. Until the development of stereotactic radiation (SBRT or stereotactic ablative radiotherapy [SABR]; herein referred to as SABR), conventionally fractionated radiation was typically used, with modest results and a significant treatment burden on patients with protracted treatment courses. With the advent of SABR, medically inoperable patients gained a treatment option with only 3 to 5 sessions and disease control approaching that of matched surgical cohorts in some series.[1–4] Percutaneous image-guided thermal ablation is also a nonsurgical option with limited toxicity and

a Department of Radiation Oncology, University of California Davis Comprehensive Cancer Center, 4501 X Street, G-140, Sacramento, CA 95817, USA; b RadiologyDepartment of Radiology, University of California, Davis, 4860 Y Street, Suite 3100, Sacramento, CA 95817, USA
* Corresponding author.
E-mail address: medaly@ucdavis.edu

Hematol Oncol Clin N Am 37 (2023) 499–512
https://doi.org/10.1016/j.hoc.2023.02.002
0889-8588/23/© 2023 Elsevier Inc. All rights reserved.

promising tumor control. Herein, we review the data for SABR and percutaneous image-guided thermal ablation in early-stage NSCLC.

WHAT IS STEREOTACTIC ABLATIVE RADIOTHERAPY?

SABR is the use of high dose per fraction, highly conformal radiation using advanced technologies for target localization, dose delivery, motion management, and image guidance to allow small target margins and steep dose gradients.[5] SABR is delivered during 1 to 5 sessions, although slightly more protracted regimens of up to 8 to 10 sessions are sometimes used for challenging anatomic scenarios with SABR-like approaches.

CLINICAL HISTORY OF STEREOTACTIC ABLATIVE RADIOTHERAPY

The earliest clinical reports using SABR for tumors of the lung were published more than 20 years ago by investigators in Sweden,[6] Japan,[7] and Germany.[8] These early reports were followed by 2 published phase I trials in 2003. Timmerman and colleagues at Indiana University enrolled 37 medically inoperable patients with T1-2 NSCLC of 7 cm or less. Patients were treated with 3 fraction SABR, starting at a dose of 24 Gy and escalating to 60 Gy in 3 fractions. Treatment was well tolerated, with dose-limiting toxicity observed in 2 patients.[9] Whyte and colleagues from Stanford University also published a phase I trial using single fraction SABR in 2003. Twenty-three patients with primary or metastatic lung tumors underwent single fraction SABR to 15 Gy without grade 3+ toxicity observed.[10]

Shortly thereafter, the first North American Cooperative Group trial using SABR in early-stage NSCLC was activated, Radiation Therapy Oncology Group (RTOG) 0236. RTOG 0236 was a single-arm phase II trial that enrolled 59 patients (55 evaluable) with T1-2N0M0, peripherally located, medically inoperable NSCLC of less than 5 cm. Patients underwent SABR to 60 Gy in 3 fractions on nonconsecutive days. At 3 years, the local (primary tumor) control (LC) was 97.6%, the local-regional control rate was 90.6%, distant recurrence was 22.1%, with overall survival (OS) of 55.8%.[11] A subsequent analysis found that given the lack of heterogeneity correction used in early SBRT trials, the delivered dose was closer to 54 Gy to 56 Gy in 3 fractions.[12] Adoption of SABR following publication of RTOG 0236 in 2010 was widespread. A timeline of the development of SABR is shown in **Fig. 1**.

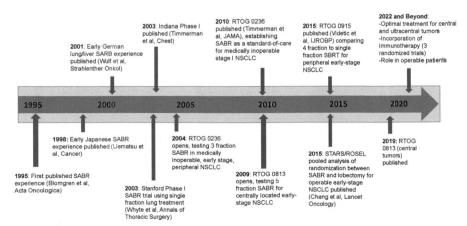

Fig. 1. Timeline of the development of SABR. Created with BioRender.com.

CLINICAL OUTCOMES FOLLOWING STEREOTACTIC ABLATIVE RADIOTHERAPY
Comparisons of Stereotactic Ablative Radiotherapy and Conventionally Fractionated Radiation

The stereotactic precision and conventional radiotherapy evaluation (SPACE) trial was a randomized phase II comparison of SABR (66 Gy in 3 fractions) and conventionally fractionated conformal radiation to 70 Gy in 35 fractions. Eighty-one enrolled patients had stage I medically inoperable NSCLC. No statistically significant difference in progression-free survival (PFS; HR = 0.85, 95% CI 0.52–1.36) or OS (HR = 0.75, 95% CI 0.43–1.30) was observed, although prognostic factors were not well balanced between the 2 arms, with more T2 tumors in the SABR arm. Toxicity was low in both arms but favored the SABR arm. The authors concluded that given the convenience of SABR as compared with conventional radiation, it should be considered the standard of care.[13] Subsequently, the CHISL trial provided a randomized phase 3 comparison of SABR and conventionally fractionated radiation with well-balanced arms.[14] The investigators randomized 101 patients with early stage, peripherally located, medically operable (or refused surgery) NSCLC between SABR to 54 Gy in 3 fractions or 48 Gy in 4 fractions, and conventionally fractionated radiation to 66 Gy in 33 fractions with a 2:1 randomization. Freedom from local treatment failure was improved in the SABR group as compared with the conventionally fractionated radiation arm (HR 0·32, 95% CI 0·13–0·77, P = .0077). Toxicity was low in both arms. In aggregate, the available prospective randomized trials suggest SABR should be the preferred radiation approach as compared with conventionally fractionated radiation due to disease control, toxicity, and patient convenience.

Comparisons of Stereotactic Ablative Radiotherapy and Surgery

Early SABR trials primarily focused on patients with medically inoperable early-stage NSCLC. However, with longer term follow-up demonstrating excellent LC at 5 years and beyond,[15–17] interest has grown in the use of SABR in medically operable populations, particularly those at higher risk of surgical complications or postsurgical decrements in pulmonary function. Several trials have attempted to prospectively randomize patients between surgery and SABR for early-stage NSCLC, which has proven challenging. Both the STARS trial (NCT00840749) and ROSEL trial (NCT00687986) were randomized phase III comparisons between lobectomy and SABR in patients with standard operative risk early-stage NSCLC, and both closed early secondary to slow accrual. A subsequent analysis pooling the 58 patients enrolled to both trials, which had similar eligibility criteria, was published. In this small, pooled analysis, 3-year OS was 95% following SABR, and 79% following lobectomy (HR 0·14, 95% CI 0·017–1·190, log-rank P = .037),[18] suggesting equipoise for future randomized prospective trials in standard-risk operable patients. A subsequent revision of the STARS trial enrolled 80 patients with operable early-stage NSCLC to a prospective, single-arm study of SABR. These patients were compared with a contemporary, protocol-specified propensity match cohort of patients treated surgically with video-assisted thoracoscopic lobectomy (VATS). OS among patients treated with SABR was 91% at 3 years and 84% at 5 years and was noninferior to the matched VATS cohort.[3]

Currently, the Veterans Affairs Lung Cancer Surgery or Stereotactic Radiotherapy (VALOR) trial is actively recruiting patients to a randomized phase 3 comparison of lobectomy and surgery within the United States Veterans Affairs system. Eligible patients have standard-operable risk disease and are fit for lobectomy (NCT02984761).

In the high-surgical risk setting, the ACOSOG Z0499 trial attempted to complete a randomized comparison of sublobar resection and SABR in patients with pulmonary, cardiac, or other risks precluding lobectomy. The study was closed due to slow accrual. However, the investigators reopened a similar concept as the JoLT-Ca STA-BLE-MATES trial and a novel "prerandomization" design is being used in which patients know their randomization before consenting to the treatment (NCT02468024). **Table 1** outlines prior and ongoing randomized trials comparing surgery and SABR for early-stage NSCLC.

TECHNICAL ASPECTS OF STEREOTACTIC ABLATIVE RADIOTHERAPY
Dose and Fractionation

For early-stage NSCLC, regimens with a biologically effective dose of at least 100 Gy_{10}, including 25 Gy to 34 Gy in a single fraction, 54 Gy to 60 Gy in 3 fractions, 48 Gy to 50 Gy in 4 fractions, and 50 Gy to 60 Gy in 5 fractions are commonly used and supported by prospective data (**Table 2**). Several randomized phase II trials have directly compared single fraction SABR to fractionated regimens with similar results. Singh and colleagues reported a randomized phase II comparison carried out at the Cleveland Clinic and Roswell Park Cancer Center. Ninety-eight medically inoperable patients with T1-2N0M0, peripherally located NSCLC were randomized between 30 Gy OK in 1 fraction and 60 Gy OK in 3 fractions. With median follow-up of 53.8 months, no significant difference in LC, PFS, or OS was noted.[19] RTOG 0915 was a randomized phase II cooperative group trial that compared 34 Gy in 1 fraction to 48 Gy in 4 fractions. Eligible patients had T1-2N0M0 peripherally located NSCLC and were medically inoperable. LC, PFS, and toxicity were similar between arms.[20]

Patient Immobilization and Motion Management

Patient immobilization is a critical component of SABR because typically small (3–7 mm) planning target volumes (PTVs) are used. Long vacuum lock bags that conform to the patient's back and sides or other rigid immobilization devise are often used. SABR planning must account for tumor motion secondary to respiratory motion. Four-dimensional computed tomography is commonly used to capture tumor motion in a single respiratory cycle to estimate the magnitude of tumor motion and allow the creation of an internal target volume (ITV) encompassing the full range of tumor positions throughout the respiratory cycles (Video 1). When tumor motion is substantial (typically more than 1 cm amplitude), measures are typically taken to either dampen this motion, track the tumor, or selectively deliver radiation during a gating window or breath hold. An additional PTV margin of approximately 5 mm is typically added to the ITV to create the final target volume (**Fig. 2**).

Stereotactic Ablative Radiotherapy Treatment Planning

A variety of treatment planning approaches can be used for SABR planning, including static noncoplanar fields, multiple dynamic conformal arcs, intensity modulated radiation, and volume modulated radiation. The key quality metrics for a SABR plan, regardless of planning technique, center around conformality of both high-dose and low-dose spillage and the ability to meet critical dose volume constraints. Normal tissues of concern with lung SABR planning include the lungs, heart, proximal bronchial tree, esophagus, great vessels, spinal cord, and brachial plexus, among others (**Fig. 3**A–D). When standard dose volume constraints are respected, toxicities following SABR are low. However, certain clinical scenarios pose higher risks of toxicity, particularly "centrally" located tumors within 2 cm of the proximal bronchial tree, and "ultracentral" tumors directly abutting the proximal bronchial tree or esophagus.

Table 1
Prospective trials comparing surgery and stereotactic ablative radiotherapy for early-stage medically operable non-small cell lung cancer

Trial	Patient Eligibility	Design	Status
STARS	T1-2aN0M0 <4 cm, fit for lobectomy	Randomized phase III comparing lobectomy to SBRT	Terminated due to poor accrual
ROSEL	T1-2aN0M0 <4 cm, fit for lobectomy	Randomized phase III comparing lobectomy to SBRT	Terminated due to poor accrual
ACOSOG Z0499	Peripheral NSCLC ≤ 3 cm; "high" surgical risk	Randomized phase III comparing sublobar resection to SBRT	Terminated due to poor accrual
SABR-TOOTH	T1-2N0M0 ≤ 3 cm, "high-risk," either lobectomy or sublobar resection	Randomized feasibility	Terminated due to poor accrual
RTOG Foundation 3502 (POSTILV)	T1N0M0 ≤ 3 cm, fit for lobectomy	Randomized phase II	Closed to accrual, no results available
JoLT-Ca STABLE-MATES	Peripheral NSCLC ≤ 4 cm; "high" surgical risk	Prerandomization design; phase III	Actively accruing
VALOR	T1-2N0M0 <5 cm, fit for lobectomy	Randomized phase III	Actively accruing

Table 2
Common stereotactic ablative radiotherapy and stereotactic ablative radiotherapy-like fractionation schemas used for early-stage non-small cell lung cancer

Number of Fractions	Dose per Fraction (Gy)	Total Dose (Gy)	Biologic Effective Dose Assuming $\alpha/\beta = 10$ in Gy_{10}
1	25	25	87.5
1	34	34	149.6
3	18	54	151.2
3	20	60	180
4	12	48	105.6
4	12.5	50	112.5
5	10	50	100
5	11	55	115.5
5	12	60	132
8	7.5	60	105

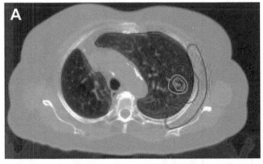

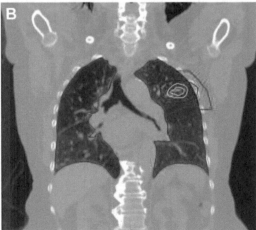

Fig. 2. Midthoracic Axial (*A*) and Coronal (*B*) CT images from a NSCLC SABR plan. The gross tumor volume is delineated in red, the ITV representing the motion envelope of the tumor as identified by 4-dimensional CT (ITV) in blue, and the PTV representing a 5-mm margin in all directions in yellow. The 50% isodose line is shown in red, highlighting the conformality of the plan. Created with BioRender.com.

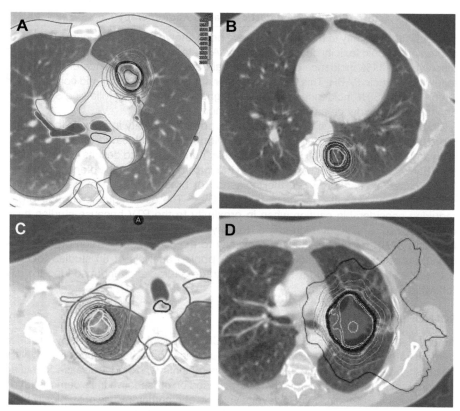

Fig. 3. Normal tissues at risk with centrally located tumors include (*A*) Great vessels, (*B*) spinal cord, (*C*) brachial plexus, and (*D*) central airways.

HIGH-RISK TREATMENT SCENARIOS
Stereotactic Ablative Radiotherapy for Centrally Located Tumors

Centrally located tumors were identified as carrying increased risks during some of the earliest SABR trials. A seminal phase II trial from Indiana University identified a 6-fold increased risk of high-grade toxicity among patients with tumors located within 2 cm of the proximal bronchial tree following 3 fraction SABR.[21] Subsequently, a seamless phase I/II trial conducted by the RTOG evaluated 5 fraction SABR with escalating doses in centrally located tumors, including both those located within 2 cm of the proximal bronchial tree and those abutting the mediastinal pleural. The rate of dose limiting toxicity, defined as any grade 3 or higher predefined toxicity occurring during the first 12 months following treatment, was 7.2%.[22] However, even with more protracted regimens, technique and dose constraints remain critical. The HILUS trial was a phase II study evaluating 8 fraction SABR-like treatments (56 Gy in 8 fractions) in patients with tumors located within 1 cm of the proximal bronchial tree.[23] Treatment-related death was seen in 10 of 65 enrolled patients, with grade 3 to 5 toxicity in 22 patients, predominantly bronchopulmonary hemorrhage. Analysis of the treatment plans showed that despite the protracted treatment course, a lack of strict dose volume constraints to airways and vessels led to high doses to these critical structures in many cases, likely causing the observed toxicity.

Other Risks Associated with Stereotactic Ablative Radiotherapy

Tumors with proximity to the chest wall have been shown to confer an increased risk of acute and chronic toxicity chest wall toxicity. A meta-analysis by Ma and colleagues[24] displayed an 11% incidence of chest wall pain and a 6.3% incidence of rib fracture following thoracic SABR. This finding is further supported by Mutter and colleagues,[25] which found a 39% incidence of grade 2 or higher chest wall pain following SABR with an increasing incidence as chest wall dose increased.

Brachial plexus injury is a rare but serious potential toxicity in apically located tumors. Apical tumors are defined as those with epicenters located above the aortic arch and injury presents with pain, paresthesia, numbness, and deficits in motor function. Earlier studies have shown that when the maximum dose to the brachial plexus in SABR cases exceeded 26 Gy, the incidence of brachial plexus toxicity was 36% compared with 11% at doses less than 26 Gy.[26] The esophagus is another organ requiring considerable caution when in proximity to the PTV because studies have demonstrated a risk of high-grade toxicity including tracheoesophageal fistula following SABR for tumors in close proximity to the esophagus.[27] High-grade pneumonitis is relatively rare following SABR. A pooled analysis of 88 studies found a 9.1% rate of grade 2+ and a 1.8% rate of grade 3+ radiation-induced lung toxicity following SABR to the thorax.[28]

ROLE OF SYSTEMIC THERAPY

Among patients with operable early-stage NSCLC, adjuvant systemic therapy has been demonstrated to provide a survival benefit for select patients. Historically, adjuvant chemotherapy was offered postoperatively to patients with nodal disease identified pathologically or for tumors larger than 4 cm, based on prospective trials demonstrating a modest survival benefit.[29–32] However, systemic chemotherapy has not typically been offered following SABR for early-stage NSCLC, both due to lack of randomized trials, and poor tolerance in the typically frail medically inoperable patient population.

However, recent phase 3 trials in operable NSCLC have demonstrated a PFS benefit to neoadjuvant[33] or adjuvant[34] immune checkpoint inhibitors (ICIs) in with surgery for resectable NSCLC, and there is an ongoing interest in the integration of ICIs with SABR for early-stage inoperable NSCLC. Currently, 3 ongoing randomized phase 3 trials are evaluating the integration of different ICIs with SABR. The PACIFIC-4 trial (NCT03833154) randomizes patients with stage I-II inoperable NSCLC between SABR followed by up to 24 months of durvalumab versus placebo. SWOG/NRG S1914 (NCT04214262) randomizes patients with node-negative NSCLC with stage I-IIA tumors up to 7 cm and at least 1 high-risk feature between neoadjuvant, concurrent, and adjuvant atezolizumab with SABR (6 months total) or SABR alone. KEYNOTE-867 (NCT03924869) randomizes patients with node negative stage I-IIA NSCLC between 12 months of concurrent and adjuvant pembrolizumab or placebo.

IMAGE-GUIDED THERMAL ABLATION TECHNIQUES FOR EARLY-STAGE NON-SMALL CELL LUNG CANCER
Overview

Thermal ablation, a minimally invasive therapy, is an alternative approach to surgery or SABR that has been reported during the past 2 decades for the treatment of early-stage NSCLC. Radiofrequency ablation (RFA), microwave ablation (MWA), and cryoablation are the 3 most prevalent techniques for thermal ablation. Other ablative techniques such as irreversible electroporation and laser-induced thermotherapy are not well established. A bronchoscopic approach may be used for ablation and has been associated with a lower rate of pneumothorax compared with the percutaneous method.[35] However, bronchoscopic ablation has not been performed on a large number of patients overall.

Ablation Modalities

RFA produces heat resulting in coagulative necrosis and cellular death. The radiofrequency electrode consists of a metal shaft with insulation and exposed tip. Voltage is generated between the radiofrequency electrode and reference electrode resulting in an electric field, which is oscillated with radiofrequency frequency.[36] Oscillation of ions in the resistive tissue media leads to heating. RFA is limited by impedance from charred tissue, low thermal conduction of lung, low electrical conductance of lung, and the heat sink effect from flowing blood in adjacent vessels.[37,38]

MWA is based on the electromagnetic field oscillation with flipping of water molecules resulting in the generation of heat.[5] MWA is less subject to the heat sink effect. MWA also allows for a greater and more expected ablation zone in less time compared with RFA.[39]

Cryoablation uses freezing and thawing to lead to tissue destruction. The technique is based on the principle of rapid expansion of pressurized gas typically argon through a narrow orifice and subsequent temperature drop.[40] Cryoablation is associated with less intraprocedural pain compared with MWA.[41] Therefore, this technique may be used for lesions involving the subpleural lung or chest wall. The method also spares

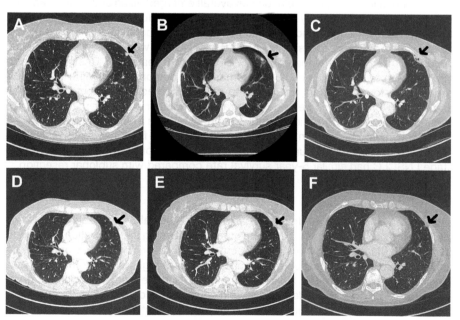

Fig. 4. Pre-MWA and post-MWA ablation axial CT images of the chest. (*A*) Preablation image demonstrating a lingular nodule as denoted by the *black arrow*. (*B*) Immediate postablation image showing the development of surrounding ground glass opacity and a small pneumothorax. (*C*) Twenty days postablation image showing increased consolidation larger than the preablation nodule with associated cavitation. (*D*) Five-month postablation image showing decreased consolidation compared with (*C*). (*E, F*) One-year (*E*) and 2-year (*F*) postablation images showing residual minimal scarring at site of prior ablation with no evidence for tumor recurrence.

tissue collagenous architecture.[42] Cryoablation can be more readily assessed with imaging during the ablation compared with other techniques.[43] There is an increased risk for hemoptysis, however, relative to other types of ablation.[44]

Ablation Procedural Complications and Imaging

Percutaneous ablation can be performed with conscious sedation or general anesthesia. Preprocedural, intraprocedural, and postprocedural computed tomography (CT) imaging is used for guidance and monitoring. Pneumothorax is a common complication and reported in up to 60% ablative procedures.[45] Pleural effusions and lung parenchymal hemorrhage also occur often with ablation. Other infrequent complications consist of bronchopleural fistula, hemothorax, seeding of tumor through the needle tract, or cryoshock with cryoablation. The ablation zone is usually larger than the preablation site of tumor on imaging. Groundglass opacity and cavitation can be seen following ablation. Examples of preablation and postablation CT images are shown in **Fig. 4**. Postablation imaging is typically performed with CT and PET/CT with increased frequency initially particularly during the first year and annually after 2 years following ablation. New or enlarging imaging findings within months after ablation particularly with nodular morphology are suspicious for residual or recurrent disease.

ABLATION FOR EARLY-STAGE NON-SMALL CELL LUNG CANCER

Percutaneous image-guided ablation has overall emerged as an alternative treatment option for patients with early-stage NSCLC, particularly for patients who cannot undergo surgical resection and have comorbid medical conditions. Multiple studies have shown promising results for the treatment of NSCLC with RFA.[46,47] Some studies suggest similar OS as compared with SABR at 2 to 3 years.[48,49] Treatment efficacy after a mean follow-up of about 4 years has been demonstrated with RFA.[50] MWA has less postoperative complications and pain compared with lobectomy.[51] Safety and efficacy of MWA has been demonstrated in another study for the treatment of early-stage NSCLC.[52] Preliminary studies suggest MWA is a cost-effective option.[20,53] Cryoablation has been shown also to be a potential option for patients with early-stage NSCLC not eligible for the surgical resection due to comorbidities.[45] Cryoablation for stage I NSCLC had similar 5-year survival rate compared with sublobar resection.[54]

SUMMARY

SABR is an established treatment of early-stage, medically inoperable NSCLC with excellent in-field tumor control. Ongoing studies are testing the integration of immunotherapy to enhance regional and distant control, and prospective studies provide guidance on dose and fractionation to minimize toxicity for high-risk anatomic scenarios. Several ongoing randomized trials are testing SABR in the medically operable population, based on preliminary data suggesting equipoise for clinical trials. Percutaneous thermal ablation, while less widely used, is also an excellent treatment option for medically inoperable lung tumors.

CLINICS CARE POINTS

- SABR over 1 to 5 fractions is a standard of care for early-stage, medically inoperable NSCLC
- Toxicity following SABR for peripheral tumors is quite low

- Dose to critical structures including proximal bronchial tree, esophagus, brachial plexus, and lungs, among others, is a critical determinant of toxicity following SABR for central tumors, and adherence to dose volume constraints is a major determinant of toxicity
- Randomized phase 3 trials testing the addition of immunotherapy to SABR for early-stage NSCLC are ongoing
- Percutaneous image-guided thermal ablation is an evidence-based treatment option for inoperable early-stage lung cancer, with modest toxicity and good tumor control
- Randomized data directly comparing SABR and percutaneous image guided thermal ablation are lacking.
- Although optimal indications for each modality are still emerging, percutaneous image guided thermal ablation may be particularly appealing for patients with tumors in previously radiated regions or with relative contraindications to radiation.

SOURCE OF FUNDING

None.

DECLARATION OF INTEREST

M.E. Daly: Research Funding: Genentech, Merck, EMD Serono. Consulting: Novocure, Boston Scientific, Astra Zeneca. P. Beagen: None. M.H. Madani: None.

ACKNOWLEDGMENTS

None.

SUPPLEMENTARY DATA

Supplementary data related to this article can be found online at https://doi.org/10.1016/j.hoc.2023.02.002.

REFERENCES

1. Dong B, Zhu X, Jin J, et al. Comparison of the outcomes of sublobar resection and stereotactic body radiotherapy for stage T1-2N0M0 non-small cell lung cancer with tumor size </= 5 cm: a propensity score matching analysis. J Thorac Dis 2020;12:5934–54.
2. Matsuo Y, Chen F, Hamaji M, et al. Comparison of long-term survival outcomes between stereotactic body radiotherapy and sublobar resection for stage I non-small-cell lung cancer in patients at high risk for lobectomy: a propensity score matching analysis. Eur J Cancer 2014;50:2932–8.
3. Chang JY, Mehran RJ, Feng L, et al. Stereotactic ablative radiotherapy for operable stage I non-small-cell lung cancer (revised STARS): long-term results of a single-arm, prospective trial with prespecified comparison to surgery. Lancet Oncol 2021;22:1448–57.
4. Grills IS, Mangona VS, Welsh R, et al. Outcomes after stereotactic lung radiotherapy or wedge resection for stage I non-small-cell lung cancer. J Clin Oncol 2010;28:928–35.
5. Videtic GMM, Donington J, Giuliani M, et al. Stereotactic body radiation therapy for early-stage non-small cell lung cancer: executive summary of an ASTRO evidence-based guideline. Pract Radiat Oncol 2017;7:295–301.

6. Blomgren H, Lax I, Naslund I, et al. Stereotactic high dose fraction radiation therapy of extracranial tumors using an accelerator. Clinical experience of the first thirty-one patients. Acta Oncol 1995;34:861–70.

7. Uematsu M, Shioda A, Tahara K, et al. Focal, high dose, and fractionated modified stereotactic radiation therapy for lung carcinoma patients: a preliminary experience. Cancer 1998;82:1062–70.

8. Wulf J, Hadinger U, Oppitz U, et al. Stereotactic radiotherapy of targets in the lung and liver. Strahlenther Onkol 2001;177:645–55.

9. Timmerman R, Papiez L, McGarry R, et al. Extracranial stereotactic radioablation: results of a phase I study in medically inoperable stage I non-small cell lung cancer. Chest 2003;124:1946–55.

10. Whyte RI, Crownover R, Murphy MJ, et al. Stereotactic radiosurgery for lung tumors: preliminary report of a phase I trial. Ann Thorac Surg 2003;75:1097–101.

11. Timmerman R, Paulus R, Galvin J, et al. Stereotactic body radiation therapy for inoperable early stage lung cancer. JAMA 2010;303:1070–6.

12. Xiao Y, Papiez L, Paulus R, et al. Dosimetric evaluation of heterogeneity corrections for RTOG 0236: stereotactic body radiotherapy of inoperable stage I-II non-small-cell lung cancer. Int J Radiat Oncol Biol Phys 2009;73:1235–42.

13. Nyman J, Hallqvist A, Lund JA, et al. Space - a randomized study of SBRT vs conventional fractionated radiotherapy in medically inoperable stage I NSCLC. Radiother Oncol 2016;121:1–8.

14. Ball D, Mai GT, Vinod S, et al. Stereotactic ablative radiotherapy versus standard radiotherapy in stage 1 non-small-cell lung cancer (TROG 09.02 CHISEL): a phase 3, open-label, randomised controlled trial. Lancet Oncol 2019;20:494–503.

15. Timmerman RD, Hu C, Michalski JM, et al. Long-term results of stereotactic body radiation therapy in medically inoperable stage I non-small cell lung cancer. JAMA Oncol 2018;4:1287–8.

16. Schonewolf CA, Heskel M, Doucette A, et al. Five-year long-term outcomes of stereotactic body radiation therapy for operable versus medically inoperable stage I non-small-cell lung cancer: analysis by operability, fractionation regimen, tumor size, and tumor location. Clin Lung Cancer 2019;20:e63–71.

17. Arnett ALH, Mou B, Owen D, et al. Long-term clinical outcomes and safety profile of SBRT for centrally located NSCLC. Adv Radiat Oncol 2019;4:422–8.

18. Chang JY, Senan S, Paul MA, et al. Stereotactic ablative radiotherapy versus lobectomy for operable stage I non-small-cell lung cancer: a pooled analysis of two randomised trials. Lancet Oncol 2015;16:630–7.

19. Singh AK, Gomez-Suescun JA, Stephans KL, et al. One versus three fractions of stereotactic body radiation therapy for peripheral stage I to II non-small cell lung cancer: a randomized, multi-institution, phase 2 trial. Int J Radiat Oncol Biol Phys 2019;105:752–9.

20. Videtic GM, Paulus R, Singh AK, et al. Long-term Follow-up on NRG Oncology RTOG 0915 (NCCTG N0927): a randomized phase 2 study comparing 2 stereotactic body radiation therapy schedules for medically inoperable patients with stage I peripheral non-small cell lung cancer. Int J Radiat Oncol Biol Phys 2019;103:1077–84.

21. Timmerman R, McGarry R, Yiannoutsos C, et al. Excessive toxicity when treating central tumors in a phase II study of stereotactic body radiation therapy for medically inoperable early-stage lung cancer. J Clin Oncol 2006;24:4833–9.

22. Bezjak A, Paulus R, Gaspar LE, et al. Safety and efficacy of a five-fraction stereotactic body radiotherapy schedule for centrally located non-small-cell lung cancer: NRG oncology/RTOG 0813 trial. J Clin Oncol 2019;37:1316–25.

23. Lindberg K, Grozman V, Karlsson K, et al. The HILUS-trial-a prospective nordic multicenter phase 2 study of ultracentral lung tumors treated with stereotactic body radiotherapy. J Thorac Oncol 2021;16:1200–10.
24. Ma JT, Liu Y, Sun L, et al. Chest wall toxicity after stereotactic body radiation therapy: a pooled analysis of 57 studies. Int J Radiat Oncol Biol Phys 2019;103:843–50.
25. Mutter RW, Liu F, Abreu A, et al. Dose-volume parameters predict for the development of chest wall pain after stereotactic body radiation for lung cancer. Int J Radiat Oncol Biol Phys 2012;82:1783–90.
26. Forquer JA, Fakiris AJ, Timmerman RD, et al. Brachial plexopathy from stereotactic body radiotherapy in early-stage NSCLC: dose-limiting toxicity in apical tumor sites. Radiother Oncol 2009;93:408–13.
27. Wang C, Rimner A, Gelblum DY, et al. Analysis of pneumonitis and esophageal injury after stereotactic body radiation therapy for ultra-central lung tumors. Lung Cancer 2020;147:45–8.
28. Zhao J, Yorke ED, Li L, et al. Simple factors associated with radiation-induced lung toxicity after stereotactic body radiation therapy of the thorax: a pooled analysis of 88 studies. Int J Radiat Oncol Biol Phys 2016;95:1357–66.
29. Arriagada R, Bergman B, Dunant A, et al. Cisplatin-based adjuvant chemotherapy in patients with completely resected non-small-cell lung cancer. N Engl J Med 2004;350:351–60.
30. Douillard JY, Rosell R, De Lena M, et al. Adjuvant vinorelbine plus cisplatin versus observation in patients with completely resected stage IB-IIIA non-small-cell lung cancer (Adjuvant Navelbine International Trialist Association [ANITA]): a randomised controlled trial. Lancet Oncol 2006;7:719–27.
31. Strauss GM, Herndon JE 2nd, Maddaus MA, et al. Adjuvant paclitaxel plus carboplatin compared with observation in stage IB non-small-cell lung cancer: CALGB 9633 with the Cancer and Leukemia Group B, Radiation Therapy Oncology Group, and North Central Cancer Treatment Group Study Groups. J Clin Oncol 2008;26:5043–51.
32. Winton T, Livingston R, Johnson D, et al. Vinorelbine plus cisplatin vs. observation in resected non-small-cell lung cancer. N Engl J Med 2005;352:2589–97.
33. Forde PM, Spicer J, Lu S, et al. Neoadjuvant nivolumab plus chemotherapy in resectable lung cancer. N Engl J Med 2022;386:1973–85.
34. Felip E, Altorki N, Zhou C, et al. Adjuvant atezolizumab after adjuvant chemotherapy in resected stage IB-IIIA non-small-cell lung cancer (IMpower010): a randomised, multicentre, open-label, phase 3 trial. Lancet 2021;398:1344–57.
35. Chan JWY, Lau RWH, Ngai JCL, et al. Transbronchial microwave ablation of lung nodules with electromagnetic navigation bronchoscopy guidance-a novel technique and initial experience with 30 cases. Transl Lung Cancer Res 2021;10:1608–22.
36. Goldberg SN. Radiofrequency tumor ablation: principles and techniques. Eur J Ultrasound 2001;13:129–47.
37. Brace CL. Radiofrequency and microwave ablation of the liver, lung, kidney, and bone: what are the differences? Curr Probl Diagn Radiol 2009;38:135–43.
38. Lu DS, Raman SS, Limanond P, et al. Influence of large peritumoral vessels on outcome of radiofrequency ablation of liver tumors. J Vasc Interv Radiol 2003;14:1267–74.
39. Poulou LS, Botsa E, Thanou I, et al. Percutaneous microwave ablation vs radiofrequency ablation in the treatment of hepatocellular carcinoma. World J Hepatol 2015;7:1054–63.

40. Erinjeri JP, Clark TW. Cryoablation: mechanism of action and devices. J Vasc Interv Radiol 2010;21:S187–91.
41. Das SK, Huang YY, Li B, et al. Comparing cryoablation and microwave ablation for the treatment of patients with stage IIIB/IV non-small cell lung cancer. Oncol Lett 2020;19:1031–41.
42. Inoue M, Nakatsuka S, Jinzaki M. Cryoablation of early-stage primary lung cancer. BioMed Res Int 2014;2014:521691.
43. Kwak K, Yu B, Lewandowski RJ, et al. Recent progress in cryoablation cancer therapy and nanoparticles mediated cryoablation. Theranostics 2022;12: 2175–204.
44. Wrobel MM, Bourgouin PP, Abrishami Kashani M, et al. Active versus passive thaw after percutaneous cryoablation of pulmonary tumors: effect on incidence, grade, and onset of hemoptysis. AJR Am J Roentgenol 2021;217:1153–63.
45. Yamauchi Y, Izumi Y, Kawamura M, et al. Percutaneous cryoablation of pulmonary metastases from colorectal cancer. PLoS One 2011;6:e27086.
46. Ambrogi MC, Fanucchi O, Dini P, et al. Wedge resection and radiofrequency ablation for stage I nonsmall cell lung cancer. Eur Respir J 2015;45:1089–97.
47. Lanuti M, Sharma A, Digumarthy SR, et al. Radiofrequency ablation for treatment of medically inoperable stage I non-small cell lung cancer. J Thorac Cardiovasc Surg 2009;137:160–6.
48. Dupuy DE, Fernando HC, Hillman S, et al. Radiofrequency ablation of stage IA non-small cell lung cancer in medically inoperable patients: results from the American College of Surgeons Oncology Group Z4033 (Alliance) trial. Cancer 2015;121:3491–8.
49. Palussiere J, Chomy F, Savina M, et al. Radiofrequency ablation of stage IA non-small cell lung cancer in patients ineligible for surgery: results of a prospective multicenter phase II trial. J Cardiothorac Surg 2018;13:91.
50. Ambrogi MC, Fanucchi O, Cioni R, et al. Long-term results of radiofrequency ablation treatment of stage I non-small cell lung cancer: a prospective intention-to-treat study. J Thorac Oncol 2011;6:2044–51.
51. Yao W, Lu M, Fan W, et al. Comparison between microwave ablation and lobectomy for stage I non-small cell lung cancer: a propensity score analysis. Int J Hyperthermia 2018;34:1329–36.
52. Nance M, Khazi Z, Kaifi J, et al. Computerized tomography-guided microwave ablation of patients with stage I non-small cell lung cancers: a single-institution retrospective study. J Clin Imaging Sci 2021;11:7.
53. Wu X, Uhlig J, Blasberg JD, et al. Microwave ablation versus stereotactic body radiotherapy for stage I non-small cell lung cancer: a cost-effectiveness analysis. J Vasc Interv Radiol 2022;33:964–971 e962.
54. Moore W, Talati R, Bhattacharji P, et al. Five-year survival after cryoablation of stage I non-small cell lung cancer in medically inoperable patients. J Vasc Interv Radiol 2015;26:312–9.

The Evolving Role for Systemic Therapy in Resectable Non-small Cell Lung Cancer

Michael J. Grant, MD[a,b,*], Gavitt A. Woodard, MD[a,c],
Sarah B. Goldberg, MD, MPH[a,b]

KEYWORDS

- Non-small cell lung cancer • Immune checkpoint inhibitors
- Lung adjuvant cisplatin evaluation • Tumor microenvironment
- Circulating tumor DNA

KEY POINTS

- Platinum-based chemotherapy is associated with prolonged overall survival (OS) for select patients with resectable non-small cell lung cancer (NSCLC); similar OS benefits are seen for neoadjuvant and adjuvant therapy based on large meta-analyses.
- Tyrosine kinase inhibitors and other targeted therapies have a clear role for patients with oncogene-driven tumors in the metastatic setting. The phase III ADAURA trial demonstrated a striking disease-free survival benefit with adjuvant osimertinib in resectable epidermal growth factor receptor (EGFR)-mutant NSCLC.
- Phase III Randomized controlled trials with anti-programmed death-1/anti-programmed death-ligand 1 agents have demonstrated efficacy in the adjuvant and neoadjuvant settings for resectable NSCLC.
- For patients with early-stage disease, adaptive management approaches involving circulating tumor DNA clearance, measurable residual disease, and pathologic response after neoadjuvant therapy are on the horizon.

INTRODUCTION

During the last 2 decades, the understanding of non-small cell lung cancer (NSCLC) has evolved from a purely histologic classification system to a more complex model synthesizing clinical, histologic, and molecular data. This is most apparent in the

[a] Yale Cancer Center, Yale University School of Medicine, 333 Cedar Street, New Haven, CT 06520, USA; [b] Department of Medicine (Medical Oncology), Yale School of Medicine, 330 Cedar Street, Rm BB 205, New Haven, CT 06520, USA; [c] Department of Surgery, Yale School of Medicine, PO Box 208028, New Haven, CT 06520, USA
* Corresponding author.
E-mail address: Michael.grant@yale.edu

Hematol Oncol Clin N Am 37 (2023) 513–531
https://doi.org/10.1016/j.hoc.2023.02.003
0889-8588/23/© 2023 Elsevier Inc. All rights reserved.

current clinical landscape of metastatic NSCLC, where molecular profiling is crucial to selecting the optimal treatment regimen for a given patient. To date, biomarker-driven targeted therapies have been approved by the United States Food and Drug Administration (FDA) for patients with metastatic NSCLC harboring specific driver alterations in *EGFR, HER2, KRAS, BRAF, MET, ALK, ROS1, RET,* and *NTRK.*[1,2] Meanwhile, various immune checkpoint inhibitors including anti-PD-1, anti-PD-L1, and anti-CTLA-4 agents have proven efficacy in diverse clinical settings for patients with advanced disease.[3] Novel targeted and immuno-oncology (IO) agents have undoubtedly contributed to improvements in NSCLC-related survival at the population level.[4] However, only in the last several years has this nuanced understanding of NSCLC permeated into the systemic management of patients with resectable tumors.

The implementation of novel adjuvant and neoadjuvant systemic therapies in early-stage, resectable NSCLC has been slower than in the metastatic setting for various reasons. For patients with NSCLC, recurrence rates are still unacceptably high, yet patients with resectable disease are often cured with surgery alone, particularly in stage I and II diseases.[5] Trials investigating novel adjuvant and neoadjuvant strategies require years of follow-up to demonstrate improvement in traditional time-to event endpoints such as OS. Across cancer types, novel systemic therapies are usually established in the metastatic setting before the adjuvant or neoadjuvant settings. This is inextricably tied to the increased risk-to-benefit tolerance for patients with incurable disease with limited treatment options versus those with disease amenable to curative-intent local therapy. Accrual to adjuvant or neoadjuvant NSCLC trials is also challenging. Among all-comers with NSCLC, only up to 25% of patients present with resectable disease.[6] This fraction is increased with modern screening efforts and resulting stage migration, yet even for many patients with resectable disease, comorbid conditions, functional status, and compromised pulmonary function preclude surgical resection.[7] Finally, the efficacy of immunotherapy and targeted therapy for NSCLC is most profound in biomarker-enriched populations, which further impedes swift patient accrual in early-stage trials.

ADJUVANT SYSTEMIC THERAPY IN NON-SMALL CELL LUNG CANCER
Adjuvant Chemotherapy in Resected Non-small Cell Lung Cancer

Many randomized trials have shown that platinum-based adjuvant chemotherapy has a small survival benefit in appropriately selected subgroups of patients with resected NSCLC.[8] A pooled analysis of 5 large clinical trials, the Lung Adjuvant Cisplatin Evaluation, demonstrated an overall 5.4% improvement in 5-year survival with adjuvant platinum-based chemotherapy.[9] With median follow-up of greater than 60 months, the OS HR was 0.89 (95% CI [0.82–0.96]). Patients were staged according to the American Joint Committee on Cancer (AJCC) sixth edition, and there was a stage gradient for benefit from cisplatin-based chemotherapy with OS HR of 1.40 (0.95–2.06) for stage IA, 0.93 (0.78–1.10) for stage IB, 0.83 (0.73–0.95) for stage II, and 0.83 (0.72–0.94). Subgroup analyses from clinical trials have demonstrated that patients with lymph node involvement or node-negative tumors 4 cm or greater have prolonged survival with adjuvant platinum-based chemotherapy, whereas those with smaller tumors do not clearly derive benefit and may in fact be harmed by this intervention.[10] Other factors such as the extent of lung resection (sub lobar vs lobectomy) and presence of high-risk pathologic features like visceral pleural invasion, lymphovascular invasion, and high tumor grade are often considered, although these factors have not been proven to predict for benefit from adjuvant chemotherapy in a prospective study.[11] Finally, DetermaRx is a 14-gene assay that has been shown to identify early-stage NSCLC tumors most at risk of recurrence following surgical resection based on tumor biology.[12] Use of this assay to identify tumors with a greater risk of recurrence and treating high-risk patients with platinum-based adjuvant chemotherapy has been shown to improve survival in prospective, nonrandomized trials.[13]

Despite its proven efficacy, the delivery of guideline-based adjuvant chemotherapy is underwhelming. In a retrospective analysis of a US-based adjuvant therapy screening protocol, only 57% of patients with stage IB ($\geq$4 cm)-IIIA (by the AJCC seventh edition staging) resected NSCLC received any adjuvant chemotherapy, many of whom neither completed 4 cycles nor received cisplatin (44% and 34%, respectively).[14]

Adjuvant Immunotherapy in Resected Non-small Cell Lung Cancer

Monoclonal antibodies against the immune checkpoint protein PD-1 and its ligand PD-L1 have contributed to unprecedented long-term survival gains in locally advanced unresectable and metastatic NSCLC.[3,15–19] The impressive activity of atezolizumab, pembrolizumab, and other anti-PD-1/PD-L1 agents in the metastatic setting spawned enthusiasm for introducing this class to the early-stage treatment landscape to improve on the modest survival benefit of platinum-based chemotherapy.[3]

IMpower010

IMpower010 was a global phase 3 trial, which randomized patients with resected AJCC seventh edition stage IB ($\geq$4 cm)-IIIA NSCLC to atezolizumab (anti-PD-L1) every 3 weeks for up to 16 cycles or best supportive care (BSC), after treatment with standard platinum-based chemotherapy.[20] The primary endpoint of disease-free survival (DFS) in patients with stage II-IIIA tumors with PD-L1 tumor proportion score (TPS) of 1% or greater was improved with atezolizumab compared with BSC with a stratified hazard ratio of 0.66 ([0.50–0.88], P = .0039). Kaplan-Meier estimates at 36 months of follow-up demonstrated that 60% of patients on the adjuvant atezolizumab arm were disease-free compared with 48.2% receiving BSC. In the stage II-IIIA population, exploratory subgroup analyses exhibited a favorable DFS trend for patients receiving atezolizumab irrespective of tumor stage, nodal status, and histology, whereas patients with a negative smoking history and those with *EGFR* and *ALK* alterations did not appear to derive benefit from adjuvant atezolizumab. With respect to PD-L1 expression levels, patients with tumor PD-L1 50% or greater benefitted most from atezolizumab treatment. Despite the overall DFS benefit in the nested PD-L1 1% or greater subgroup, the hazard ratio for those with tumor PD-L1 1% to 49% was more modest, whereas patients with PD-L1 of 0% did not seem to derive meaningful benefit (**Table 1**). Atezolizumab resulted in grade 3 to 4 immune-related adverse events in 8% of patients.

The US FDA approved adjuvant atezolizumab for patients with resected AJCC seventh edition stage II-IIIA tumors with PD-L1 TPS of 1% or greater after administration of platinum-based chemotherapy. Subsequently, an interim analysis of IMPower010 was presented at the IASLC World Conference of Lung Cancer in 2022, with median follow-up of 46 months.[21] In the PD-L1 50% or greater subgroup, a clinically meaningful OS benefit with adjuvant atezolizumab was demonstrated, with OS HR 0.43 (0.24–0.78). There was a trend toward improved OS in the PD-L1 1% or greater subgroup with OS HR 0.72 (0.49–1.03), which included and seems to be driven by the PD-L1 50% or greater subgroup given the OS HR for the PD-L1 of 1% to 49% population was 0.95 (0.59–1.54). Notably, there was a trend toward harm in patients with PD-L1 of 0% (OS HR 1.36 [0.93–1.99]). Therefore, adjuvant atezolizumab seems to be

Table 1
Phase III adjuvant immunotherapy trials in resectable non-small cell lung cancer

Trial	Primary Efficacy Population	Treatment Arms	Number of Patients	DFS HR (95% CI)	OS HR (95% CI)
PEARLS NCT02504372 [22]	Stage IB (≥4 cm)-IIIA, PD-L1+ resectable NSCLC	Pembrolizumab (×18) vs placebo	590 (pembrolizumab) 587 (placebo)	All PD-L1: 0.76 (0.63–0.91) PD-L1 0%: 0.78 (0.58–1.03) PD-L1 1%–49%: 0.67 (0.48–0.92) PD-L1 ≥50%: 0.82 (0.57–1.18)	0.87 (0.67–1.15)[a]
IMPOWER-010 NCT02486718 [20,21]	Stage II-IIIA resectable NSCLC	Atezolizumab (×16) vs BSC	507 (atezolizumab) 498 (BSC)	All PD-L1: 0.66 (0.50–0.88) PD-L1 0%: 0.97 (0.72–1.31) PD-L1 1%–49%: 0.87 (0.60–1.26) PD-L1 ≥50%: 0.43 (0.27–0.68)	0.72 (0.49–1.03)[b]

Abbreviations: BSC, best supportive care; CI, confidence interval; DFS, disease-free survival; HR, hazard ratio; OS, overall survival.
[a] Data immature at an interim analysis with median follow-up 36 mo.
[b] Data immature at an interim analysis with median follow-up of 46 mo.

most efficacious in those with high PD-L1 expression ($\geq$50%), and for patients with PD-L1 of 1% to 49%, treatment should be considered on an individualized basis.

PEARLS/KEYNOTE-091. The EORTC-1416-LCG/ETOP8-15 study, also known as PEARLS/KEYNOTE-091, was a global, placebo-controlled phase III clinical trial of pembrolizumab every 3 weeks for up to 18 cycles as adjuvant therapy for patients with resected early-stage NSCLC.[22] Similar to IMPower010, eligible patients had AJCC seventh edition stage IB ($\geq$4 cm)-IIIA resected NSCLC, and most patients (86%) had completed standard-of-care adjuvant platinum-doublet chemotherapy. The coprimary endpoints were DFS in the overall population and DFS in the PD-L1 high population (TPS$\geq$50%). In the overall population, the stratified DFS hazard ratio was 0.76 (0.63–0.91) demonstrating the benefit of pembrolizumab over placebo. Interestingly, and discordant with the results from the PD-L1 high population in IMPower010, pembrolizumab did not lead to a significant DFS benefit for patients with tumor PD-L1 50% or greater (see **Table 1**). Exploratory subgroup analyses demonstrated more pronounced benefit in patients who had received adjuvant chemotherapy, and those with active smoking history, stage II disease, *EGFR*-mutated tumors (n = 73), nonsquamous histology, and tumor PD-L1 of 1% to 49%. Treatment-related adverse events were experienced by 15% of patients on the pembrolizumab arm compared with 4% on the placebo arm.

At the time of this writing, adjuvant pembrolizumab is under review by the US FDA for the treatment of patients with resected stage IIA-IIIA NSCLC irrespective of tumor PD-L1 status. In addition to the perplexing DFS results in the PD-L1 high subgroup, patients with squamous NSCLC and those with stage IIIA tumors did not seem to derive benefit from adjuvant pembrolizumab, while those with *EGFR* mutations unexpectedly did. The latter finding highlights an important limitation of this study, which is the lack of relevant biomarker testing required for enrollment. Only 43% and 37% of patients were tested for *EGFR* and *ALK* limiting the ability to draw meaningful conclusions from these subgroups despite knowledge that these NSCLC genotypes have limited sensitivity to anti-PD-1/PD-L1 agents in the metastatic setting.[23,24]

Ongoing investigation
Ongoing trials have been designed to answer outstanding questions in the adjuvant immunotherapy setting. The phase III ALCHEMIST Chemo-IO trial (NCT04267848) randomizes patients with resected AJCC seventh edition stage IB ($\geq$4 cm)-IIIA to adjuvant concurrent or sequential chemotherapy and pembrolizumab. In patients with detectable circulating tumor DNA (ctDNA), or measurable residual disease positive, after surgical resection and standard preoperative or postoperative chemotherapy, the phase III MERMAID-2 study is investigating adjuvant durvalumab versus placebo, with DFS as the primary endpoint. This approach is somewhat analogous to the recent data for therapy selection based on ctDNA detection in stage II colon cancer.[25]

Adjuvant Tyrosine Kinase Inhibitors in Resected Non-small Cell Lung Cancer

EGFR TKIs
Early attempts to bring first-generation EGFR inhibitors into the adjuvant setting for *EGFR* mutant tumors, including ADJUVANT-CTONG1104 (gefitinib) and EVAN (erlotinib), were not successful in significantly changing practice.[26–31] Compared with first-generation and second-generation EGFR TKIs, the third-generation EGFR inhibitor osimertinib further prolonged survival, enhanced *EGFR* mutant selectivity, including against T790 M, increased blood-brain-barrier penetration, and was better tolerated by patients with lower rates of adverse events and treatment

discontinuation.[32–35] Such considerations spurred the investigation of osimertinib in the adjuvant setting.

ADAURA

The landmark phase III ADAURA trial investigated adjuvant osimertinib versus placebo for 3 years duration after resection and adjuvant chemotherapy (if appropriate) for patients with AJCC seventh edition stage IB-IIIA NSCLC harboring *EGFR* exon 19 deletions or L858 R mutations.[36] With nearly 2 years of follow-up, there was a remarkable 83% reduction in risk of disease recurrence or death associated with osimertinib in the patients with stage II-IIIA disease (DFS HR = 0.17, 99.06% CI [0.11–0.26] $P < .001$). In the overall population, the DFS HR was 0.20 (99.12% CI [0.14–0.30] $P < .001$). Patients who did not receive adjuvant chemotherapy derived significant benefit from osimertinib as well, and this benefit was seen in all stage strata (IB, II, IIIA).[37] Arguably the most striking finding from these early data was the impressive 82% relative risk reduction in CNS recurrence (DFS HR = 0.18, 95% CI [0.10–0.33], $P < .001$) attributable to adjuvant osimertinib. Updated results from this trial were presented at the ESMO Congress 2022 with 50% data maturity at median follow-up of 44.2 months for the osimertinib arm.[38] Although a large DFS benefit persists, from 36 to 48 months, the Kaplan Meier plot is characterized by a narrowing distance between the osimertinib and placebo curves related to a steeper decline in the osimertinib curve. Longer follow-up and OS results will shed light on the significance of this observation, to determine whether adjuvant osimertinib is benefitting patients by delaying recurrence, including in critical sites such as CNS, or truly increasing the fraction of patients with early-stage EGFR mutant NSCLC who are cured of their disease. Regardless, adjuvant osimertinib has been approved by the FDA and is widely considered a new standard of care for patients with resected early-stage NSCLC harboring classical *EGFR* mutations.

Ongoing investigation

Although adjuvant TKI trials are beset by slow accrual due to the relative rarity of some driver alterations, these efforts are necessary to establish the role of TKIs and other targeted therapies in patients with resected NSCLC. In the National Cancer Institute's ALCHEMIST trials, patients are screened for *EGFR* and *ALK* alterations and if present, randomized to erlotinib or crizotinib versus placebo after resection ± standard adjuvant therapy.[39] Adjuvant alectinib is being investigated in the phase III ALINA trial (NCT03456076).[36,40] Trials investigating adjuvant selpercatinib for *RET* rearranged NSCLC and perioperative capmatinib for NSCLC harboring a *MET* exon 14 skipping mutation or *MET* amplification are also underway.[41,42]

NEOADJUVANT SYSTEMIC THERAPY IN NON-SMALL CELL LUNG CANCER
Neoadjuvant Chemotherapy in Resectable Non-small Cell Lung Cancer

When delivered preoperatively, platinum-based chemotherapy also prolongs survival for patients with resectable AJCC seventh edition stage IB (≥4 cm)-IIIA NSCLC. In a meta-analysis published in 2014 including 12 trials and more than 2000 patients, neoadjuvant chemotherapy followed by resection was associated with a 5% absolute 5-year survival advantage compared with resection alone (45% vs 40%, respectively).[43] Unfortunately, adequately powered randomized controlled trials comparing neoadjuvant against adjuvant platinum-based chemotherapy for resectable NSCLC do not exist. A large meta-analysis, published in 2009, which included 32 RCTs with and 10,000 patients demonstrated that hazard ratios for OS comparing postoperative chemotherapy to surgery alone (0.80 [0.74–0.87], $P < .001$) and preoperative chemotherapy (0.81 [0.68–0.97], $P < .024$) were remarkably similar for patients with early-stage NSCLC.[44] Results from retrospective comparisons are mixed, but historically, the adjuvant chemotherapy approach has been heavily favored.[45,46] This poor uptake of neoadjuvant chemotherapy is at least partially attributable to the low rates of pathologic complete response, an early endpoint associated with survival outcomes in resected NSCLC.[47]

Neoadjuvant Immunotherapy in Resectable Non-small Cell Lung Cancer

An attractive feature of the neoadjuvant approach, especially relevant for IO-containing regimens, is the ability to deliver therapy with an intact tumor and an abundant source of tumor antigens.[48] T-cells within the tumor microenvironment (TME), which may already be primed to tumor antigen, can expand in situ when exposed to PD-1 pathway inhibition. In the case of up-front surgical resection, T-cells within the TME are extracted along with other integral components of the antitumor immune response (eg, antigen presenting cells in the TME or regional lymph nodes).

Several small trials and one larger study have investigated anti-PD-1/PD-L1 monotherapy in resectable NSCLC (**Table 2**).[49] Pathologic complete response rates range from 0% to 15% while major pathologic response rates (defined as $\geq$90% pathologic regression at resection) range from 14% to 45%. Although established biomarkers and predictive patient characteristics in the metastatic setting are likely to be useful in patient-selection for neoadjuvant immunotherapy, patients with PD-L1-negative tumors and lack of smoking history have been reported to achieve pathologic complete responses as well.[49] One downside to neoadjuvant anti-PD-1/PD-L1 monotherapy is that a subset of patients does not achieve initial disease control with immunotherapy and instead experience primary progression or even hyperprogression. This has been evident in clinical trials investigating this class in the first-line metastatic setting.[50–54] However, when there is a window for surgery in a patient with resectable early-stage disease, the potential for nonresponse is especially undesirable. One strategy to maximize the proportion of responding patients has been to use combination regimens.

In the phase II NEOSTAR study, major pathologic response (mPR) and pathologic complete response (pCR) rates were numerically higher for nivolumab plus ipilimumab compared with nivolumab monotherapy (see **Table 2**). Seven patients did not undergo surgical resection on trial. Five of these patients were on the neoadjuvant nivolumab plus ipilimumab arm although not all instances of surgical cancellation or study discontinuation were related to progression or treatment-related toxicity.

In the first-line metastatic setting, combination chemoimmunotherapy regimens are associated with the highest response rates across trials in this space.[3] Moreover, given the widespread experience with and predictable toxicity of these regimens, there was strong interest for investigation in the neoadjuvant space (see **Table 2**). Among the first trials to report efficacy and safety results for neoadjuvant chemoimmunotherapy was a phase II study investigating 2 cycles of neoadjuvant carboplatin, nab-paclitaxel, and atezolizumab for patients with resectable AJCC seventh edition stage IB-IIIA tumors of 4 cm or greater.[55] The mPR rate was 57% while 33% of patients achieved a pCR. There was a trend toward prolonged DFS in patients with mPR at the time of resection (34.5 months) compared with those with less than mPR, in which DFS was 14.3 months. Neoadjuvant therapy did not lead to any surgical delays and 13% of enrolled patients were not surgically treated due to the lack of R0 resection potential. Similarly, the randomized phase II NADIM II trial investigated 3 cycles of neoadjuvant carboplatin, paclitaxel, and nivolumab followed by 6 months of adjuvant nivolumab in patients with resectable stage IIIA NSCLC.[56] Strikingly, 83% of patients who underwent surgery achieved mPR, with 63% achieving pCR. Although most

Table 2
Phase II and III clinical trials investigating neoadjuvant immunotherapy in resectable non-small cell lung cancer

Trial	Population	Experimental Regimen	Phase	N	mPR	pCR	EFS/DFS/RFS/PFS (95% CI)	OS (95% CI)	Grade ≥3 TRAEs
NEOSTAR NCT03158129 [64]	Stage I-IIIA resectable NSCLC	Nivolumab (×3) Nivolumab (×3) plus ipilimumab (×1)	II II	23 21	22% 38%	9% 29%	Median RFS NR Median RFS NR	Median OS NR Median OS NR	13% 10%
IONESCO NCT03030131 [83]	Stage IB (≥4 cm)-IIIA (non-N2) resectable NSCLC	Durvalumab (×3)	II	46	17%	7%	12-mo DFS: 78% (63–88)	12-mo OS: 89% (76–95)	0%
PRINCEPS NCT02994576 [84]	stage I (≥2 cm)-IIIA (non-N2) resectable NSCLC	Atezolizumab (×1)	II	30	14%	0%	Not Reported	Not Reported	0%
LCMC3 NCT02927301 [85]	Stage IB-IIIB (T3N2 or T4 by size) resectable NSCLC	Atezolizumab (×2)	II	181	16%	4%	36-mo DFS (resected patients only): 72% (62–79)	36-mo OS (resected patients only): 80% (71–87)	11%
Shu et al [55] 2020 NCT02716038	Stage IB-IIIA resectable NSCLC	Atezolizumab plus carboplatin and nab-paclitaxel (×4)	II	30	57%	33%	Median DFS 18 mo (14-NR)	Median OS NR (28-NR)	91%
NADIM II NCT03081689 [57,64]	Stage IIIA resectable NSCLC	Nivolumab plus carboplatin and paclitaxel (×3)[a]	II	46	74%	56%	36-mo PFS: 70% (54–81)	36-mo OS: 82% (67–91)	30%
CheckMate-816 NCT02998528 [56]	Stage IB (≥4 cm)-IIIA resectable NSCLC	Nivolumab plus histology-selected platinum doublet (×3)	III	179 (Nivolumab arm)	37%	24%	Median EFS 32 mo (30-NR); 24-mo EFS: 64%	Median OS NR; 24-mo OS 83%	34%

Abbreviations: CI, confidence interval; DFS, disease-free survival; EFS, event-free survival; mPR, major pathologic response; NR, not reached; OS, overall survival; pCR, pathologic complete response; PFS, progression-free survival; RFS, recurrence-free survival; TRAE, treatment related adverse events.

[a] Surgery followed by 6 mo of adjuvant nivolumab in NADIM

patients experienced treatment-related adverse events (with 30% grade $\geq$3) with neoadjuvant therapy, none led to treatment discontinuation or delay/cancellation of surgery. This trial has now reported 81.9% (95% CI, 66.8–90.6) 3-year survival in the intention-to-treat population.[57] Of note, PD-L1 expression, tumor mutational burden, and radiographic response were not predictive of OS but patients had improved PFS and OS if ctDNA was undetectable after the neoadjuvant phase, even when patients with undetectable levels at baseline were excluded.

Checkmate-816

The Checkmate-816 study is the first phase III study comparing neoadjuvant chemo-immunotherapy with chemotherapy for patients with early-stage NSCLC. In this trial, patients with resectable AJCC seventh edition stage IB ($\geq$4 cm)-IIIA NSCLC were ran-domized to receive 3 cycles of histology-selected platinum doublet chemotherapy $\pm$ nivolumab, with the primary study outcomes of pCR rate and event-free survival. Although patients with known *EGFR* mutations and *ALK* rear-rangements were excluded, biomarker testing was not required outside of Asian countries, where *EGFR* testing was mandated.

The addition of neoadjuvant nivolumab did not seem to delay surgery or cause surgical cancellations. In fact, 83% of those treated with nivolumab and chemotherapy were able to undergo definitive surgery compared with 75% of patients treated with chemotherapy alone. Immune-related adverse events were experienced by 20% of patients receiving nivolumab, including pneumonitis, type I diabetes, hypophysitis, and adrenal insufficiency, most of which were grade 1 or 2 (17%). Potential concerns that neoadjuvant immunotherapy would induce tissue inflammation and make surgical resections technically more challenging were disproven. Exploratory outcomes related to surgery revealed that patients receiving neoadjuvant nivolumab and chemo-therapy were more likely to have an R0 resection (83% vs 78%), less likely to require pneumonectomy (17% vs 25%), and less likely to require conversion to thoracotomy (11% vs 16%). Operative times were shorter in patients treated with nivolumab (185 minutes vs 213 minutes) and there were no differences in postoperative compli-cations or hospital length-of-stay.[56]

As for efficacy, the primary endpoint of pCR rate was significantly higher in the nivo-lumab arm compared with chemotherapy alone (24% vs 2%; Odds ratio = 13.94, [99% CI, 3.49–55.75]). Nivolumab also led to significantly longer median event-free survival (EFS) compared with chemotherapy alone (31.6 months vs 20.8 months; EFS HR 0.63; [97.38% CI, 0.43–0.91]). Notable benefit was experienced by patients with clinical stage IIIA tumors receiving nivolumab with EFS HR 0.54 [95% CI, 0.37–0.80] as well as in the PD-L1 50% or greater subgroup (EFS HR = 0.24 [0.10–0.61]. OS results are immature but the early data demonstrates an impressive trend toward prolonged OS favoring the nivolumab arm. Based on the pCR and EFS coprimary endpoint results, nivolumab plus chemotherapy was US FDA-approved in patients with resectable stage II-IIIA NSCLC. Considering the impressive results presented to-date, immunotherapy-containing neoadjuvant regimens have been practice chang-ing and generated substantial excitement in the early-stage setting for patients with NSCLC.

Neoadjuvant Targeted Therapy in Resectable Non-small Cell Lung Cancer

Given the impressive and durable disease control afforded by various targeted thera-pies in metastatic NSCLC, neoadjuvant targeted approaches hold significant promise in biomarker-selected populations. That said, the available data for neoadjuvant EGFR TKIs has been surprisingly underwhelming. First-generation EGFR TKIs have resulted in mPR rates from 10% to 24% and pCR rate of 0% in the context of neoadjuvant trials.[58,59] The question remains whether these early endpoints used in chemotherapy and immunotherapy neoadjuvant trials apply similarly to TKI-treated tumors. Additionally, these trials used relatively short durations of preoperative TKI exposure and included early-generation TKIs that we now know to be inferior to osimertinib in the metastatic setting.[32] Neoadjuvant osimertinib is under investigation in the phase III NeoADAURA (NCT04351555).[60] Several other TKIs and small molecule inhibitors are being actively investigated in the neoadjuvant setting for early-stage, driver-mutant NSCLC (eg, NCT05015010, NCT05118854, NCT04926831). Moreover, the LCMC4 LEADER neoadjuvant screening trial (NCT04712877) will screen patients with resectable stage IA2-IIIA (AJCC eighth edition) lung cancer for actionable alterations for potential enrollment onto genomically matched neoadjuvant-targeted therapy arms.[61] Large, practical trials such as this may take time to produce results but ultimately will clarify the role for neoadjuvant-targeted therapies in NSCLC-harboring driver alterations.

PREOPERATIVE/PERIOPERATIVE VERSUS POSTOPERATIVE SYSTEMIC THERAPY

Surgery followed by adjuvant chemotherapy, rather than neoadjuvant therapy followed by surgery, has been the preferred approach for many patients with resectable NSCLC.[46] The delivery of neoadjuvant chemotherapy is associated with the risk of disease progression during therapy, and potentially results in a missed opportunity to perform a curative surgical resection. However, whether delivered preoperatively or postoperatively, chemotherapy contributes modestly to early-stage NSCLC cure rates.[9,43] Now, that immunotherapies and targeted therapies have entered the early-stage treatment landscape in parallel with biomarkers for patient selection, the optimal sequencing of systemic therapy and surgery for a given patient is unknown. Given the OS benefit of platinum-based chemotherapy for patients with AJCC eighth edition stage II-IIIA NSCLC, we offer chemotherapy to all patients who are platinum-eligible and stand to benefit based on cancer stage and pathologic features, and additionally we consider immunotherapy or targeted therapy based on tumor and patient characteristics.

For EGFR mutant NSCLC, the results of the ADAURA trial were practice changing.[36] Patients with stage IB-IIIA (AJCC seventh edition) EGFR mutant tumors (L858 R or exon 19 deletions) that are resectable should receive 3 years of adjuvant osimertinib after chemotherapy if indicated (**Fig. 1**). The data are not yet strong enough for neoadjuvant EGFR TKIs to be widely recommended, although ongoing trials such as NeoADAURA will further elucidate this approach. As for the other targetable driver alterations in NSCLC, ongoing trials previously discussed in this review seek to clarify the role for these highly effective therapies in the early-stage setting. Currently, we do not routinely prescribe targeted therapy in the neoadjuvant or adjuvant settings (other than adjuvant osimertinib) but we do seek to enroll patients on clinical trials using neoadjuvant or adjuvant therapy whenever possible.

As for immunotherapy in early-stage NSCLC, the decision to pursue neoadjuvant versus adjuvant therapy has sparked contentious debate, which remains unresolved. Two available IO-containing treatment approaches for patients with EGFR/ALK wild-type, resectable stage II-IIIA (AJCC eighth edition) NSCLC are based on phase III data and are depicted in **Fig. 1**. These are as follows: (1) 3 cycles of neoadjuvant nivolumab-based chemoimmunotherapy followed by surgery based on the CheckMate-816 trial or (2) up-front surgery followed by 4 cycles of platinum doublet and subsequently, 1 year of adjuvant atezolizumab based on the IMPower-010 trial.[20,56]

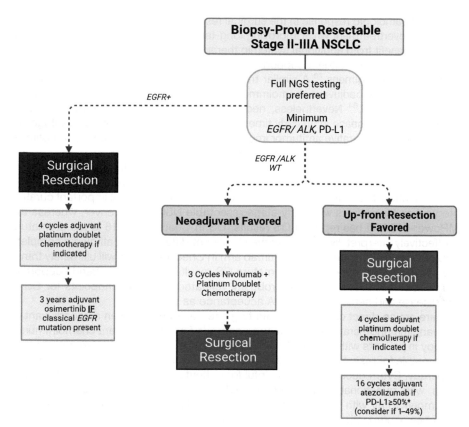

Fig. 1. Approach to perioperative therapy for patients with resectable NSCLC in 2022. WT, wild type. * tumor PD-L1 expression.

According to retrospective data, patients treated with neoadjuvant chemotherapy are more likely to complete intended cycles and receive full dose therapy with lower rates of grade 3 or more toxicity.[45] Other theoretical benefits include the potential for preoperative tumor downstaging, mitigation of surgical extent, and interrogation of tumor biology based on the pathologic treatment effect. Therefore, as more effective systemic therapies and predictive biomarkers have emerged in NSCLC, there has been an explosion of interest in neoadjuvant treatment strategies.

The preclinical and practical advantages of neoadjuvant chemoimmunotherapy provide a compelling rationale for this strategy. Preclinical studies using triple-negative breast cancer models demonstrate superior long-term efficacy of neoadjuvant immunotherapy compared to adjuvant immunotherapy, which is related to peripheral evidence of a more potent antitumor immune response.[62] The robust induction of antitumor immunity has been demonstrated in translational studies with melanoma and NSCLC with immunotherapy or chemoimmunotherapy regimens.[49,63,64] Similarly, neoadjuvant immunotherapy will allow for more deliberate translational study of novel biomarkers of response (eg, Tumor-associated neoantigen burden), mechanisms of anti-PD-1/PD-L1 resistance or persistence, radiographic and pathologic response correlation, pseudoprogression and the recently described "nodal immune flare" phenomenon.[49,65–67] As demonstrated in breast cancer, neoadjuvant therapy also allows for the development of paradigms involving tailored adjuvant therapy based on the degree of pathologic response in the surgical resection specimen.[68,69] This approach minimizes overtreatment while improving long-term outcomes in a subset of patients who may benefit from additional systemic therapy. Results from the PRADO study in high-risk stage III melanoma support this adaptable response-driven approach for immunotherapy regimens.[70] A similar trial may help to clarify the need for adjuvant nivolumab after neoadjuvant chemoimmunotherapy for stage IIIA NSCLC as studied in the NADIM trial.[64] Nevertheless, neoadjuvant chemoimmunotherapy addresses micrometastatic disease at an early timepoint, and has other potential advantages of expansion of preoperative antitumor immune response and enabling time to optimize patients for surgery with preoperative exercise training.[71]

Inevitable drawbacks of neoadjuvant systemic therapy are the potential to delay surgery or miss the patient's "window" for surgical resection. The IMPower-010 approach offers the fastest time to surgery, which remains the most important curative intervention for patients with early-stage resectable NSCLC. Moreover, whereas the IMPower-010 trial has reported OS results, OS in CheckMate-816 is too premature to effectively interpret. We think that the significant difference in pathologic complete response and EFS favoring the nivolumab arm in CheckMate-816 will ultimately translate into an OS benefit—and the immature OS results show a clear trend supporting this notion—but these are not yet robustly validated surrogate endpoints for OS in this disease and setting despite FDA acceptance as such.[72]

There are no direct comparison data to guide decisions between a neoadjuvant or adjuvant immunotherapy treatment approach. We favor neoadjuvant chemoimmunotherapy in patients with resectable stage II-IIIA NSCLC in whom cytoreduction would be favorable for resection and in tumors with a higher likelihood of benefit from immunotherapy. Cytoreduction may be helpful for patients with stage II and III tumors, patients with questionable R0 resection potential, and for those likely to require pneumonectomy with large tumors or with mediastinal nodal involvement. Neoadjuvant chemoimmunotherapy should not be initiated for patients who are borderline surgical candidates or patients with stage IIIA disease with low likelihood for R0 resection based on clinical staging. High PD-L1 ($\geq$50%) expression, significant smoking history, and EGFR/ALK (and possibly other non-IO-responsive oncogenes) wild-type status are factors that would positively influence the decision to use a neoadjuvant chemoimmunotherapy approach for a given patient because these patient subsets have a higher chance of benefit from immunotherapy. For patients with unresectable stage IIIA NSCLC, the PACIFIC regimen of concurrent chemotherapy and radiation followed by 1 year of consolidation durvalumab represents a highly effective regimen with impressive long-term survival data in this population.[19,73]

ADDITIONAL CONSIDERATIONS AND FUTURE DIRECTIONS

Accompanying all the recent changes to the early-stage NSCLC treatment landscape is a great deal of uncertainty (**Fig. 2**). Although we have focused on perioperative systemic therapy in this review, radiation is another effective treatment modality for NSCLC and may synergize with immunotherapy.[74] After the negative results of the Lung ART and PORT-C trials, which demonstrated no benefit of postoperative radiotherapy (PORT) for patients with pathologic N2+ stage IIIA NSCLC, routine PORT for these patients has largely fallen out of favor.[75,76] However, these trials had notable flaws and in select patients at high risk for mediastinal relapse or those with positive margins, PORT may still have a role.[77] In the context of novel systemic neoadjuvant and adjuvant therapies, the role for PORT and other forms of perioperative radiotherapy is not clear. The ADAURA and IMPower-010 studies did not allow for

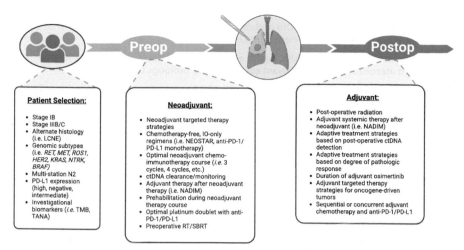

Patient Selection:

- Stage IB
- Stage IIIB/C
- Alternate histology (i.e. LCNE)
- Genomic subtypes (i.e. RET, MET, ROS1, HER2, KRAS, NTRK, BRAF)
- Multi-station N2
- PD-L1 expression (high, negative, intermediate)
- Investigational biomarkers (i.e. TMB, TANA)

Neoadjuvant:

- Neoadjuvant targeted therapy strategies
- Chemotherapy-free, IO-only regimens (i.e. NEOSTAR, anti-PD-1/PD-L1 monotherapy)
- Optimal neoadjuvant chemo-immunotherapy course (i.e. 3 cycles, 4 cycles, etc.)
- ctDNA clearance/monitoring
- Adjuvant therapy after neoadjuvant therapy (i.e. NADIM)
- Prehabilitation during neoadjuvant therapy course
- Optimal platinum doublet with anti-PD-1/PD-L1
- Preoperative RT/SBRT

Adjuvant:

- Post-operative radiation
- Adjuvant systemic therapy after neoadjuvant (i.e. NADIM)
- Adaptive treatment strategies based on post-operative ctDNA detection
- Adaptive treatment strategies based on degree of pathologic response
- Duration of adjuvant osimertinib
- Adjuvant targeted therapy strategies for oncogene-driven tumors
- Sequential or concurrent adjuvant chemotherapy and anti-PD-1/PD-L1

Fig. 2. Open questions, ongoing considerations, and future directions for perioperative therapy in resectable non-small cell lung cancer. ctDNA, circulating tumor DNA; IO, immuno-oncology; LCNE, large cell neuroendocrine; SBRT, stereotactic body radiation therapy; TANA, tumor-associated neoantigens; TMB, tumor mutational burden. **Figs. 1** and **2** created with BioRender.com.

PORT, and although CheckMate-816 did, very few patients on either arm received adjuvant radiation.[20,36,56] Novel combination strategies combining perioperative immunotherapy with radiation are under investigation.[78]

A role for utilizing ctDNA to measure residual disease in early-stage NSCLC is emerging as well. Multiple studies have demonstrated the prognostic significance of ctDNA dynamics in early-stage NSCLC, yet the implications for guiding therapy have not been defined as in other diseases such as stage II colon cancer.[79–82] In CheckMate-816, 46% of patients achieving preoperative ctDNA clearance with nivolumab plus chemotherapy were found to have a pCR compared with 13% with chemotherapy alone.[56] Moreover, no patients with detectable preoperative ctDNA achieved pCR on the nivolumab arm. Reliably detecting ctDNA in patients with a limited disease burden preoperatively or residual micrometastases postoperatively remains a challenge for ctDNA-based approaches, which may have limited sensitivity in these settings.[79] Adaptive trial designs utilizing ctDNA detection as a patient-selection biomarker for adjuvant therapy are ongoing (NCT04385368).

We have entered a new era for early-stage NSCLC in which precision approaches and novel systemic therapies will undoubtedly contribute to declining rates of relapse and disease-specific mortality. Experience with these agents in the metastatic setting should help with their swift transition into the early-stage setting. The last few years have been triumphant for advancing therapeutics in lung cancer and we anticipate even more profound advances in the years to come.

CLINICS CARE POINTS

- Despite advances in immunotherapy and targeted therapy for NSCLC, cisplatin-based chemotherapy should be offered to eligible patients with AJCC eighth edition stage IIA-III resected NSCLC, given the survival benefit—albeit modest—in this setting.

- Adjuvant osimertinib prolongs DFS and central nervous system DFS for patients with *EGFR*-mutant (L858 R and exon 19 deletion) NSCLC.
- For patients with stage II-IIIA (AJCC eighth edition) resected NSCLC with PD-L1 1% or greater, adjuvant atezolizumab after adjuvant chemotherapy prolongs DFS.
- The benefit of adjuvant atezolizumab in the PD-L1 1% or greater population is driven by the PD-L1 50% or greater subgroup, in which adjuvant atezolizumab also prolongs OS based on an interim analysis of the IMPower-010 trial.
- The addition of nivolumab to neoadjuvant platinum-based chemotherapy leads to a profound increase in pathologic complete response and a significant improvement in event-free survival over neoadjuvant chemotherapy alone, for resectable NSCLC.

REFERENCES

1. Tan AC, Tan DSW. Targeted therapies for lung cancer patients with oncogenic driver molecular alterations. J Clin Onco 2022;40(6):611–25.
2. Li BT, Smit EF, Goto Y, et al. Trastuzumab Deruxtecan in HER2-Mutant Non-Small-Cell Lung Cancer. N Engl J Med 2022;386(3):241–51.
3. Grant MJ, Herbst RS, Goldberg SB. Selecting the optimal immunotherapy regimen in driver-negative metastatic NSCLC. Nat Rev Clin Oncol 2021;18(10):625–44.
4. Howlader N, Forjaz G, Mooradian MJ, et al. The Effect of Advances in Lung-Cancer Treatment on Population Mortality. N Engl J Med 2020;383(7):640–9.
5. Goldstraw P, Chansky K, Crowley J, et al. The IASLC Lung Cancer Staging Project: Proposals for Revision of the TNM Stage Groupings in the Forthcoming (Eighth) Edition of the TNM Classification for Lung Cancer. J Thorac Oncol 2016;11(1):39–51.
6. Datta D, Lahiri B. Preoperative evaluation of patients undergoing lung resection surgery. Chest 2003;123(6):2096–103.
7. Vachani A, Carroll NM, Simoff MJ, et al. Stage Migration and Lung Cancer Incidence After Initiation of Low-Dose Computed Tomography Screening. J Thorac Oncol 2022;17(12):P1355–64.
8. Woodard GA, Li A, Boffa DJ. Role of adjuvant therapy in T1-2N0 resected non–small cell lung cancer. J Thorac Cardiovasc Surg 2022;163(5):1685–92.
9. Pignon JP, Tribodet H, Scagliotti GV, et al. Lung adjuvant cisplatin evaluation: a pooled analysis by the LACE Collaborative Group. J Clin Oncol 2008;26(21):3552–9.
10. Strauss GM, Herndon JE 2nd, Maddaus MA, et al. Adjuvant paclitaxel plus carboplatin compared with observation in stage IB non-small-cell lung cancer: CALGB 9633 with the Cancer and Leukemia Group B, Radiation Therapy Oncology Group, and North Central Cancer Treatment Group Study Groups. J Clin Oncol 2008;26(31):5043–51.
11. Pathak R, Goldberg SB, Canavan M, et al. Association of Survival With Adjuvant Chemotherapy Among Patients With Early-Stage Non-Small Cell Lung Cancer With vs Without High-Risk Clinicopathologic Features. JAMA Oncol 2020;6(11):1741–50.
12. Kratz JR, He J, Van Den Eeden SK, et al. A practical molecular assay to predict survival in resected non-squamous, non-small-cell lung cancer: development and international validation studies. Lancet 2012;379(9818):823–32.
13. Woodard GA, Kratz JR, Haro G, et al. Molecular Risk Stratification is Independent of EGFR Mutation Status in Identifying Early-Stage Non-Squamous Non-Small

Cell Lung Cancer Patients at Risk for Recurrence and Likely to Benefit From Adjuvant Chemotherapy. Clin Lung Cancer 2021;22(6):587–95.

14. Kehl KL, Zahrieh D, Yang P, et al. Rates of Guideline-Concordant Surgery and Adjuvant Chemotherapy Among Patients With Early-Stage Lung Cancer in the US ALCHEMIST Study (Alliance A151216). JAMA Oncol 2022;8(5):717–28.

15. Garon EB, Hellmann MD, Rizvi NA, et al. Five-Year Overall Survival for Patients With Advanced NonSmall-Cell Lung Cancer Treated With Pembrolizumab: Results From the Phase I KEYNOTE-001 Study. J Clin Oncol 2019;37(28):2518–27.

16. Borghaei H, Gettinger S, Vokes EE, et al. Five-Year Outcomes From the Randomized, Phase III Trials CheckMate 017 and 057: Nivolumab Versus Docetaxel in Previously Treated Non-Small-Cell Lung Cancer. J Clin Oncol 2021;39(7):723–33.

17. Reck M, Rodriguez-Abreu D, Robinson AG, et al. Five-Year Outcomes With Pembrolizumab Versus Chemotherapy for Metastatic Non-Small-Cell Lung Cancer With PD-L1 Tumor Proportion Score >/= 50. J Clin Oncol 2021;39(21):2339–49.

18. Garassino MC, Gadgeel SM, Speranza G, et al. 973MO KEYNOTE-189 5-year update: First-line pembrolizumab (pembro) + pemetrexed (pem) and platinum vs placebo (pbo) + pem and platinum for metastatic nonsquamous NSCLC. Ann Oncol 2022;33:S992–3.

19. Spigel DR, Faivre-Finn C, Gray JE, et al. Five-Year Survival Outcomes From the PACIFIC Trial: Durvalumab After Chemoradiotherapy in Stage III Non-Small-Cell Lung Cancer. J Clin Oncol 2022;40(12):1301–11.

20. Felip E, Altorki N, Zhou C, et al. Adjuvant atezolizumab after adjuvant chemotherapy in resected stage IB-IIIA non-small-cell lung cancer (IMpower010): a randomised, multicentre, open-label, phase 3 trial. Lancet 2021;398(10308):1344–57.

21. Wakelee H, Altorki N, Felip E, et al. PL03.09 IMpower010:Overall Survival Interim Analysis of a Phase III Study of Atezolizumab vs Best Supportive Care in Resected NSCLC. J Thorac Oncol 2022;17(9, Supplement):S2.

22. O'Brien M, Paz-Ares L, Marreaud S, et al. Pembrolizumab versus placebo as adjuvant therapy for completely resected stage IB-IIIA non-small-cell lung cancer (PEARLS/KEYNOTE-091): an interim analysis of a randomised, triple-blind, phase 3 trial. Lancet Oncol 2022;23(10):1274–86.

23. Mazieres J, Drilon A, Lusque A, et al. Immune checkpoint inhibitors for patients with advanced lung cancer and oncogenic driver alterations: results from the IMMUNOTARGET registry. Ann Oncol 2019;30(8):1321–8.

24. Gainor JF, Shaw AT, Sequist LV, et al. EGFR Mutations and ALK Rearrangements Are Associated with Low Response Rates to PD-1 Pathway Blockade in Non-Small Cell Lung Cancer: A Retrospective Analysis. Clin Cancer Res 2016;22(18):4585–93.

25. Tie J, Lo SN, Gibbs P. Circulating Tumor DNA Guiding Adjuvant Therapy in Colon Cancer. Reply N Engl J Med 2022;387(8):760.

26. Zhong WZ, Wang Q, Mao WM, et al. Gefitinib versus vinorelbine plus cisplatin as adjuvant treatment for stage II-IIIA (N1-N2) EGFR-mutant NSCLC (ADJUVANT/CTONG1104): a randomised, open-label, phase 3 study. Lancet Oncol 2018;19(1):139–48.

27. Pennell NA, Neal JW, Chaft JE, et al. SELECT: A Phase II Trial of Adjuvant Erlotinib in Patients With Resected Epidermal Growth Factor Receptor-Mutant Non-Small-Cell Lung Cancer. J Clin Oncol 2019;37(2):97–104.

28. Kelly K, Altorki NK, Eberhardt WE, et al. Adjuvant Erlotinib Versus Placebo in Patients With Stage IB-IIIA Non-Small-Cell Lung Cancer (RADIANT): A Randomized, Double-Blind, Phase III Trial. J Clin Oncol 2015;33(34):4007–14.

29. Yue D, Xu S, Wang Q, et al. Updated Overall Survival and Exploratory Analysis From Randomized, Phase II EVAN Study of Erlotinib Versus Vinorelbine Plus Cisplatin Adjuvant Therapy in Stage IIIA Epidermal Growth Factor Receptor+ Non-Small-Cell Lung Cancer. J Clin Oncol 2022;JCO2200428. https://doi.org/10.1200/JCO.22.00428.

30. He J, Su C, Liang W, et al. Icotinib versus chemotherapy as adjuvant treatment for stage II-IIIA EGFR-mutant non-small-cell lung cancer (EVIDENCE): a randomised, open-label, phase 3 trial. Lancet Respir Med 2021;9(9):1021–9.

31. Tada H, Mitsudomi T, Misumi T, et al. Randomized Phase III Study of Gefitinib Versus Cisplatin Plus Vinorelbine for Patients With Resected Stage II-IIIA Non-Small-Cell Lung Cancer With EGFR Mutation (IMPACT). J Clin Oncol 2022; 40(3):231 41.

32. Ramalingam SS, Vansteenkiste J, Planchard D, et al. Overall Survival with Osimertinib in Untreated, EGFR-Mutated Advanced NSCLC. N Engl J Med 2020; 382(1):41–50.

33. Janne PA, Yang JC, Kim DW, et al. AZD9291 in EGFR inhibitor-resistant non-small-cell lung cancer. N Engl J Med 2015;372(18):1689–99.

34. Colclough N, Chen K, Johnstrom P, et al. Preclinical Comparison of the Blood-brain barrier Permeability of Osimertinib with Other EGFR TKIs. Clin Cancer Res 2021;27(1):189–201.

35. Soria JC, Ohe Y, Vansteenkiste J, et al. Osimertinib in Untreated EGFR-Mutated Advanced Non-Small-Cell Lung Cancer. N Engl J Med 2018;378(2):113–25.

36. Wu YL, Tsuboi M, He J, et al. Osimertinib in Resected EGFR-Mutated Non-Small-Cell Lung Cancer. N Engl J Med 2020;383(18):1711–23.

37. Wu YL, John T, Grohe C, et al. Postoperative Chemotherapy Use and Outcomes From ADAURA: Osimertinib as Adjuvant Therapy for Resected EGFR-Mutated NSCLC. J Thorac Oncol 2022;17(3):423–33.

38. Tsuboi M, Wu YL, Grohe C, et al. LBA47 Osimertinib as adjuvant therapy in patients (pts) with resected EGFR-mutated (EGFRm) stage IB-IIIA non-small cell lung cancer (NSCLC): Updated results from ADAURA. Ann Oncol 2022;33: S1413–4.

39. Govindan R, Mandrekar SJ, Gerber DE, et al. ALCHEMIST Trials: A Golden Opportunity to Transform Outcomes in Early-Stage Non-Small Cell Lung Cancer. Clin Cancer Res 2015;21(24):5439–44.

40. Solomon BJ, Ahn JS, Barlesi F, et al. ALINA: A phase III study of alectinib versus chemotherapy as adjuvant therapy in patients with stage IB–IIIA anaplastic lymphoma kinase-positive (ALK+) non-small cell lung cancer (NSCLC). J Clin Oncol 2019;37(15_suppl):TPS8569.

41. Tsuboi M, Goldman JW, Wu YL, et al. LIBRETTO-432, a phase III study of adjuvant selpercatinib or placebo in stage IB-IIIA RET fusion-positive non-small-cell lung cancer. Future Oncol 2022;18(28):3133–41.

42. Lee JM, Awad MM, Saliba TR, et al. Neoadjuvant and adjuvant capmatinib in resectable non–small cell lung cancer with MET exon 14 skipping mutation or high MET amplification: GEOMETRY-N trial. J Clin Oncol 2022;40(16_suppl): TPS8590.

43. Group NM-aC. Preoperative chemotherapy for non-small-cell lung cancer: a systematic review and meta-analysis of individual participant data. Lancet 2014; 383(9928):1561–71.

44. Lim E, Harris G, Patel A, et al. Preoperative versus postoperative chemotherapy in patients with resectable non-small cell lung cancer: systematic review and

indirect comparison meta-analysis of randomized trials. J Thorac Oncol 2009; 4(11):1380–8.

45. Brandt WS, Yan W, Zhou J, et al. Outcomes after neoadjuvant or adjuvant chemotherapy for cT2-4N0-1 non-small cell lung cancer: A propensity-matched analysis. J Thorac Cardiovasc Surg 2019;157(2):743–753 e3.

46. MacLean M, Luo X, Wang S, et al. Outcomes of neoadjuvant and adjuvant chemotherapy in stage 2 and 3 non-small cell lung cancer: an analysis of the National Cancer Database. Oncotarget 2018;9(36):24470–9.

47. Hellmann MD, Chaft JE, William WN Jr, et al. Pathological response after neoadjuvant chemotherapy in resectable non-small-cell lung cancers: proposal for the use of major pathological response as a surrogate endpoint. Lancet Oncol 2014; 15(1):e42–50.

48. Topalian SL, Taube JM, Pardoll DM. Neoadjuvant checkpoint blockade for cancer immunotherapy. Science 2020;367:6477.

49. Forde PM, Chaft JE, Pardoll DM. Neoadjuvant PD-1 Blockade in Resectable Lung Cancer. N Engl J Med 2018;379(9):e14.

50. Reck M, Rodriguez-Abreu D, Robinson AG, et al. Pembrolizumab versus Chemotherapy for PD-L1-Positive Non-Small-Cell Lung Cancer. N Engl J Med 2016; 375(19):1823–33.

51. Mok TSK, Wu YL, Kudaba I, et al. Pembrolizumab versus chemotherapy for previously untreated, PD-L1-expressing, locally advanced or metastatic non-small-cell lung cancer (KEYNOTE-042): a randomised, open-label, controlled, phase 3 trial. Lancet 2019;393(10183):1819–30.

52. Herbst RS, Giaccone G, de Marinis F, et al. Atezolizumab for First-Line Treatment of PD-L1-Selected Patients with NSCLC. N Engl J Med Oct 1 2020;383(14): 1328–39.

53. Carbone DP, Reck M, Paz-Ares L, et al. First-Line Nivolumab in Stage IV or Recurrent Non–Small-Cell Lung Cancer. New Engl J Med 2017;376(25):2415–26.

54. Rizvi NA, Cho BC, Reinmuth N, et al. Durvalumab With or Without Tremelimumab vs Standard Chemotherapy in First-line Treatment of Metastatic Non–Small Cell Lung Cancer: The MYSTIC Phase 3 Randomized Clinical Trial. JAMA Oncol 2020;6(5):661–74.

55. Shu CA, Gainor JF, Awad MM, et al. Neoadjuvant atezolizumab and chemotherapy in patients with resectable non-small-cell lung cancer: an open-label, multicentre, single-arm, phase 2 trial. Lancet Oncol 2020;21(6):786–95.

56. Forde PM, Spicer J, Lu S, et al. Neoadjuvant Nivolumab plus Chemotherapy in Resectable Lung Cancer. N Engl J Med 2022;386(21):1973–85.

57. Provencio M, Serna-Blasco R, Nadal E, et al. Overall Survival and Biomarker Analysis of Neoadjuvant Nivolumab Plus Chemotherapy in Operable Stage IIIA Non-Small-Cell Lung Cancer (NADIM phase II trial). J Clin Oncol 2022;40(25): 2924–33.

58. Zhong WZ, Chen KN, Chen C, et al. Erlotinib Versus Gemcitabine Plus Cisplatin as Neoadjuvant Treatment of Stage IIIA-N2 EGFR-Mutant Non-Small-Cell Lung Cancer (EMERGING-CTONG 1103): A Randomized Phase II Study. J Clin Oncol 2019;37(25):2235–45.

59. Zhang Y, Fu F, Hu H, et al. Gefitinib as neoadjuvant therapy for resectable stage II-IIIA non-small cell lung cancer: A phase II study. J Thorac Cardiovasc Surg Feb 2021;161(2):434–442 e2.

60. Tsuboi M, Weder W, Escriu C, et al. Neoadjuvant osimertinib with/without chemotherapy versus chemotherapy alone for EGFR-mutated resectable non-small-cell lung cancer: NeoADAURA. Future Oncol Nov 2021;17(31):4045–55.

61. Sepesi B, Jones DR, Meyers BF, et al. LCMC LEADER neoadjuvant screening trial: LCMC4 evaluation of actionable drivers in early-stage lung cancers. J Clin Oncol 2022;40(16_suppl):TPS8596.

62. Liu J, Blake SJ, Yong MC, et al. Improved Efficacy of Neoadjuvant Compared to Adjuvant Immunotherapy to Eradicate Metastatic Disease. Cancer Discov 2016; 6(12):1382–99.

63. Blank CU, Rozeman EA, Fanchi LF, et al. Neoadjuvant versus adjuvant ipilimumab plus nivolumab in macroscopic stage III melanoma. Nat Med 2018;24(11): 1655–61.

64. Cascone T, William WN Jr, Weissferdt A, et al. Neoadjuvant nivolumab or nivolumab plus ipilimumab in operable non-small cell lung cancer: the phase 2 randomized NEOSTAR trial. Nat Med 2021;27(3):504–14.

65. Gupta RG, Li F, Roszik J, et al. Exploiting Tumor Neoantigens to Target Cancer Evolution: Current Challenges and Promising Therapeutic Approaches. Cancer Discov 2021;11(5):1024–39.

66. Sehgal K, Portell A, Ivanova EV, et al. Dynamic single-cell RNA sequencing identifies immunotherapy persister cells following PD-1 blockade. J Clin Invest 2021; 131(2). https://doi.org/10.1172/JCI135038.

67. Cascone T, Weissferdt A, Godoy MCB, et al. Nodal immune flare mimics nodal disease progression following neoadjuvant immune checkpoint inhibitors in non-small cell lung cancer. Nat Commun 2021;12(1):5045.

68. Masuda N, Lee SJ, Ohtani S, et al. Adjuvant Capecitabine for Breast Cancer after Preoperative Chemotherapy. N Engl J Med 2017;376(22):2147–59.

69. von Minckwitz G, Huang CS, Mano MS, et al. Trastuzumab Emtansine for Residual Invasive HER2-Positive Breast Cancer. N Engl J Med Feb 14 2019;380(7): 617–28.

70. Reijers ILM, Menzies AM, van Akkooi ACJ, et al. Personalized response-directed surgery and adjuvant therapy after neoadjuvant ipilimumab and nivolumab in high-risk stage III melanoma: the PRADO trial. Nat Med Jun 2022;28(6):1178–88.

71. Cavalheri V, Granger C. Preoperative exercise training for patients with non-small cell lung cancer. Cochrane Database Syst Rev 2017;6:CD012020.

72. Walia A, Haslam A, Prasad V. FDA validation of surrogate endpoints in oncology: 2005-2022. J Cancer Policy 2022;34:100364.

73. Senan S, Ozguroglu M, Daniel D, et al. Outcomes with durvalumab after chemoradiotherapy in stage IIIA-N2 non-small-cell lung cancer: an exploratory analysis from the PACIFIC trial. ESMO Open 2022;7(2):100410.

74. Sharabi AB, Lim M, DeWeese TL, et al. Radiation and checkpoint blockade immunotherapy: radiosensitisation and potential mechanisms of synergy. Lancet Oncol 2015;16(13):e498–509.

75. Hui Z, Men Y, Hu C, et al. Effect of Postoperative Radiotherapy for Patients With pIIIA-N2 Non-Small Cell Lung Cancer After Complete Resection and Adjuvant Chemotherapy: The Phase 3 PORT-C Randomized Clinical Trial. JAMA Oncol 2021;7(8):1178–85.

76. Le Pechoux C, Pourel N, Barlesi F, et al. Postoperative radiotherapy versus no postoperative radiotherapy in patients with completely resected non-small-cell lung cancer and proven mediastinal N2 involvement (Lung ART): an open-label, randomised, phase 3 trial. Lancet Oncol 2022;23(1):104–14.

77. Canova S, Arcangeli S, Cortinovis DL. A Cast of Shadow on Postoperative Radiotherapy for pIIIA-N2 Non-Small Cell Lung Cancer? JAMA Oncol 2022. https://doi.org/10.1001/jamaoncol.2022.4442.

78. Altorki NK, McGraw TE, Borczuk AC, et al. Neoadjuvant durvalumab with or without stereotactic body radiotherapy in patients with early-stage non-small-cell lung cancer: a single-centre, randomised phase 2 trial. Lancet Oncol 2021; 22(6):824–35.
79. Li N, Wang B-X, Li J, et al. Perioperative circulating tumor DNA as a potential prognostic marker for operable stage I to IIIA non–small cell lung cancer. Cancer 2022;128(4):708–18.
80. Xia L, Mei J, Kang R, et al. Perioperative ctDNA-Based Molecular Residual Disease Detection for Non-Small Cell Lung Cancer: A Prospective Multicenter Cohort Study (LUNGCA-1). Clin Cancer Res 2022;28(15):3308–17.
81. Gale D, Heider K, Ruiz-Valdepenas A, et al. Residual ctDNA after treatment predicts early relapse in patients with early-stage non-small cell lung cancer. Ann Oncol 2022;33(5):500–10.
82. Tie J, Cohen JD, Lahouel K, et al. Circulating Tumor DNA Analysis Guiding Adjuvant Therapy in Stage II Colon Cancer. N Engl J Med 2022;386(24):2261–72.
83. Wislez M, Mazieres J, Lavole A, et al. Neoadjuvant durvalumab for resectable non-small-cell lung cancer (NSCLC): results from a multicenter study (IFCT-1601 IONESCO). J ImmunoTherapy Cancer 2022;10(10):e005636.
84. Besse B, Adam J, Cozic N, et al. 1215O - SC Neoadjuvant atezolizumab (A) for resectable non-small cell lung cancer (NSCLC): Results from the phase II PRINCEPS trial. Ann Oncol 2020;31:S794–5.
85. Chaft JE, Oezkan F, Kris MG, et al. Neoadjuvant atezolizumab for resectable non small cell lung cancer: an open-label, single arm phase II trial. Nat Med 2022; 28(10):2155–61.

Locally Advanced Lung Cancer

Sarah Oh, PharmD[a], George N. Botros[a], Milan Patel[a], Missak Haigentz, MD[b],
Eshan Patel, MD[c], Iaonnis Kontopidis, MD[d], John Langenfeld, MD[b],
Matthew P. Deek, MD[a], Salma K. Jabbour, MD[a,*]

KEYWORDS

- Locally advanced lung cancer • Non–small cell lung cancer
- Unresectable non–small cell lung cancer • Immune checkpoint inhibitor
- Immunotherapy • Chemoradiation therapy • Radiotherapy

KEY POINTS

- Overall and progression-free survival remains modest in patients with unresectable, locally advanced lung cancer, despite standard-of-care management with concurrent chemoradiation followed by consolidative durvalumab immunotherapy.
- New treatment approaches to improve survival outcomes involve concurrent administration of immunotherapy with chemoradiotherapy or consolidation with novel or targeted agents , though there is an associated increased risk of overlapping toxicity.
- Studies involving next-generation immunotherapy and targeted therapy with chemoradiotherapy are underway to better define the standard of care for patients with programmed death ligand 1–negative tumors, oncogenic driver mutations, toxicity leading to discontinuation, or limited performance status.
- Refinement of radiation techniques may mitigate treatment-related toxicity and optimize efficacy of current treatment strategies.

INTRODUCTION

Lung cancer is the leading cause of cancer mortality worldwide, with non–small cell lung cancer (NSCLC) accounting for 82% of all lung cancer diagnoses.[1] If feasible, surgical resection is the standard of care (SoC) for early stage local disease;

[a] Department of Radiation Oncology, Rutgers Cancer Institute of New Jersey, Rutgers Robert Wood Johnson Medical School, Rutgers University, New Brunswick, NJ, USA; [b] Division of Thoracic Oncology, Rutgers Cancer Institute of New Jersey, Rutgers Robert Wood Johnson Medical School, Rutgers University, New Brunswick, NJ, USA; [c] Division of Medical Oncology, Rutgers Cancer Institute of New Jersey, New Brunswick, NJ, USA; [d] Department of Surgery, Robert Wood Johnson University Hospital, Rutgers Robert Wood Johnson Medical School, New Brunswick, NJ, USA
* Corresponding author. Rutgers Cancer Insitute of New Jersey, 195 Little Albany Street, New Brunswick, NJ 08901.
E-mail address: jabbousk@cinj.rutgers.edu

Hematol Oncol Clin N Am 37 (2023) 533–555
https://doi.org/10.1016/j.hoc.2023.02.007
0889-8588/23/© 2023 Elsevier Inc. All rights reserved.

however, approximately one-fifth of patients with NSCLC present with unresectable, locally advanced Stage III disease at the time of diagnosis.[2,3] Resectability in non-small cell lung cancer is determined by staging, tumor location, lung function, and patient comorbidities. Tumors that are large (>7 cm), located deep in the lungs, or that invade into adjacent structures or organs (T4), or multistation mediastinal or extrathoracic (ie, supraclavicular) lymph nodes (N2/N3), may not be eligible for complete surgical resection. Surgery is also not recommended in patients with poor lung function, coagulopathy, or other medical conditions that increase their risk for perioperative and postoperative complications including death (ie, recent cardiac events, such as cardiac stent placement).[4] The prognosis for unresectable, locally advanced NSCLC (LA-NSCLC) historically had been suboptimal, with 5-year overall survival (OS) ranging between 20% and 32% using definitive concurrent chemoradiotherapy (cCRT).[5,6]

Immune checkpoint inhibition (ICI) has since transformed the management of unresectable, locally advanced lung cancer, with 5-year OS now reaching 43% using cCRT followed by 1 year of durvalumab.[7] Despite this shift in treatment paradigm, OS remains modest, with disease recurrence limiting life expectancy. Moreover, patients with PD-L1 negative tumors, low tumor mutational burden (TMB), and certain oncogenic driver mutations, namely epidermal growth factor (EGFR), may not derive as much benefit from consolidation durvalumab.[8,9] Many patients are also not eligible due to disease progression, toxicities of cCRT, or other reasons.[10] As such, the optimal timing and combination of cCRT, immunotherapy, and/or targeted therapy are being investigated to further improve survival outcomes in patients with LA-NSCLC.

This review summarizes historical data that galvanized new research efforts, as well as ongoing clinical trials that address the challenges of current therapeutic approaches for unresectable, locally advanced lung cancer.

SEQUENTIAL VERSUS CONCURRENT CHEMORADIATION THERAPY

Thoracic radiation therapy (TRT) alone has demonstrated OS benefit for inoperable lung cancer by providing local tumor control.[11,12] By contrast, chemotherapy provides a systemic cytotoxic effect and offers radiosensitizing benefit. Together, the synergistic effect of chemoradiotherapy achieves greater tumor response compared with radiotherapy or chemotherapy alone.[13,14] The ideal time to pair chemotherapy with RT became the basis of many early studies.[15,16] A 2010 meta-analysis evaluated 6 trials (n = 1205) and concluded that cCRT achieved superior OS advantage over sequential chemoradiotherapy (sCRT) (hazard ratio [HR], 0.84; 95% confidence interval [CI], 0.74–0.95; $P = .004$), with a 4.5% absolute benefit (10.6%–15.1%) at 5 years.[5] Furthermore, cCRT improved rates of locoregional progression (HR, 0.77; 95% CI, 0.62–0.95; $P = .01$), with a 6.1% absolute decrease (35.0%–28.9%) at 5 years. There was, however, no statistically significant difference in progression-free survival (PFS) or distant progression. Survival advantages have been observed with multiple platinum-doublet regimens, with a 2022 meta-analysis reporting a higher 3-year OS and simultaneously lower toxicity with cisplatin and pemetrexed.[17–20] cCRT improved OS but at the cost of increased toxicity, specifically acute grade 3 to 4 esophageal toxicity from 4% to 18%, compared with sCRT (relative risk, 4.9; 95% CI, 3.1–7.8; $P < .001$).[5] Furthermore, the more synchronized the initiation of chemotherapy and radiation, the more likely it is for the patient to achieve a benefit.[21] An analysis of the National Cancer Database found that non-concurrent initiation of chemotherapy and radiation therapy (RT) can result in significant decrements in survival rates.[21] Although cCRT has proved more efficacious than sCRT in most patient populations, there remain opportunities to further improve prognoses and reduce toxicity profiles.

Strategies for Concurrent Chemoradiotherapy Optimization and Toxicity Reduction

To improve local tumor control with cCRT, the RTOG (Radiation Therapy Oncology Group) 0617, a 2 × 2 factorial designed trial, randomized patients (n = 544) to standard 60 Gy or high-dose 74 Gy TRT to investigate the potential benefit of dose escalation, as well as assess a benefit to the integration of cetuximab, an anti-EGFR antibody.[6] TRT dose escalation, however, did not increase and in fact was associated with lower median OS (28.7 vs 20.3 months, 60 Gy vs 74 Gy; P = .0072), 5-year OS (32.1% vs 23%; P = .004), and PFS (18.3% vs 13%; P = .055). TRT dose escalation was also associated with higher treatment-related grade 3 or higher dysphagia (3.2% vs 12.1%; P = .0005) and esophagitis (5.0% vs 17.4%; P < .0001). These findings solidified 60 Gy at 2 Gy per fraction over a 6-week period as the SoC radiation regimen.[2] There was also no statistically significant benefit to the addition of cetuximab in patients with EGFR mutation–positive tumors, defined as an H-score greater than or equal to 200 by EGFR immunohistochemistry staining, but possibly a numerical benefit.

RTOG 0617 also elucidated the impact of TRT dose–related toxicity on survival outcomes. It was the first phase III trial to use intensity-modulated RT (IMRT), a high-precision technique in which the intensity of radiation beams varies to conform to the contours of the tumor, thereby minimizing injury to adjacent critical structures.[22–24] Secondary analyses showed that IMRT was associated with both lower cardiac irradiation and lower mortality, compared with 3-dimensional radiation planning. Radiation-induced heart disease and mortality had been thought to take decades to develop, but this trial showed that radiation dose to the heart was an independent predictor of OS, suggesting that TRT-related cardiotoxicity was not only a late but also dose-dependent toxicity.[6,24]

Similarly, esophageal toxicity was also shown to be a consequence of TRT dose escalation. Despite the use of IMRT to minimize off-target toxicity, severe esophagitis can be a challenging toxicity in some cases.[23] IMRT contralateral esophagus-sparing technique (CEST) involves contouring the esophagus as an avoidance structure. The effectiveness of this strategy, however, remains unclear. One phase I clinical trial found that CEST reduced esophageal toxicity without compromising target coverage, with no patients experiencing grade 3 or higher esophagitis despite radiation dose of 70 Gy at a tumor within 1 cm of the esophagus.[25,26] On the other hand, another phase III trial in the setting of palliative radiotherapy showed this strategy reduced incidence of symptomatic esophagitis, most evidently in patients receiving a higher RT dose but did not significantly improve esophageal quality of life.[27] The results of these 2 studies suggest that the extent of benefit seen with CEST may depend on the RT dose. Ongoing and future studies will clarify the safety discoveries of RTOG 0617 and add to the growing knowledge of radiation dose–related toxicity on prognosis.

Thoracic RT can also potentiate myelosuppression and induce radiation pneumonitis (RP). A secondary analysis of the RTOG 0617 trial showed that higher radiation dose to immune cells was also an independent risk factor for shorter OS and local PFS, suggesting that preservation of lymphocytes is critical for tumor control.[28] Lymphocytes are radiosensitive cells, with DNA fragmentation occurring at doses as low as 0.5 Gy.[29] Specifically with TRT, irradiation of blood-carrying structures, such as the heart, lung, and large blood vessels, can injure circulating lymphocytes, causing lymphopenia, which, if severe, is associated with poor OS.[30] **Figs. 1–6** depict the

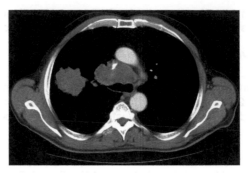

Fig. 1. Baseline CT chest with contrast.

baseline scans, radiotherapy plans, and follow-up imaging of a patient with stage IIIB NSCLC with enlarged mediastinal lymph nodes who experienced grade 2 pneumonitis following chemoradiation (carboplatin, paclitaxel, 60 Gy). The patient was treated with prednisone. Moreover, the recent use of consolidative immunotherapy in SoC can be associated with an additive incidence of immune-related adverse events (irAE) and pneumonitis.[31] Although some prospective studies showed that both cCRT alone and with consolidative ICI therapy worsened pulmonary toxicity, other studies found that the incidence of grade 2 or higher RP did not differ significantly between consolidation durvalumab and cCRT alone.[32–35] In addition, prospective studies suggest that the toxicities of combining checkpoint inhibitors with cCRT are within expected, historical rates of pneumonitis.[36,37] Further investigation is needed to better understand how to mitigate the immune-related effects of current first-line therapies.

Advancements in radiation technology have greatly contributed to the reduction of treatment-related toxicity. Stereotactic body radiotherapy (SBRT), or stereotactic ablative radiotherapy (SABR), is a high-precision technique that reduces toxicity to the mediastinum by delivering a high dose per fraction within a shorter treatment duration, as opposed to general TRT dose escalation.[38–42] In patients with nonoperative, early stage lung cancer, SBRT/SABR achieves high rates of local control with apparent similarity in long-term survival rates compared with surgery. Preliminary success has jumpstarted ongoing phase II and III clinical trials on SBRT/SABR boost or monotherapy in locally advanced lung cancer to evaluate its efficacy and safety with CRT or ICI.[43,44] Local relapse continues to be a challenge in locally advanced lung cancer, with relapse rates ranging between 20% and 50%, despite use of SoC

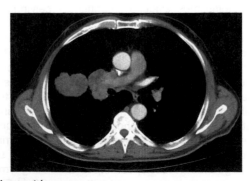

Fig. 2. Baseline CT chest with contrast.

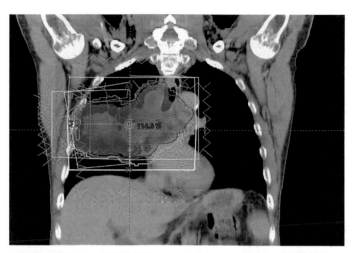

Fig. 3. Coronal CT simulation with 100% coverage.

consolidation durvalumab.[42,43] SBRT/SABR as boost or monotherapy has demonstrated lower toxicity without compromising oncologic endpoints for late-stage NSCLC as well.[44,45] Proton beam therapy (PBT) has also been shown to reduce irradiation dose to the heart and lungs, possibly sparing more heart volume compared with IMRT.[46,47] NRG/RTOG 1308 is an ongoing trial investigating the survival and toxicity advantages of using PBT over conventional RT for inoperable stage II to IIIB NSCLC (ClinicalTrials.gov NCT01993810). For locally advanced inoperable NSCLC, chemoradiation followed by durvalumab remains the SoC with ongoing efforts to optimize the toxicity and efficacy of this therapy.

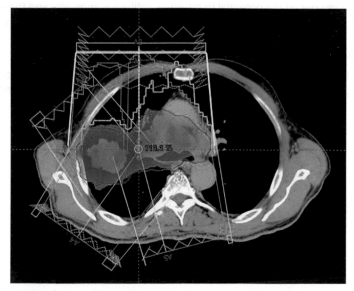

Fig. 4. Axial CT simulation with 100% coverage.

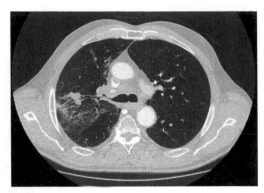

Fig. 5. 3-month follow-up with early changes on CT scan.

ROLE OF IMMUNOTHERAPY
Rationale for Immunotherapy

Despite definitive cCRT, historically, survival outcomes were limited, as median PFS remained limited at 8 months, and only 20% to 30% of patients were alive at 5 years.[5,6] High rates of relapse led to studies evaluating consolidation chemotherapy, but they failed to demonstrate definitive benefit.[48,49] The still suboptimal survival rates highlighted the need for new pharmacological options.

ICIs became the subject of LA-NSCLC research interest after their success in patients with advanced lung cancer.[36] Cancer cells evade the immune system by mimicking ligands of immune checkpoints and preventing cytotoxic CD8+ T-cell–mediated killing.[50] Preclinical evidence suggests that chemoradiation triggers tumor cell death and subsequent release of immunogenic antigens, which upregulates the immune response, namely PD-L1 expression in tumor cells.[50–53] ICIs further restore the immune antitumor response against remaining cancer cells by blocking the checkpoint ligands.[54] The synergistic utility of this combination therapy had been demonstrated in mouse models of lung cancer.[55,56] Together, chemoradiation and immunotherapy posed the potential to improve antitumor immunity and therefore survival outcomes, albeit at risk of irAEs, in patients with locally advanced lung cancer.

PACIFIC Trial

The phase III PACIFIC trial evaluated consolidation with durvalumab, a PD-L1 checkpoint inhibitor, against placebo in patients with unresectable stage III NSCLC and Eastern

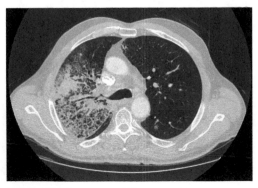

Fig. 6. 5-month follow-up with changes on CT scan.

Cooperative Oncology Group (ECOG)/World Health Organization PS score 0 or 1, whose disease had not worsened after at least two cycles of platinum-doublet–based cCRT.[8] A total of seven hundred thirteen patients were randomized in a 2:1 ratio to receive durvalumab (10 mg/kg, once every 2 weeks for up to 12 months) (n = 476) or placebo (n = 237) within 6 weeks of cCRT completion; 26.8% of patients also received induction chemotherapy, and 92.4% of patients received RT dose between 54 and 66 Gy. The initial results revolutionized the SoC for this patient population. Compared with placebo (cCRT alone), consolidation durvalumab prolonged median PFS (16.8 months vs 5.6 months; stratified HR, 0.52, 95% CI, 0.42–0.65; $P < .001$) and OS (not reached vs 28.7 months, stratified HR, 0.68, 99.73% CI, 0.48–0.997; $P = .0025$).[8,57] The 5-year PFS and OS updates demonstrated sustained benefit, with median PFS of 16.9 months on durvalumab versus 5.6 months on placebo (stratified HR, 0.55, 95% CI, 0.45–0.68) and median OS of 47.5 months versus 29.1 months, respectively (stratified HR, 0.72, 95% CI, 0.59–0.89).[7] The estimated 5-year PFS and OS rates of 33.1% and 42.9%, respectively, with durvalumab were massive improvements from the historical rates that had been seen with cCRT alone (19.0% and 33.4%, respectively).

Consolidation with durvalumab was well tolerated, with a treatment-related discontinuation rate of 15.4% compared with 9.8% with placebo.[8] The most frequent adverse events owing to discontinuation of therapy were pneumonitis, radiation pneumonitis, or pneumonia. Toxicity was mostly low grade, and the incidence of grade 3 or 4 pneumonitis or radiation pneumonitis (3.4% vs 2.6%) and pneumonia (4.4% vs 3.8%) was similar between treatment arms and lower than the rates observed with consolidation chemotherapy. Of note, the trial excluded patients who experience early pneumonitis after cCRT, limiting the generalizability of the safety results. Overall, the results of the PACIFIC trial showed the clinical benefit of consolidation durvalumab after cCRT.

The PACIFIC trial was impactful in establishing consolidation immunotherapy after platinum-based cCRT as SoC for unresectable stage III NSCLC with ECOG PS of 0 to 1 and no disease progression after chemoradiation.[2] Although the United States Food and Drug Administration (FDA) approved an expanded indication for durvalumab in NSCLC irrespective of PD-L1 tumor expression, the European Medicines Agency (EMA) reserved its use to patients with PD-L1 greater than or equal to 1% because an unplanned post-hoc analysis failed to show survival advantage in the subgroup with PD-L1 less than 1%.[54] The FDA stood by its decision, as the analysis was unplanned and PD-L1 status was not an inclusion criterion in the trial. In addition to tumor PD-L1 status, the role of biomarkers to guide treatment planning is another area for further investigation. The PACIFIC trial showed that early initiation of ICI therapy within 14 days of the end of cCRT improved survival outcomes, which could be a suggestion of synergy with cCRT or possibly patients with less toxicity from cCRT having the ability to initiate durvalumab sooner.[8] The trial saw a favorable survival advantage with durvalumab across all prespecified subgroups except in patients with EGFR mutations (HR, 0.76, 95% CI, 0.35–1.64) (compared with wild-type EGFR status, HR, 0.47, 95% CI, 0.35–0.60).[8] With still suboptimal 5-year OS and PFS rates in some patients, but particularly for those with ECOG PS 2 status, PD-L1 negative, and/or EGFR mutation–positive tumors, recent years have ushered in an era of immunotherapy and targeted therapy research to optimize current SoC.

Concurrent Immunotherapy with Chemoradiotherapy

Other trials evaluated the optimal timing—concurrent versus consolidation—of various PD-L1 inhibitors in relation to the recommended cCRT regimen. The phase II DETERRED and phase I/II NICOLAS trials assessed atezolizumab and nivolumab, respectively, with cCRT (**Table 1**).[58,59] In addition, a phase I trial by Jabbour and

Table 1
Comparison of efficacy and safety data of RTOG 0617 trial, PACIFIC trial, and completed trials on consolidation versus concurrent immunotherapy

Trial Name	Phase	N =	Notable Eligibility Criteria	Chemotherapy Regimen	Arm 1	Arm 2	Arm 3	Median Follow-up	Survival Data	Safety Data
RTOG 0617	III	544	ECOG/WHO PS 0 or 1	Carboplatin/paclitaxel	cCRT with 60 Gy ± cetuximab	cCRT with 74 Gy ± cetuximab	N/A	5.1 y	Median OS, 28.7 vs 20.3 mo; 5-y OS, 23% vs 32.1%; 5-y PFS, 18.3% vs 13%	Grade ≥3 pneumonitis, 7% vs 4%
PACIFIC	III	709	ECOG/WHO PS 0 or 1	Platinum-based doublet (with etoposide, vinblastine, vinorelbine, paclitaxel or docetaxel, or pemetrexed)	cCRT + durvalumab (10 mg/kg, every 2 wk for 12 mo)	cCRT + placebo	N/A	14.5 mo; 5-y update: 34.2 mo (all patients); 61.6 mo (censored patients)	Median PFS, 16.8 vs 5.6 mo; 12-mo PFS, 55.7% vs 34.4%; Median PFS, 16.9 vs 5.6 mo; Median OS, 47.5 vs 29.1 mo; Estimated 5-y PFS, 33.1% vs 19.0%; Estimated 5-y OS, 42.9% vs 33.4%	Grade ≥3 pneumonitis, 4.4% vs 3.8%
DETERRED	II	40	ECOG/WHO PS 0-2	Carboplatin/paclitaxel	Part 1: cCRT, followed by consolidation chemotherapy + atezolizumab (every 3 wk for 2 cycles), followed by maintenance atezolizumab (for 1 y)	Part 2: cCRT + atezolizumab, followed same consolidation and maintenance regimens as in part 1	N/A	Part 1: 22.5 mo; Part 2: 15.1 mo	Part 1: median PFS, 18.6 mo; median OS, 22.8 mo; Part 2: median PFS, 13.2 mo; median OS, not reached	Part 1: grade ≥3 pneumonitis, 0%; Part 2: grade ≥3 pneumonitis, 3%
NICOLAS	II	79	ECOG/WHO PS 0 or 1	Cisplatin or carboplatin combined with either vinorelbine, etoposide, or pemetrexed	cCRT + nivolumab (360 mg, 3-wk cycle), followed by nivolumab	N/A	N/A	21.0 mo; 32.6 mo (extended)	12-mo PFS, 53.7%; median PFS, 12.7 mo; Median OS, 38.8 mo; 2-y OS, 63.7%; ORR, 73.4%	Grade ≥3 pneumonitis, 11.7%

Study	Phase	N	ECOG/WHO PS	Chemotherapy	Treatment arms			Follow-up	Results	Safety
Jabbour, et al.	I	21	ECOG/WHO PS 0 or 1	Carboplatin and paclitaxel	Cohort 1: Full-dose pembrolizumab (200 mg every 3 wk) 2–6 wk after CRT	Cohort 2: reduced dose pembrolizumab (100 mg every week) starting day 29 of CRT Cohort 3: full-dose pembrolizumab starting day 29 of CRT	Cohort 4: reduced dose pembrolizumab starting day 1 of CRT Cohort 5: full dose of pembrolizumab starting day 1 of CRT	16.0 mo	Received ≥1 dose of pembrolizumab: median PFS, 18.7 mo; 12-mo PFS, 69.7% Received ≥1 dose of pembrolizumab: median PFS, 21.0 mo	All cohorts: grade ≥3 pneumonitis, 9.5%; grade ≥3 irAEs, 18%
KEYNOTE-799	II	216	ECOG/WHO PS 0 or 1	Cohort A: Carboplatin/ paclitaxel Cohort B: Cisplatin/ pemetrexed	Cohort A: 1 cycle of chemotherapy + pembrolizumab (200 mg) on day 1 of a 3-wk cycle, followed by chemotherapy (weekly for 6 wk) + 2 cycles of pembrolizumab (every 3 wk) + TRT	Cohort B: cCRT + pembrolizumab, followed by pembrolizumab	N/A	Cohort A: 1.1 y Cohort B: 1.5 y	Cohort A: ORR, 70.5%; ORR in PD-L1 <1%, 66.7%; ORR in PD-L1 ≥1%, 77.3%; estimated 12-mo PFS, 67.1%; estimated 12-mo OS, 81.3% Cohort B: ORR, 70.6%; ORR in PD-L1 <1%, 78.6%; ORR in PD-L1 ≥1%, 72.5%; estimated 12-mo PFS, 71.6%; estimated 12-mo OS, 87.0%	Cohort A: grade ≥3 pneumonitis, 8.0%; grade ≥3 irAEs, 14.3% Cohort B: grade ≥3 pneumonitis, 6.9%; grade ≥3 irAEs, 8.8%

colleagues and the phase II KEYNOTE-799 trial evaluated concurrent pembrolizumab plus CRT, as consolidation pembrolizumab had demonstrated delay in time to metastatic disease or death in the phase II LUN 14 to 179 trial (see **Table 1**).[36,37,60] All 3 ICIs amplified antitumor activity when combined with cCRT. Although an increased rate of pneumonitis was observed with concurrent PD-L1 inhibition during cCRT, most cases resolved with high-dose corticosteroid treatment.[36] In sum, the safety and survival outcomes of these trials were comparable with those of the PACIFIC trial and thus support further investigation of concurrent immunotherapy and cCRT.

In addition, these studies expanded the generalizability of the results to more patient populations. For example, the inclusion criteria of the NICOLAS trial represented a greater proportion of patients with stage IIIB disease.[59] The nonrandomized phase II KEYNOTE-799 trial also provided more information about the use of ICI for PD-L1 status less than 1%, although PD-L1 expression was not available in all patients (n=155 patients), 32% of whom had PD-L1 less than 1%.[37] The trial studied concurrent pembrolizumab in 2 cohorts, patients with squamous or nonsquamous histology (n = 112) and those with nonsquamous histology only (n = 102). Cohort A received one cycle of systemic carboplatin/paclitaxel and pembrolizumab 3 weeks before radiotherapy initiation, followed by radiotherapy with chemotherapy once weekly for 6 weeks integrated with 2 cycles of pembrolizumab. Cohort B received 3 cycles of cisplatin/pemetrexed, pembrolizumab every 3 weeks, and TRT during the second and third cycles. The objective response rate (ORR) was 70.5% (95% CI, 61.2% to 78.8%) and 70.6% (95% CI, 60.7% to 79.2%) in cohorts A and B, respectively,[37] which is comparable with ORR of 73.4% with concurrent nivolumab[59] and higher than the historical ORR of 36% to 55% with cCRT alone.[19,61,62] The 2-year update showed ORR ranging between 71.4% and 75.5% and 2-year OS of approximately 70% and 80%, as well as median PFS of 30.6 months and not reached yet, in cohorts A and B, respectively.[63] Importantly, response was observed irrespective of disease stage, tumor histologic type, and PD-L1 expression, whereas the PACIFIC trial did not see major benefit in PD-L1 less than 1% status.[7,37]

The PACIFIC-2 trial is investigating the potential PFS benefit of concurrent durvalumab during cCRT compared with placebo (ClinicalTrials.gov NCT03519971), whereas phase III ECOG-ACRIN EA5181 trial is comparing it with consolidation durvalumab alone (ClinicalTrials.gov NCT04092283) (**Table 2**). Similarly, the KEYLYNK-012 and CheckMate 73L are also asking similar questions.[64,65] These ongoing trials and others will hopefully strengthen the current evidence for concurrent cCRT and ICI therapy.

Other Novel Therapies in the Consolidation after Chemoradiation

The success of a single immunotherapeutic agent generated interest in the potential survival advantage of dual immunotherapy. The phase II COAST trial built on the PACIFIC trial and randomized patients (n = 189) to durvalumab alone or in combination with oleclumab, an anti-CD73 agent, or monalizumab, an anti-NKG2A agent, as consolidation therapy post-cCRT.[66] At median follow-up of 11.5 months, combination with oleclumab or monalizumab showed higher ORR (30.0% and 35.5%, respectively, vs 17.9%) and prolonged 12-month PFS (62.6% and 72.7%, respectively, vs 33.9%), compared with consolidation durvalumab alone, with similar safety profiles across arms (grade ≥3 treatment adverse events; 40.7% and 27.9%, respectively, vs 39.4%). Of note, the durvalumab arm grossly underperformed in the COAST trial compared with the PACIFIC trial, possibly owing to a higher proportion of older patients or those with stage IIIB/C disease. Furthermore, 46 out of 66 participants (60.7%) in the durvalumab arm discontinued treatment, 26 (56.5%) of whom discontinued due to confirmed disease progression. Similarly, approximately 50% of

Table 2
Ongoing trials on consolidation versus concurrent immunotherapy

Trial Name	Phase	N =	Notable Eligibility Criteria	Chemotherapy Regimen	Arm 1	Arm 2	Median Follow-Up	Survival Data	Safety Data
PACIFIC-2	III	328	ECOG/WHO PS 0 or 1	Platinum-based doublet (with cisplatin/etoposide, carboplatin/cisplatin, pemetrexed/carboplatin, or pemetrexed/carboplatin)	cCRT + durvalumab (beginning day 1 until progression)	cCRT + placebo	Ongoing study	Ongoing study	Ongoing study
EA5181	III	660	ECOG/WHO PS 0 or 1	Cisplatin/etoposide, cisplatin/ pemetrexed, carboplatin/ paclitaxel	cCRT + durvalumab (70 mg, every 2 wk), followed by durvalumab (1500 kg, every 4 wk for 1 y)	cCRT, followed by durvalumab	Ongoing study	Ongoing study	Ongoing study

participants in the durvalumab plus oleclumab and durvalumab plus monalizumab arms discontinued treatment, approximately 50% due to confirmed disease progression. Rates of pneumonitis (18.6% and 16.4%, respectively, vs 16.7%) and discontinuation rates (15.3% and 14.8%, respectively, vs 16.7%) were also similar across arms, suggesting that dual combination immunotherapy is safe and effective. Clinical benefit was apparent among patients with unknown PD-L1 status and PD-L1 greater than or equal to 1% but was unclear for PD-L1 less than 1% due to limited number of patients in this subgroup. The phase III PACIFIC-9 trial is building on the design and results of the COAST trial and investigating outcomes in different tumor PD-L1 expression levels (ClinicalTrials.gov NCT05221840). Further evaluation is required to include consolidation intensification with dual ICI into treatment guidelines.

Dual Checkpoint Inhibition in Locally Advanced NSCLC

The phase II BTCRC-LUN 16 to 081 trial also explored dual ICI along with a shorter duration of therapy, specifically nivolumab, an anti-PD1, and ipilimumab, anti-CTLA4, as consolidation treatment post-cCRT for 6 months (**Table 3**).[67] Patients (n = 105) were randomized to receive nivolumab alone or nivolumab with ipilimumab, both after cCRT. Despite a shorter treatment duration, both treatment arms demonstrated 18-month PFS (63.7% and 67.6%, respectively), comparable with historical efficacy data (30% and 44% with CRT alone and consolidation durvalumab, respectively). Median PFS was 25.8 and 25.4 months, respectively, and estimated 18- and 24-month OS were 82.1% and 76.6% and 85.5% and 82.8%, respectively. The safety data, however, showed higher incidence of grade 3 or higher treatment-related adverse events (trAEs) (52.9% vs 38.9%) including pneumonitis (17.6% vs 9.3%) with the combination regimen compared with nivolumab alone. Liveringhouse et al. found higher incidence of pulmonary toxicity was seen in a phase I/II trial studying conurrent ipilimumab with cCRT followed by maintenance nivolumab.[68] In fact, the trial was discontinued early due to unacceptable toxicity, with 16 out of 19 (84%) patients experiencing grade ≥3 treatment-related toxicity, mostly pulmonary, and 14 (74%) patients discontinuing treatment because of the adverse events. . Numerous ongoing trials are investigating various consolidation immunotherapeutic combinations (**Table 3**). As therapies continued to be developed for patients with locally advanced NSCLC, there is a continuinung need for further research into minimizing toxicity risk.

Limitations of Current Standard of Care

Despite advancements in radiation technology and pharmacotherapy, real-world evidence suggests that about up to half of patients with locally advanced lung cancer are ineligible for SoC therapy, owing to toxicity from both cCRT and ICI.[69] Durvalumab toxicity leading to early discontinuation has been associated with inferior PFS and OS outcomes, whereas later discontinuation may provide similar tumor control as 1 year of durvalumab.[70,71] Further research is needed to identify toxicity mitigation strategies and optimal ICI treatment duration to improve treatment experience and survival outcomes in this population.

In patients unable to tolerate cCRT, sCRT can serve as an alternative for this subgroup. Many studies have been conducted and are currently underway to understand the safety and efficacy of sCRT with ICI. The phase II PACIFIC-6 trial assessed safety of consolidation durvalumab in patients (n = 117) with no progression after sCRT and found that this regimen was generally well tolerated, with grade 3 or 4 possible related adverse event incidence of 4.3% (95% CI, 1.4%–9.7%).[72] The study also found median PFS of 10.9 months, 12-month PFS of 49.6%, median OS of 25.0 months, and

Table 3
Completed and ongoing trials on consolidative combination immunotherapy

Trial Name	Phase	N =	Notable Eligibility Criteria	Chemotherapy Regimen	Arm 1	Arm 2	Arm 3	Median Follow-Usp	Survival Data	Safety Data
COAST	II	189	ECOG/WHO PS 0 or 1	Platinum-based cCRT	Durvalumab (1500 mg, every 4 wk for 12 mo)	Durvalumab + oleclumab (3000 mg, every 2 wk on days 1 and 15 for cycles 1 and 2, then every 4 wk on days 1 of cycle 3)	Durvalumab + monalizumab (750 mg, every 2 wk on days 1 and 15 of each cycle)	11.5 mo	ORR, 17.9% vs 30.0% vs 35.5% 12-mo PFS, 33.9% vs 62.6% vs 72.7%	Grade 3/4 pneumonitis, 0% vs 0% vs 1.5%
BTCRC-LUN 16-081	II	105	ECOG/WHO PS 0 or 1	Platinum-based cCRT	Nivolumab (480 mg, every 4 wk for 6 cycles)	Nivolumab (240 mg, every 2 wk) + ipilimumab (1 mg/kg, every 6 wk for 4 cycles)	N/A	Arm 1: 24.5 mo Arm 2: 24.1 mo	18-mo PFS, 62.3% vs 67%; median PFS, 25.8 vs 25.4 mo Median OS, not reached on either arm; 18-mo OS, 82.1% vs 85.5%; 24-mo OS, 76.6% vs 82.8%	Grade ≥3 pneumonitis, 9.3% vs 15.7%
PACIFIC-8	III	860	ECOG/WHO PS 0 or 1; documented PD-L1, EGFR, and ALK status	Platinum-based cCRT	Durvalumab + domvanalimab (every 4 wk for 12 mo)	Durvalumab + placebo	N/A	Ongoing study	Ongoing study	Ongoing study
PACIFIC-9	III	999	ECOG/WHO PS 0 or 1; documented PD-L1, EGFR, and ALK status	Platinum-based cCRT	Durvalumab (every 4 wk) + oleclumab (every 2 wk of cycles 1 and 2, then every 4 wk for 12 mo)	Durvalumab + monalizumab (every 4 wk for 12 mo)	Durvalumab + placebo	Ongoing study	Ongoing study	Ongoing study
SKYSCRAPER-03	III	800	ECOG/WHO PS 0 or 1; known PD-L1 result	Platinum-based cCRT	Tiragolumab (840 mg) + atezolizumab (1680 mg, every 4 wk)	Durvalumab (10 mg/kg, every 2 wk)	N/A	Ongoing study	Ongoing study	Ongoing study

(continued on next page)

Table 3
(continued)

Trial Name	Phase	N =	Notable Eligibility Criteria	Chemotherapy Regimen	Arm 1	Arm 2	Arm 3	Median Follow-Usp	Survival Data	Safety Data
KEYLYNK-012	III	870	ECOG/WHO PS 0 or 1	Platinum-based cCRT	cCRT + pembrolizumab (200 mg, every 3 wk), followed by pembrolizumab + placebo	cCRT + pembrolizumab followed by pembrolizumab + olaparib (300 mg, twice daily for 1 y)	cCRT, followed by durvalumab (10 mg/kg every 2 wk)	Ongoing study	Ongoing study	Ongoing study
CheckMate 73L	III	888	ECOG/WHO PS 0 or 1	Platinum-based cCRT	cCRT + nivolumab (360 mg, every 3 wk), followed by nivolumab + ipilimumab (1 mg/kg, every 6 wk for 1 y)	cCRT + nivolumab, followed by nivolumab	cCRT, followed by durvalumab (10 mg/kg, every 2 wk)	Ongoing study	Ongoing study	Ongoing study

12-month OS of 84.1%, which are comparable with the 12-month PFS and OS of 55.7% and 83.1%, respectively, from the PACIFIC trial. Of note, there were patients, albeit only 3 (2.6%), with ECOG PS 2 included in the study, a patient population that was excluded in the PACIFIC trial, even though up to 14% of patients fall in this subgroup.[73] The phase II SPRINT trial also assesses a chemotherapy-free regimen for patients with locally advanced NSCLC and PD-L1 tumor proportion score greater than or equal to 50%.[74] Initial results showed actuarial 1-year PFS of 74% and OS of 95%, with limited grade 3 AEs, in patients (n = 25) who received fluorodeoxyglucose (FDG)-PET/computed tomography (CT), induction pembrolizumab, restaging FDG-PET/CT, dose-painted TRT, and consolidation pembrolizumab. Image-guided TRT plus ICI without chemotherapy may serve as a promising and safe treatment modification for this patient subgroup. In addition, the SWOG S1933 (ClinicalTrials.gov NCT04310020) and DUART (ClinicalTrials.gov NCT04249362) phase II trials are ongoing studies investigating hypofractionated TRT followed by atezolizumab in patients with ECOG PS 2 and different doses of TRT alone plus durvalumab in patients ineligible for chemotherapy, respectively. The phase I ARCHON-1 trial (ClinicalTrials.gov NCT03801902) is investigating accelerated hypofractionated radiation therapy (ARCT) versus conventionally fractionated radiation therapy, combined with durvalumab. For patients who cannot tolerate cCRT, the PACIFIC-5 trial is assessing the efficacy and safety of consolidation durvalumab after cCRT versus sCRT (ClinicalTrials.gov NCT03706690). These studies will hopefully clarify the role of ICI for patients relying on sCRT.

PERSONALIZED, GENOTYPE-DIRECTED THERAPY

The treatment strategies discussed thus far demonstrate less clear benefit in patients with tumors expressing certain oncogenic driver gene mutations, which account for up to 60% of lung adenocarcinomas. Thus, prompt identification of mutations and personalized treatment approaches, as is routinely incorporated for patients with advanced stage disease, are critical for improving prognosis in these patient populations. Targeted therapy has provided durable responses in advanced disease, and combinations of therapy with cCRT need to be further investigated for curative intent in locally advanced disease.[75]

Epidermal Growth Factor Receptor Mutation–Positive Tumors

High EGFR-sensitizing mutation (L858 R, Exon 19 deletion) frequency is observed in approximately 20% of Caucasian and 50% of Asian patients with NSCLC adenocarcinoma, with higher incidence among nonsmokers.[76] Patients with EGFR mutations experience inferior survival rates compared with those with EGFR-negative tumors when treated with cCRT alone.[77] The RTOG 0617 trial was a 2 × 2 factorial design that investigated the role of cetuximab, an anti-EGFR antibody. The initial data showed that patients with high EGFR H-score greater than or equal to 200 who received cetuximab exhibited increased median OS (42.0 months, 95% CI 20.6–not reached) compared with those who did not (21.2 months, 95% CI 17.2–29.2) (HR 1.72, 95% CI 1.04–2.84; P = .032). The 5-year update, however, revealed that cetuximab benefit was no longer clinically significant, although the outcomes were still numerically better for patients with high H-scores, with a median OS of 2.9 years with cetuximab versus 1.8 years without (P = .14).[6]

The introduction of newer generation, central nervous system (CNS)-active EGFR tyrosine kinase inhibitors (TKI), namely osimertinib, has since improved survival outcomes in patients with advanced stage disease, leading to investigations of this agent in curative-intent settings.[78,79] The phase III ADAURA trial randomized patients with resected EGFR-positive lung cancer to receive adjuvant osimertinib (n = 339) or placebo (n = 343) and found that 98% of patients receiving osimertinib were alive without CNS disease at 24 months, as opposed to 85% in the placebo group (HR, 0.18; 95% CI, 0.10–0.33).[80] Moreover, 89% of patients receiving osimertinib were disease-free at 24 months, compared with 52% in the placebo group (HR, 0.20; 95% CI, 0.14–0.30; P < .001). Of note, the disease-free survival rate with placebo was lower than that historically seen in the LACE meta-analysis, possibly owing to the lack of PET staging.[81] This study limitation may have resulted in the understaging of patients, thereby yielding an advantage to osimertinib over placebo.

Furthermore, EGFR TKIs have been coadministered with RT, with or without chemotherapy, given their potential radiosensitizing effect, but at an increased risk of overlapping toxicity of pneumonitis.[48,82] A retrospective analysis of patients who had received concurrent EGFR-TKI plus once-daily conventionally fractionated TRT (n = 85) versus cCRT (n = 129) showed that the former group was significantly more likely to develop pneumonitis, with ipsilateral lung volume receiving greater than or equal to 30 (ilV30), total lung volume receiving greater than or equal to 20, and chronic obstructive pulmonary disease comorbidity being risk predictors.[82] Another retrospective study reported 1-year PFS of 84.4% and median PFS of 30.3 months in patients with advanced, EGFR-mutated lung adenocarcinoma who were treated with EGFR-TKI and RT.[83] In addition, a single-arm, phase II trial evaluated concurrent EGFR-TKI and RT in patients (n = 10) with EGFR-positive, stage IV NSCLC and found 1-year PFS of 57.1% and median PFS of 13 months, with grade 3 or higher radiation pneumonitis of 20%, which resolved with corticosteroid therapy.[84] Although these studies demonstrated that EGFR-TKI combined with RT was efficacious and tolerable, the results have a wide variability, possibly owing to the studies' lack of randomization and small sample sizes. Further studies are required to confirm these findings. The recent phase III SINDAS trial randomized patients with EGFR-mutated oligometastatic NSCLC to receive a first-generation EGFR-TKI only (n = 65) or upfront radiotherapy (25–40 Gy in 5 fractions) before TKI (n = 68).[85] The trial was interrupted prematurely after demonstrating remarkable efficacy results, with median PFS of 12.5 versus 20.2 months (HR, 0.22; 95% CI, 0.17–0.46; P < .001) and median OS of 17.6 versus 25.5 months (HR, 0.44; 95% CI 0.28–0.68; P < .001) with TKI only versus TKI with RT, respectively. Incidence of symptomatic grade 3 or 4 pneumonitis was 6% in the TKI with RT arm, compared with 1.5% with TKI only. Of note, brain metastasis was an exclusion criterion, despite its prevalence in EGFR-mutated NSCLC. The phase III LAURA trial is investigating the potential PFS benefit of consolidation osimertinib in patients with EGFR-positive tumors and whose disease has not progressed following platinum-based chemoradiation (ClinicalTrials.gov NCT03521154). A phase II study is also underway to assess the safety and efficacy of concurrent RT and almonertinib, a newer third-generation EGFR-TKI, in EGFR-mutated LA-NSCLC (ClinicalTrials.gov NCT04636593).

Although EGFR-targeted therapy has become first-line therapy for patients with advanced stage EGFR-mutated lung cancer leading to trials of these agents with definitive thoracic radiotherapy, the role of ICI in this setting remains unclear. A post-hoc exploratory analysis of the PACIFIC trial found that PFS (11.2 vs 10.9 months; HR, 0.91; 95% CI, 0.39–2.13) and OS (46.8 vs 43 months; HR, 1.02; 95% CI, 0.39–2.63) did not improve with consolidation durvalumab compared with placebo in this subgroup of patients with EGFR-mutated NSCLC.[86] Likewise, multiple retrospective studies concluded against the use of durvalumab in this population, given the heightened incidence of pneumonitis without any survival advantage.[87–89] Furthermore, risk of severe irAEs and interstitial lung disease is exacerbated when combining osimertinib and durvalumab, both sequentially and concomitantly.[90] In fact, the European Society for Medical Oncology (ESMO) does not recommend consolidation ICI therapy after curative-intent chemoradiation in EGFR-positive disease.[91] Prospective studies, such as the LAURA trial, will hopefully clarify the use and timing of EGFR-targeted therapy in this subgroup population.

SUMMARY

Although effective and safe, the current SoC of consolidation durvalumab after cCRT seems to have the greatest benefit to patients with PD-L1–positive tumors, without oncogenic driver mutations, and good PS. Even among patients with good PS who can tolerate durvalumab consolidation therapy, locoregional and distant relapse is a common obstacle. These challenges have generated multiple ongoing clinical trials to build on the current treatment paradigm and improve prognoses for more patients with inoperable, locally advanced lung cancer.

CLINICS CARE POINTS

- Consolidative immunotherapy after concurrent chemoradiotherapy is the SoC in unresectable, locally advanced lung cancer, based on the results of the phase III PACIFIC trial.
- Further advancements are still needed, however, to reduce the risk of distant relapse, as disease progression remains a challenge even with the current SoC.
- Concurrent immunotherapy with chemoradiation may safely and effectively prolong survival, based on the phase I Jabbour and colleagues phase II DETERRED, phase I/II NICOLAS, and phase II KEYNOTE-799 trials.
- The results of the phase II COAST trial suggest that consolidation with dual immunotherapy provides better survival outcomes compared with a single immunotherapeutic agent and require further study.
- Treatment personalization remains an unmet need for patients with PD-L1–negative tumors, oncogenic driver mutations, toxicity leading to discontinuation, or limited PS, and studies involving new targeted therapies and radiation techniques are underway to improve prognosis in these patient populations.

DISCLOSURE

The authors have no financial disclosures to declare and no conflicts of interest to report.

REFERENCES

1. Siegel RL, Miller KD, Fuchs HE, et al. Cancer statistics, 2022. CA Cancer J Clin 2022;72(1):7–33.
2. Ettinger DS, Wood DE, Aisner DL, et al. NCCN Guidelines Insights: Non-Small Cell Lung Cancer, Version 2.2021. J Natl Compr Canc Netw 2021;19(3):254–66.
3. National Cancer Institute. Cancer stat facts: lung and bronchus. Available at: https://seer.cancer.gov/statfacts/html/lungb.html. Accessed 21 July 2022.

4. Suzuki S, Goto T. Role of Surgical Intervention in Unresectable Non-Small Cell Lung Cancer. J Clin Med 2020;9(12). https://doi.org/10.3390/jcm9123881.

5. Auperin A, Le Pechoux C, Rolland E, et al. Meta-analysis of concomitant versus sequential radiochemotherapy in locally advanced non-small-cell lung cancer. J Clin Oncol 2010;28(13):2181–90.

6. Bradley JD, Hu C, Komaki RR, et al. Long-Term Results of NRG Oncology RTOG 0617: Standard- Versus High-Dose Chemoradiotherapy With or Without Cetuximab for Unresectable Stage III Non-Small-Cell Lung Cancer. J Clin Oncol 2020;38(7):706–14.

7. Spigel DR, Faivre-Finn C, Gray JE, et al. Five-Year Survival Outcomes From the PACIFIC Trial: Durvalumab After Chemoradiotherapy in Stage III Non-Small-Cell Lung Cancer. J Clin Oncol 2022;40(12):1301–11.

8. Antonia SJ, Villegas A, Daniel D, et al. Durvalumab after Chemoradiotherapy in Stage III Non-Small-Cell Lung Cancer. N Engl J Med 2017;377(20):1919–29.

9. Lebow ES, Shepherd A, Eichholz JE, et al. Analysis of Tumor Mutational Burden, Progression-Free Survival, and Local-Regional Control in Patents with Locally Advanced Non-Small Cell Lung Cancer Treated With Chemoradiation and Durvalumab. JAMA Netw Open 2023;6(1):e2249591.

10. Shaverdian N, Offin MD, Rimner A, et al. Utilization and factors precluding the initiation of consolidative durvalumab in unresectable stage III non-small cell lung cancer. Radiother Oncol 2020;144:101–4.

11. Roswit B, Patno ME, Rapp R, et al. The survival of patients with inoperable lung cancer: a large-scale randomized study of radiation therapy versus placebo. Radiology 1968;90(4):688–97.

12. Perez CA, Stanley K, Rubin P, et al. A prospective randomized study of various irradiation doses and fractionation schedules in the treatment of inoperable non-oat-cell carcinoma of the lung. Preliminary report by the Radiation Therapy Oncology Group. Cancer 1980;45(11):2744–53.

13. Chen Y, Peng X, Zhou Y, et al. Comparing the benefits of chemoradiotherapy and chemotherapy for resectable stage III A/N2 non-small cell lung cancer: a meta-analysis. World J Surg Oncol 2018;16(1):8.

14. Hung MS, Wu YF, Chen YC. Efficacy of chemoradiotherapy versus radiation alone in patients with inoperable locally advanced non-small-cell lung cancer: A meta-analysis and systematic review. Medicine (Baltim) 2019;98(27):e16167.

15. Dillman RO, Herndon J, Seagren SL, et al. Improved survival in stage III non-small-cell lung cancer: seven-year follow-up of cancer and leukemia group B (CALGB) 8433 trial. J Natl Cancer Inst 1996;88(17):1210–5.

16. Curran WJ Jr, Paulus R, Langer CJ, et al. Sequential vs. concurrent chemoradiation for stage III non-small cell lung cancer: randomized phase III trial RTOG 9410. J Natl Cancer Inst 2011;103(19):1452–60.

17. Albain KS, Crowley JJ, Turrisi AT 3rd, et al. Concurrent cisplatin, etoposide, and chest radiotherapy in pathologic stage IIIB non-small-cell lung cancer: a Southwest Oncology Group phase II study, SWOG 9019. J Clin Oncol 2002;20(16):3454–60.

18. Belani CP, Choy H, Bonomi P, et al. Combined chemoradiotherapy regimens of paclitaxel and carboplatin for locally advanced non-small-cell lung cancer: a randomized phase II locally advanced multi-modality protocol. J Clin Oncol 2005;23(25):5883–91.

19. Senan S, Brade A, Wang LH, et al. PROCLAIM: Randomized Phase III Trial of Pemetrexed-Cisplatin or Etoposide-Cisplatin Plus Thoracic Radiation Therapy

Followed by Consolidation Chemotherapy in Locally Advanced Nonsquamous Non-Small-Cell Lung Cancer. J Clin Oncol 2016;34(9):953–62.

20. Zheng Q, Min S, Zhou Y. A network meta-analysis for efficacies and toxicities of different concurrent chemoradiotherapy regimens in the treatment of locally advanced non-small cell lung cancer. BMC Cancer 2022;22(1):674.

21. Deek MP, Kim S, Beck R, et al. Variations in Initiation Dates of Chemotherapy and Radiation Therapy for Definitive Management of Inoperable Non-Small Cell Lung Cancer Are Associated With Decreases in Overall Survival. Clin Lung Cancer 2018;19(4):e381–90.

22. Movsas B, Hu C, Sloan J, et al. Quality of Life Analysis of a Radiation Dose-Escalation Study of Patients With Non-Small-Cell Lung Cancer: A Secondary Analysis of the Radiation Therapy Oncology Group 0617 Randomized Clinical Trial. JAMA Oncol 2016;2(3):359–67.

23. Chun SG, Hu C, Choy H, et al. Impact of Intensity-Modulated Radiation Therapy Technique for Locally Advanced Non-Small-Cell Lung Cancer: A Secondary Analysis of the NRG Oncology RTOG 0617 Randomized Clinical Trial. J Clin Oncol 2017;35(1):56–62.

24. Verma V, Simone CB 2nd, Werner-Wasik M. Acute and Late Toxicities of Concurrent Chemoradiotherapy for Locally-Advanced Non-Small Cell Lung Cancer. Cancers 2017;9(9). https://doi.org/10.3390/cancers9090120.

25. Al-Halabi H, Paetzold P, Sharp GC, et al. A Contralateral Esophagus-Sparing Technique to Limit Severe Esophagitis Associated With Concurrent High-Dose Radiation and Chemotherapy in Patients With Thoracic Malignancies. Int J Radiat Oncol Biol Phys 2015;92(4):803–10.

26. Kamran SC, Yeap BY, Ulysse CA, et al. Assessment of a Contralateral Esophagus-Sparing Technique in Locally Advanced Lung Cancer Treated With High-Dose Chemoradiation: A Phase 1 Nonrandomized Clinical Trial. JAMA Oncol 2021;7(6):910–4.

27. Louie AV, Granton PV, Fairchild A, et al. Palliative Radiation for Advanced Central Lung Tumors With Intentional Avoidance of the Esophagus (PROACTIVE): A Phase 3 Randomized Clinical Trial. JAMA Oncol 2022;8(4):1–7.

28. Jin JY, Hu C, Xiao Y, et al. Higher Radiation Dose to the Immune Cells Correlates with Worse Tumor Control and Overall Survival in Patients with Stage III NSCLC: A Secondary Analysis of RTOG0617. Cancers 2021;13(24). https://doi.org/10.3390/cancers13246193.

29. Heylmann D, Rodel F, Kindler T, et al. Radiation sensitivity of human and murine peripheral blood lymphocytes, stem and progenitor cells. Biochim Biophys Acta 2014;1846(1):121–9.

30. Abravan A, Faivre-Finn C, Kennedy J, et al. Radiotherapy-Related Lymphopenia Affects Overall Survival in Patients With Lung Cancer. J Thorac Oncol 2020;15(10):1624–35.

31. Arroyo-Hernandez M, Maldonado F, Lozano-Ruiz F, et al. Radiation-induced lung injury: current evidence. BMC Pulm Med 2021;21(1):9.

32. Shaverdian N, Lisberg AE, Bornazyan K, et al. Previous radiotherapy and the clinical activity and toxicity of pembrolizumab in the treatment of non-small-cell lung cancer: a secondary analysis of the KEYNOTE-001 phase 1 trial. Lancet Oncol 2017;18(7):895–903.

33. Theelen W, Peulen HMU, Lalezari F, et al. Effect of Pembrolizumab After Stereotactic Body Radiotherapy vs Pembrolizumab Alone on Tumor Response in Patients With Advanced Non-Small Cell Lung Cancer: Results of the PEMBRO-RT Phase 2 Randomized Clinical Trial. JAMA Oncol 2019;5(9):1276–82.

34. Shaverdian N, Thor M, Shepherd AF, et al. Radiation pneumonitis in lung cancer patients treated with chemoradiation plus durvalumab. Cancer Med 2020;9(13): 4622–31.

35. Saito S, Abe T, Kobayashi N, et al. Incidence and dose-volume relationship of radiation pneumonitis after concurrent chemoradiotherapy followed by durvalumab for locally advanced non-small cell lung cancer. Clin Transl Radiat Oncol 2020; 23:85–8.

36. Jabbour SK, Berman AT, Decker RH, et al. Phase 1 Trial of Pembrolizumab Administered Concurrently With Chemoradiotherapy for Locally Advanced Non-Small Cell Lung Cancer: A Nonrandomized Controlled Trial. JAMA Oncol 2020; 6(6):848–55.

37. Jabbour SK, Lee KH, Frost N, et al. Pembrolizumab Plus Concurrent Chemoradiation Therapy in Patients With Unresectable, Locally Advanced, Stage III Non-Small Cell Lung Cancer: The Phase 2 KEYNOTE-799 Nonrandomized Trial. JAMA Oncol 2021. https://doi.org/10.1001/jamaoncol.2021.2301.

38. Chen Y, Gao M, Huang Z, et al. SBRT combined with PD-1/PD-L1 inhibitors in NSCLC treatment: a focus on the mechanisms, advances, and future challenges. J Hematol Oncol 2020;13(1):105.

39. Chang JY, Mehran RJ, Feng L, et al. Stereotactic ablative radiotherapy for operable stage I non-small-cell lung cancer (revised STARS): long-term results of a single-arm, prospective trial with prespecified comparison to surgery. Lancet Oncol 2021;22(10):1448–57.

40. Timmerman RD, Paulus R, Pass HI, et al. Stereotactic Body Radiation Therapy for Operable Early-Stage Lung Cancer: Findings From the NRG Oncology RTOG 0618 Trial. JAMA Oncol 2018;4(9):1263–6.

41. Timmerman RD, Hu C, Michalski JM, et al. Long-term Results of Stereotactic Body Radiation Therapy in Medically Inoperable Stage I Non-Small Cell Lung Cancer. JAMA Oncol 2018;4(9):1287–8.

42. Timmerman R, Paulus R, Galvin J, et al. Stereotactic body radiation therapy for inoperable early stage lung cancer. JAMA 2010;303(11):1070–6.

43. Alcibar OL, Nadal E, Romero Palomar I, et al. Systematic review of stereotactic body radiotherapy in stage III non-small cell lung cancer. Transl Lung Cancer Res 2021;10(1):529–38.

44. Williams TM, Welliver MX, Brownstein JM, et al. A phase II trial of primary tumor SBRT boost prior to concurrent chemoradiation for locally-advanced non-small cell lung cancer (LA-NSCLC). Int J Radiat Oncol Biol Phys 2021;111(3):S90.

45. Luke JJ, Lemons JM, Karrison TG, et al. Safety and Clinical Activity of Pembrolizumab and Multisite Stereotactic Body Radiotherapy in Patients With Advanced Solid Tumors. J Clin Oncol 2018;36(16):1611–8.

46. Baumann BC, Mitra N, Harton JG, et al. Comparative Effectiveness of Proton vs Photon Therapy as Part of Concurrent Chemoradiotherapy for Locally Advanced Cancer. JAMA Oncol 2020;6(2):237–46.

47. Liao Z, Lee JJ, Komaki R, et al. Bayesian Adaptive Randomization Trial of Passive Scattering Proton Therapy and Intensity-Modulated Photon Radiotherapy for Locally Advanced Non-Small-Cell Lung Cancer. J Clin Oncol 2018;36(18): 1813–22.

48. Puri S, Saltos A, Perez B, et al. Locally Advanced, Unresectable Non-Small Cell Lung Cancer. Curr Oncol Rep 2020;22(4):31.

49. Wang X, Ding X, Kong D, et al. The effect of consolidation chemotherapy after concurrent chemoradiotherapy on the survival of patients with locally advanced non-small cell lung cancer: a meta-analysis. Int J Clin Oncol 2017;22(2):229–36.

50. Malhotra J, Jabbour SK, Aisner J. Current state of immunotherapy for non-small cell lung cancer. Transl Lung Cancer Res 2017;6(2):196–211.
51. Vatner RE, Cooper BT, Vanpouille-Box C, et al. Combinations of immunotherapy and radiation in cancer therapy. Front Oncol 2014;4:325.
52. Sharabi AB, Lim M, DeWeese TL, et al. Radiation and checkpoint blockade immunotherapy: radiosensitisation and potential mechanisms of synergy. Lancet Oncol 2015;16(13):e498–509.
53. Zeng J, See AP, Phallen J, et al. Anti-PD-1 blockade and stereotactic radiation produce long-term survival in mice with intracranial gliomas. Int J Radiat Oncol Biol Phys 2013;86(2):343–9.
54. Higgins KA, Puri S, Gray JE. Systemic and Radiation Therapy Approaches for Locally Advanced Non-Small-Cell Lung Cancer. J Clin Oncol 2022;40(6):576–85.
55. Gong X, Li X, Jiang T, et al. Combined Radiotherapy and Anti-PD-L1 Antibody Synergistically Enhances Antitumor Effect in Non-Small Cell Lung Cancer. J Thorac Oncol 2017;12(7):1085–97.
56. Deng L, Liang H, Burnette B, et al. Irradiation and anti-PD-L1 treatment synergistically promote antitumor immunity in mice. J Clin Invest 2014;124(2):687–95.
57. Antonia SJ, Villegas A, Daniel D, et al. Overall Survival with Durvalumab after Chemoradiotherapy in Stage III NSCLC. N Engl J Med 2018;379(24):2342–50.
58. Lin SH, Lin Y, Yao L, et al. Phase II Trial of Concurrent Atezolizumab With Chemoradiation for Unresectable NSCLC. J Thorac Oncol 2020;15(2):248–57.
59. Peters S, Felip E, Dafni U, et al. Progression-Free and Overall Survival for Concurrent Nivolumab With Standard Concurrent Chemoradiotherapy in Locally Advanced Stage IIIA-B NSCLC: Results From the European Thoracic Oncology Platform NICOLAS Phase II Trial (European Thoracic Oncology Platform 6-14). J Thorac Oncol 2021;16(2):278–88.
60. Durm GA, Jabbour SK, Althouse SK, et al. A phase 2 trial of consolidation pembrolizumab following concurrent chemoradiation for patients with unresectable stage III non-small cell lung cancer: Hoosier Cancer Research Network LUN 14-179. Cancer 2020;126(19):4353–61.
61. Ahn JS, Ahn YC, Kim JH, et al. Multinational Randomized Phase III Trial With or Without Consolidation Chemotherapy Using Docetaxel and Cisplatin After Concurrent Chemoradiation in Inoperable Stage III Non-Small-Cell Lung Cancer: KCSG-LU05-04. J Clin Oncol 2015;33(24):2660–6.
62. Choy H, Schwartzberg LS, Dakhil SR, et al. Phase 2 study of pemetrexed plus carboplatin, or pemetrexed plus cisplatin with concurrent radiation therapy followed by pemetrexed consolidation in patients with favorable-prognosis inoperable stage IIIA/B non-small-cell lung cancer. J Thorac Oncol 2013;8(10):1308–16.
63. Reck M, Lee KH, Frost N, et al. Two-year update from KEYNOTE-799: Pembrolizumab plus concurrent chemoradiation therapy (cCRT) for unresectable, locally advanced, stage III NSCLC. J Clin Oncol 2022;40(16_suppl):8508.
64. Jabbour SK, Cho BC, Bria E, et al. Rationale and Design of the Phase III KEYLYNK-012 Study of Pembrolizumab and Concurrent Chemoradiotherapy Followed by Pembrolizumab With or Without Olaparib for Stage III Non-Small-Cell Lung Cancer. Clin Lung Cancer 2022;23(6):e342–6.
65. De Ruysscher D, Ramalingam S, Urbanic J, et al. CheckMate 73L: A Phase 3 Study Comparing Nivolumab Plus Concurrent Chemoradiotherapy Followed by Nivolumab With or Without Ipilimumab Versus Concurrent Chemoradiotherapy Followed by Durvalumab for Previously Untreated, Locally Advanced Stage III Non-Small-Cell Lung Cancer. Clin Lung Cancer 2022;23(3):e264–8.

66. Herbst RS, Majem M, Barlesi F, et al. COAST: An Open-Label, Phase II, Multidrug Platform Study of Durvalumab Alone or in Combination With Oleclumab or Monalizumab in Patients With Unresectable, Stage III Non-Small-Cell Lung Cancer. J Clin Oncol 2022;JCO2200227. https://doi.org/10.1200/JCO.22.00227.

67. Durm GA, Mamdani H, Althouse SK, et al. Consolidation nivolumab plus ipilimumab or nivolumab alone following concurrent chemoradiation for patients with unresectable stage III non-small cell lung cancer: BTCRC LUN 16-081. J Clin Oncol 2022;40(16_suppl):8509.

68. Liveringhouse CL, Latifi K, Asous AG, et al. Dose Limiting Pulmonary Toxicity in a Phase 1/2 Study of Radiation and Chemotherapy with Ipilimumab Followed by Nivolumab for Patients With Stage 3 Unresectable Non-Small Cell Lung Cancer. Int J Radial Oncol Biol Phys 2023. https://doi.org/10.1016/j.ijrobp.2023.01.006. S0360-3016(23)00046-9.

69. Al-Shamsi HO, Al Farsi A, Ellis PM. Stage III non-small-cell lung cancer: Establishing a benchmark for the proportion of patients suitable for radical treatment. Clin Lung Cancer 2014;15(4):274–80.

70. Shaverdian N, Offin M, Shepherd AF, et al. Association Between the Early Discontinuation of Durvalumab and Poor Survival in Patients With Stage III NSCLC. JTO Clin Res Rep 2021;2(7):100197.

71. Bryant AK, Sankar K, Zhao L, et al. De-escalating adjuvant durvalumab treatment duration in stage III non-small cell lung cancer. Eur J Cancer 2022;171:55–63.

72. Garassino MC, Mazieres J, Reck M, et al. 108MO Safety and efficacy outcomes with durvalumab after sequential chemoradiotherapy (sCRT) in stage III, unresectable NSCLC (PACIFIC-6). Ann Oncol 2022;33:S81–2.

73. Ryan KJ, Skinner KE, Fernandes AW, et al. Real-world treatment patterns among patients with unresected stage III non-small-cell lung cancer. Future Oncol 2019; 15(25):2943–53.

74. Ohri N, Jolly S, Cooper BT, et al. The Selective Personalized Radioimmunotherapy for Locally Advanced NSCLC Trial (SPRINT): Initial results. J Clin Oncol 2022;40(16_suppl):8510.

75. Olmedo ME, Cervera R, Cabezon-Gutierrez L, et al. New horizons for uncommon mutations in non-small cell lung cancer: BRAF, KRAS, RET, MET, NTRK, HER2. World J Clin Oncol 2022;13(4):276–86.

76. Shi Y, Au JS, Thongprasert S, et al. A prospective, molecular epidemiology study of EGFR mutations in Asian patients with advanced non-small-cell lung cancer of adenocarcinoma histology (PIONEER). J Thorac Oncol 2014;9(2):154–62.

77. Park SE, Noh JM, Kim YJ, et al. EGFR Mutation Is Associated with Short Progression-Free Survival in Patients with Stage III Non-squamous Cell Lung Cancer Treated with Concurrent Chemoradiotherapy. Cancer Res Treat 2019; 51(2):493–501.

78. Lee HJ, Jeong GH, Li H, et al. Efficacy and safety of epidermal growth factor receptor-tyrosine kinase inhibitor (EGFR-TKI) monotherapy for advanced EGFR-mutated non-small cell lung cancer: systematic review and meta-analysis. Eur Rev Med Pharmacol Sci 2021;25(20):6232–44.

79. Liu L, Bai H, Seery S, et al. Efficacy and safety of treatment modalities across EGFR selected/unselected populations with non-small cell lung cancer and brain metastases: A systematic review and Bayesian network meta-analysis. Lung Cancer 2021;158:74–84.

80. Wu YL, Tsuboi M, He J, et al. Osimertinib in Resected EGFR-Mutated Non-Small-Cell Lung Cancer. N Engl J Med 2020;383(18):1711–23.

81. Gyawali B, West HJ. Lessons From ADAURA on Adjuvant Cancer Drug Trials: Evidence, Ethics, and Economics. J Clin Oncol 2021;39(3):175–7.
82. Yang X, Mei T, Yu M, et al. Symptomatic Radiation Pneumonitis in NSCLC Patients Receiving EGFR-TKIs and Concurrent Once-daily Thoracic Radiotherapy: Predicting the Value of Clinical and Dose-volume Histogram Parameters. Zhongguo Fei Ai Za Zhi 2022;25(6):409–19.
83. Wang Y, Yu W, Shi J, et al. Evaluating the Efficacy of EGFR-TKIs Combined With Radiotherapy in Advanced Lung Adenocarcinoma Patients With EGFR Mutation: A Retrospective Study. Technol Cancer Res Treat 2022;21. https://doi.org/10.1177/15330338221100358. 15330338221100358.
84. Zheng L, Wang Y, Xu Z, et al. Concurrent EGFR-TKI and Thoracic Radiotherapy as First-Line Treatment for Stage IV Non-Small Cell Lung Cancer Harboring EGFR Active Mutations. Oncol 2019;24(8):1031-e612.
85. Wang XS, Bai YF, Verma V, et al. Randomized Trial of First-Line Tyrosine Kinase Inhibitor With or Without Radiotherapy for Synchronous Oligometastatic EGFR-Mutated NSCLC. J Natl Cancer Inst 2022. https://doi.org/10.1093/jnci/djac015.
86. Naidoo J, Antonia SJ, Wu Y-L, et al. Durvalumab (durva) after chemoradiotherapy (CRT) in unresectable, stage III, EGFR mutation-positive (EGFRm) NSCLC: A post hoc subgroup analysis from PACIFIC. J Clin Oncol 2022;40(16_suppl):8541.
87. Ross HJ, Kozono DE, Urbanic JJ, et al. Phase II trial of atezolizumab before and after definitive chemoradiation for unresectable stage III NSCLC. J Clin Oncol 2018;36(15_suppl):TPS8585.
88. Hellyer JA, Aredo JV, Das M, et al. Role of Consolidation Durvalumab in Patients With EGFR- and HER2-Mutant Unresectable Stage III NSCLC. J Thorac Oncol 2021;16(5):868–72.
89. Wang CC, Chiu LC, Ju JS, et al. Durvalumab as Consolidation Therapy in Post-Concurrent Chemoradiation (CCRT) in Unresectable Stage III Non-Small Cell Lung Cancer Patients: A Multicenter Observational Study. Vaccines (Basel) 2021;9(10). https://doi.org/10.3390/vaccines9101122.
90. Ahn MJ, Cho BC, Ou X, et al. Osimertinib Plus Durvalumab in Patients With EGFR-Mutated, Advanced NSCLC: A Phase 1b, Open-Label, Multicenter Trial. J Thorac Oncol 2022;17(5):718–23.
91. Passaro A, Leighl N, Blackhall F, et al. ESMO expert consensus statements on the management of EGFR mutant non-small-cell lung cancer. Ann Oncol 2022;33(5):466–87.

First-Line Treatment of Driver-Negative Non–Small Cell Lung Cancer

So Yeon Kim, MD*, Scott Gettinger, MD

KEYWORDS

- Driver-negative advanced non–small cell lung cancer • Smoker • Never-smoker
- Immunotherapy • Chemoimmunotherapy • PD-L1

KEY POINTS

- PD1 axis inhibitor therapy with pembrolizumab, atezolizumab, or cemiplimab monotherapy continue to be standard first-line treatment options for driver-negative (*EGFR/ALK/ROS* WT) high PD-L1 ($\geq$50%) NSCLC with prior smoking history. In patients with high tumor burden or rapidly progressive disease, chemotherapy may be added to immunotherapy.
- For patients with PD-L1 less than 50% driver-negative NSCLC or for patients with PD-L1 greater than or equal to 50% driver-negative NSCLC with no prior smoking history, chemoimmunotherapy is the preferred treatment.
- For patients with PD-L1 less than 1% driver-negative NSCLC, chemoimmunotherapy is standard first-line treatment.
- An alternative to first-line chemoimmunotherapy for advanced NSCLC is combination immunotherapy with nivolumab and ipilimumab.

INTRODUCTION

The treatment paradigm for the management of driver-negative (*EGFR/ALK/ROS* WT) advanced non–small cell lung cancer (NSCLC) shifted in 2016 with the introduction of immune checkpoint inhibitors (ICI). Historically, treatment of advanced NSCLC was largely palliative, with response rates of only 20% to 30% and a median survival of 8 to 10 months with platinum-doublet chemotherapy regardless of the chemotherapy backbone.[1–3] In 2008, histology-specific treatment was widely adapted, after superior overall survival (OS) was demonstrated with pemetrexed chemotherapy relative to gemcitabine-based chemotherapy in adenocarcinoma and large cell tumors.[4] This differential treatment response was attributed to biologic differences in the expression of

Section of Medical Oncology, Department of Internal Medicine, Yale Cancer Center, Yale School of Medicine, New Haven, CT, USA
* Corresponding author.
E-mail address: soyeon.kim@yale.edu

Hematol Oncol Clin N Am 37 (2023) 557–573
https://doi.org/10.1016/j.hoc.2023.02.008
0889-8588/23/© 2023 Elsevier Inc. All rights reserved.

thymidylate synthase, which plays a key role in DNA synthesis, and is more highly expressed in squamous cell cancers.[5] Bevacizumab, a vascular endothelial cell growth factor antagonist, also demonstrated a 2-month OS improvement when added to carboplatin/paclitaxel and is an option for nonsquamous histology.[6–11] Its use is limited to nonsquamous cell histology, however, based on fatal hemoptysis seen with squamous histology.[8,9] Following bevacizumab, nab-paclitaxel was developed to reduce paclitaxel-associated hypersensitivity reactions,[12] and was evaluated against paclitaxel based on its improved drug transcytosis.[13] Nab-paclitaxel demonstrated similar OS compared with paclitaxel in all comers, but improved OS in patients greater than or equal to 70 years of age (19.9 months vs 10.4 months for paclitaxel; hazard ratio [HR], 0.583), with reduced incidence of grade greater than or equal to 3 peripheral neuropathy[14] relative to paclitaxel and thus may be a favorable chemotherapy backbone in older patients.

First discovered in 1992, programmed cell death protein 1 (PD-1) is a protein expressed on activated T cells, B cells, and natural killer cells.[15] On binding of PD-1 to PD-L1 (also known as B7-H1/CD274), which is expressed on tumor cells and macrophages, activated T cells undergo apoptosis, exhaustion, and/or anergy leading to tumor-cell-mediated immune evasion and proliferation.[16] Blockade of the PD-1/PD-L1 axis normalizes dysregulated effector T cells, allowing antigen-specific T cells to regain their cytotoxic function and is the biologic basis of ICI.[17] PD-L1 is a widely accepted biomarker that affects treatment selection in driver-negative advanced NSCLC. In this review, we outline the most recent updates in the first-line treatment of advanced NSCLC with no driver alterations, with the goal of providing a practical guideline for clinicians based on PD-L1 biomarker-directed therapy.

PD-L1 GREATER THAN OR EQUAL TO FIFTY PERCENT

ICI monotherapy is one established standard of care in patients with advanced NSCLC with PD-L1 greater than or equal to 50%. The phase 3 KEYNOTE-024,[18] KEYNOTE-042,[19] IMpower110,[20] and EMPOWER-Lung01[21] trials all have demonstrated superior OS with pembrolizumab, atezolizumab, and cemiplimab monotherapy, respectively, relative to platinum-doublet chemotherapy, in treatment-naive patients with advanced NSCLC with high PD-L1 expression. Despite differences in PD-L1 antibody assays used to define PD-L1 expression (PD-L1 $\geq$50% by tumor cells by PD-L1 immunohistochemistry [IHC] 22c3 pharmDx assay [Dako] with pembrolizumab[18] and cemiplimab[21]; PD-L1 $\geq$50% by tumor cells or $\geq$10% by tumor-infiltrating immune cells by SP142 IHC [Ventana] with atezolizumab[20]), the HR for OS were largely similar among compounds, with HR for OS rate at 6 months of 0.60 (95% confidence interval [CI], 0.41–0.89; P = 0.005) for pembrolizumab in KEYNOTE-024,[18] HR for OS of 0.69 (95% CI, 0.56–0.85; P = 0.0003) for pembrolizumab in KEYNOTE-042[19] (TPS $\geq$50%), HR of 0.59 (95% CI, 0.40–0.89; P = 0.01) for atezolizumab in IMpower110,[20] and HR of 0.57 (95% CI, 0.42–0.77; P = 0.0002) for cemiplimab in EMPOWER-Lung01 (**Table 1**).[21] Based on these studies, PD-L1 IHC 22c3 and SP142 assays have been approved as companion diagnostics for pembrolizumab (22c3, in April 2020), cemiplimab (22c3, in February 2021), and atezolizumab (SP142, in June 2020). Within the PD-L1 greater than or equal to 50% population, higher PD-L1 expression has also been associated with superior outcomes with PD-1 inhibitor, with longer median OS observed within PD-L1 greater than or equal to 90% versus 50% to 89% populations (not reached vs 15.9 months in PD-L1 50%–89%; HR, 0.39; 95% CI, 0.21–0.70; P = 0.002).[22] This observation was supported by a 3-year follow-up of a larger cohort of 396 patients (30.2 vs 16.9 months in PD-L1 50%–89%; HR, 0.66; P < 0.01)[23]

Table 1
First-line phase III randomized immunotherapy monotherapy versus chemotherapy trials and their primary outcomes, including their updated overall survival outcome

Immunotherapy Monotherapy	Therapy (N)	Primary End Point	Primary Outcome				Updated Analysis			
			IO-Therapy (mo)	Control (mo)	HR (95% CI)	P Value	IO-Therapy (mo)	Control (mo)	HR (95% CI)	P Value
KEYNOTE-024 PD-L1 ≥50%	Pembrolizumab (154) vs platinum-doublet (151)	PFS	10.3 (6.7–NR)	6.0 (4.2–6.2)	0.50 (0.37–0.68)	<0.001	5-y OS: 26.3 (18.3–40.4)	13.4 (9.4–18.3)	0.62 (0.48–0.81)	NA
KEYNOTE-042 PD-L1 ≥1%	Pembrolizumab (637) vs platinum-doublet (637)	OS PD-L1 ≥50%: PD-L1 ≥20%: PD-L1 ≥1%:	20.0 (15.4–24.9) 17.7 (15.3–22.1) 16.7 (13.9–19.7)	12.2 (10.4–14.2) 13.0 (11.6–15.3) 12.1 (11.3–13.3)	0.69 (0.56–3.85) 0.77 (0.64–0.92) 0.81 (0.71–0.93)	0.0003 0.0020 0.0018	5-y OS: 20.0 (15.9–24.2) 18.0 (15.5–21.5) 16.4 (14.0–19.6)	12.2 (10.4–14.6) 13.0 (11.6–15.3) 12.1 (11.3–13.3)	0.68 (0.57–0.81) 0.75 (0.64–0.87) 0.79 (0.70–0.89)	NA NA NA
IMpower110 PD-L1 ≥1% TC or IC	Atezolizumab (277) vs Platinum-doublet (277)	OS High: High-intermediate: intermediate: Any:	20.2 (16.5–NR) 18.2 (13.3–NR) 17.5 (12.8–23.1)	13.1 (7.4–16.5) 14.9 (10.8–16.6) 14.1 (11.0–16.6)	0.59 (0.40–0.89) 0.72 (0.52–0.99) 0.83 (0.65–1.07)	0.01 0.04 NA	2-y OS: 20.2 (17.2–27.9) 19.9 (17.2–25.3) 18.9 (13.4–23.0)	14.7 (7.4–17.7) 16.1 (12.6–18.0) 14.7 (11.2–16.5)	0.76 (0.54–1.09) 0.87 (0.66–1.14) 0.85 (0.69–1.04)	0.3091 0.1070 (descriptive only)
EMPOWER-Lung01 PD-L1 ≥50%	Cemiplimab (356) vs platinum-doublet (354)	OS PD-L1 ≥50% Any PD-L1 (ITT) PFS PD-L1 ≥50% Any PD-L1 (ITT)	NR (17.9–NR) 22.1 (17.7–NR) 8.2 (6.1–8.8) 6.2 (4.5–8.3)	14.2 (11.2–17.5) 14.3 (11.7–19.2) 5.7 (4.5–6.2) 5.6 (4.5–6.1)	0.57 (0.42–0.77) 0.68 (0.53–0.87) 0.54 (0.43–0.68) 0.59 (0.49–0.72)	0.0002 0.0022 <0.0001 <0.0001	NA	NA	NA	NA

In KEYNOTE-024, KEYNOTE-042, and EMPOWER-Lung01, PD-L1 expression was defined by 22C3 assay. In IMpower110: High: PD-L1 expression (SP142 IHC) TC ≥50% or IC ≥10%; high-intermediate: PD-L1 expression (SP142 IHC) TC ≥5% or IC ≥5%; any: PD-L1 expression (SP142 IHC) TC ≥1% or IC ≥1%.

Abbreviations: HR, hazard ratio; IO, immunotherapy; ITT, intent on-to-treat; N, number of patients in each cohort; NA, not available; NR, not-reached; OS, overall survival; PFS, progression-free survival.

suggesting PD-L1 to be a continuous rather than a categorical predictive biomarker of immunotherapy response.

With multiple ICI approved for PD-L1 greater than or equal to 50% patients with advanced NSCLC in the first-line setting, a network meta-analysis sought to compare ICI monotherapies, and a trend toward highest OS benefit relative to chemotherapy was observed with cemiplimab, followed by atezolizumab, then pembrolizumab.[24] There were no statistically significant differences among the drugs and given limitations with cross-trial comparisons, including the primary end point in KEYNOTE-024 being progression-free survival (PFS) and not OS, pembrolizumab, atezolizumab, and cemiplimab are all suitable first-line treatment options for PD-L1 greater than or equal to 50%. Although nivolumab and durvalumab are also PD-1/PD-L1 axis inhibitors, neither drug met its primary end point of PFS or OS in the phase 3 CheckMate-026[25] and phase 3 MYSTIC trial,[26] respectively, and are not Food and Drug Administration (FDA) approved for ICI monotherapy in the first-line setting.

Based on the improved tolerance of immunotherapy compared with chemotherapy, in which less grade greater than or equal to 3 treatment-related adverse events have been observed with pembrolizumab (26.6% vs 53.3%),[18] atezolizumab (30.1% vs 52.5%),[20] and cemiplimab (28% vs 39%) relative to chemotherapy,[21] ICI may be a more preferred treatment option for older patients or patients with poor performance status (PS). The phase 2 PePS2 trial[27] and the phase 3 IPSOS trial[28] sought to evaluate this hypothesis and have prospectively demonstrated safety and efficacy of atezolizumab and pembrolizumab in patients with PS greater than or equal to 2, who have been excluded from prior ICI monotherapy studies. In the single-arm multicenter PePS2 trial, single-agent pembrolizumab in patients with PS of 2 and PD-L1 greater than or equal to 50% in the first-line setting demonstrated a durable clinical response (complete response, partial response, and stable disease until approximately 18 weeks) of 44.6% at a median follow-up of 10 months with tolerable safety profile.[27] In the phase 3 IPSOS trial, which randomized atezolizumab monotherapy against single-agent chemotherapy (vinorelbine or gemcitabine) in older patients (age ≥70) with PS greater than or equal to 2 not eligible for platinum-doublets in the first-line setting, patients who received atezolizumab monotherapy demonstrated improved OS (10.3 vs 9.2 with chemotherapy; HR, 0.78; 95% CI, 0.63–0.97; $P = 0.028$) and decreased grade 3 to 4 treatment-related adverse events (16.3% vs 33.3%) compared with those who received single-agent chemotherapy.[28] Based on these two trials, single-agent pembrolizumab or atezolizumab are safe and effective regimens for elderly patients (age ≥70) and/or for patients with PS greater than or equal to 2.

Whether the addition of a checkpoint inhibitor or chemotherapy to PD-1/PD-L1 monotherapy in patients with PD-L1 greater than or equal to 50% can further improve clinical outcomes has been evaluated in two studies, both of which favored ICI monotherapy. In the phase 3 KEYNOTE-598 trial, which randomized patients with PD-L1 high driver-negative NSCLC to pembrolizumab/ipilimumab (CTLA-4 inhibitor) or pembrolizumab/placebo, no differences in OS (21.4 months vs 21.9 months for pembrolizumab/placebo; HR, 1.08; 95% CI, 0.85–1.37; $P = 0.74$) or PFS (8.2 months vs 8.4 months for pembrolizumab/placebo; HR, 1.06; 95% CI, 0.86–1.30; $P = 0.72$) were observed.[29] In fact, the combination ICI cohort demonstrated a higher incidence of grade greater than or equal to 3 treatment-related toxicity (62.4% vs 50.2% in the pembrolizumab-placebo group), including greater incidence of colitis, pneumonitis, adrenal insufficiency, and myocarditis, demonstrating only added toxicity without survival benefit with combination ICI in previously untreated PD-L1 greater than or equal to 50% advanced NSCLC.[29] Although no randomized trial has compared the addition of chemotherapy to ICI monotherapy versus ICI monotherapy in previously untreated PD-L1 greater than or equal to 50% advanced NSCLC, the FDA conducted an exploratory pooled analysis of 12 randomized trials evaluating ICI alone versus chemoimmunotherapy in this subpopulation.[30] Although superior PFS and ORR were observed in the chemoimmunotherapy cohort, with the exception of patients greater than or equal to 75 years of age, this PFS benefit did not translate into an OS benefit (25.0 months vs 20.9 months with ICI monotherapy; HR, 0.82; 95% CI, 0.62–1.08), and single-agent immunotherapy remains the treatment of choice within the PD-L1 high-advanced NSCLC.[30]

PD-L1 LESS THAN FIFTY PERCENT

For patients with driver-negative advanced NSCLC with PD-L1 less than 50%, combination chemoimmunotherapy is the preferred treatment of choice in patients with acceptable PS. Multiple phase 3 trials, including KEYNOTE-189,[31] KEYNOTE-407,[32] and IMpower150,[33] have demonstrated statistically significant superior OS with combination chemoimmunotherapy to platinum-doublet therapy regardless of PD-L1 stratification (**Table 2**). Although KEYNOTE-042 demonstrated superior OS with pembrolizumab monotherapy relative to chemotherapy in PD-L1 greater than or equal to 1%, and pembrolizumab is FDA-approved for use as monotherapy in PD-L1 greater than or equal to 1%, the OS benefit was likely largely driven by PD-L1 greater than or equal to 50%[19] and the addition of chemotherapy in PD-L1 1% to 49% is recommended. These results subsequently led to the FDA approval of pembrolizumab with chemotherapy in August 2018 (nonsquamous) and October 2018 (squamous) regardless of PD-L1 expression, and of atezolizumab with bevacizumab-chemotherapy (nonsquamous) in December 2018. In KEYNOTE-189 and IMpower150, PD-L1 was observed to be a possible predictive biomarker and demonstrated improved OS and PFS HR, respectively, with higher PD-L1 expression.[31,33] The updated 5-year OS data for KEYNOTE-189[34] and KEYNOTE-407[35] demonstrated sustained superior OS with combination chemoimmunotherapy compared with chemotherapy alone (OS 22.0 months vs 10.6 months for chemotherapy; HR, 0.60; 95% CI, 0.50–0.72 for KEYNOTE-189; OS 17.2 months vs 11.6 months for chemotherapy; HR, 0.71; 95% CI, 0.59–0.85 for KEYNOTE-407).[34]

Key trial differences among the KEYNOTE-189, KEYNOTE-407, and IMpower150 were the inclusion of bevacizumab to the platinum-doublet, atezolizumab/bevacizumab/carboplatin/paclitaxel (ABCP) versus bevacizumab/carboplatin/paclitaxel (BCP), and the inclusion of EGFR/ALK-mutated patients who progressed after first-line tyrosine kinase inhibitor in IMpower150.[33] Despite up to 33% of EGFR patients and up to 57% of ALK patients demonstrating high PD-L1 greater than or equal to 50%,[36] patients with EGFR/ALK mutations have largely demonstrated resistance to immunotherapy[37–39] and thus have been excluded in most KEYNOTE studies. This discordance between PD-L1 expression and immunotherapy resistance is attributed to the upregulation of PD-L1 driven by mutant EGFR and EML4-ALK fusion in contrast to the adaptive upregulation of PD-L1 in driver-negative NSCLC.[40–42] Although PFS benefit with the addition of atezolizumab to chemotherapy was observed in IMpower150 in the EGFR/ALK cohort (9.7 months vs 6.1 months; HR, 0.59; 95% CI, 0.37–0.94),[33] the small sample size (n = 108) precludes a definitive conclusion and ABCP is currently only FDA-approved in the EGFR/ALK WT setting.

Following IMpower150, atezolizumab was also FDA-approved in October 2019 with carboplatin/nab-paclitaxel backbone (without bevacizumab) for nonsquamous histology after clinically meaningful OS benefit was observed with atezolizumab/

Table 2
First-line phase III randomized combination chemoimmunotherapy versus chemotherapy or combination immunotherapy versus chemotherapy trials and their primary outcomes, including their updated overall survival outcome

Chemoimmunotherapy (N) / Therapy	Primary End Point	Primary Outcome				Updated Analysis			
		IO-Therapy (mo)	Control (mo)	HR (95% CI)	P Value	IO-Therapy (mo)	Control (mo)	HR (95% CI)	P Value
KEYNOTE-189 *Nonsquamous* Pembrolizumab (410) + platinum-doublet vs platinum-doublet + PI (206)	OS PFS	NR 8.8 (7.6–9.2)	11.3 (8.7–15.1) 4.9 (4.7–5.5)	0.49 (0.38–0.64) 0.52 (0.43–0.64)	<0.001 <0.001	5-y: 22.0 (19.5–24.5) 9.0 (8.1–10.4)	10.6 (8.7–13.6) 4.9 (4.7–5.5)	0.60 (0.50–0.72) 0.50 (0.42–0.60)	NA NA
KEYNOTE-407 *Squamous* Pembrolizumab (278) + platinum-doublet vs platinum-doublet + PI (281)	OS PFS	15.9 (13.2–NR) 6.4 (6.2–8.3)	11.3 (9.5–14.8) 4.8 (4.3–5.7)	0.64 (0.49–0.85) 0.56 (0.45–0.70)	<0.001 <0.001	5-y: 17.2 (14.4–19.7) 8.0 (6.3–8.5)	11.6 (10.1–13.7) 5.1 (4.3–6.0)	0.71 (0.59–0.85) 0.62 (0.52–0.74)	NA NA
IMpower150 *Nonsquamous* ABCP (356) vs BCP (336)	PFS WT WT/Teff-high OS (WT)	8.3 (7.7–9.8) 11.3 (9.1–13.0) 19.2 (17.0–23.8)	6.8 (6.0–7.1) 6.8 (5.9–7.4) 14.7 (13.3–16.9)	0.62 (0.52–0.74) 0.51 (0.38–0.68) 0.78 (0.64–0.96)	<0.001 <0.001 0.02	3-y: 8.4 (not reported) Not reported 19.5 (17.0–22.2)	6.8 (not reported) Not reported 14.7 (12.9–17.1)	0.57 (0.48–0.67) Not reported 0.80 (0.67–0.95)	NA NA NA
IMpower130 *Nonsquamous* A + CnP (451) vs CnP (228)	ITT-WT PFS OS	7.0 (6.2–7.3) 18.6 (16–21.2)	5.5 (4.4–5.9) 13.9 (12.0–18.7)	0.64 (0.54–0.77) 0.79 (0.64–0.98)	<0.0001 0.033	NA	NA	NA	NA
IMpower131 *Squamous* A + CP (338) vs A + CnP (343) vs CnP (340) PFS, OS reported for A + CnP vs. CnP	PFS OS	6.3 (5.7–7.1) 14.2 (12.3–16.8)	5.6 (5.5–5.7) 13.5 (12.2–15.1)	0.71 (0.60–0.85) 0.88 (0.73–1.05)	0.0001 0.1581	NA	NA	NA	NA
CheckMate 9LA Platinum-doublet (2C) + ipilimumab/ nivolumab (361) vs platinum-doublet (4C) (358)	OS	14.1 (13.2–16.2)	10.7 (9.5–12.4)	0.69 (96.71% CI, 0.55–0.87)	0.00065	3-y: 15.8	11.0	0.74 (0.62–0.87)	NA
EMPOWER-Lung 3 Cemiplimab + platinum-doublet (312) vs platinum-doublet + Placebo (154)	OS	21.9 (15.5–NR)	13.0 (11.9–16.1)	0.71 (0.53–0.93)	0.014	NA	NA	NA	NA

POSEIDON	Durvalumab ± tremelimumab/ platinum-doublet vs platinum-doublet	PFS	5.5 (4.7-6.5)	4.8 (4.6-5.8)	0.74 (0.62-0.89)	0.0009	NA	NA	NA	NA
		OS	13.3 (11.4-14.7)	11.7 (10.5-13.1)	0.86 (0.72-1.02)	0.0758				
	Durvalumab/ platinum-doublet (338) vs platinum-doublet (337)	OS (ad hoc)	15.0 (8.2-23.8)	10.7 (6.0-14.9)	0.55 (0.30-1.03)	NA				
	Durvalumab/tremelimumab/ platinum-doublet vs platinum-doublet		13.7 (7.2-26.5)	8.7 (5.1-NE)	0.43 (0.16-1.25)	NA				
	STK11 mutant (31 vs. 22)									
	KEAP1 mutant (22 vs. 6)									
	Nonsquamous									
	Any histology									
Combination immunotherapy										
CheckMate 227 Part 1a	Ipilimumab/nivolumab (396) vs nivolumab ± platinum-doublet vs platinum-doublet (397) Ipilimumab/nivolumab vs platinum-doublet	OS PD-L1 ≥ 1%	17.1 (15.0-20.1)	14.9 (12.7-16.7)	0.79 (0.65-0.96)	0.007	5-y (part 1a): 17.1 (15.0-20.2)	14.9 (12.7-16.7)	0.77 (0.66-0.91)	NA

In KEYNOTE-189, KEYNOTE-407, and EMPOWER-Lung 3, PD-L1 expression was defined by 22c3 assay. In IMpower150, IMpower130, IMpower131, PD-L1 was defined by expression in tumor cells (TC) and tumor infiltrating immune cells (IC) by SP142 PD-L1 immunohistochemistry (IHC). In CheckMate 9LA and CheckMate 227, PD-L1 expression was defined by 28-8 antibody.

Abbreviations: 2C, 2 cycles; 4C, 4 cycles; A + CnP, atezolizumab/carboplatin/nab-paclitaxel; A + CP, atezolizumab/carboplatin/paclitaxel; ABCP, atezolizumab/bevacizumab/carboplatin/paclitaxel; BCP, bevacizumab/carboplatin/paclitaxel; CnP, carboplatin/nab-paclitaxel; CP, carboplatin/paclitaxel; HR, hazard ratio; IO, immunotherapy; ITT, intention-to-treat; N, number of patients in each cohort; NA, not available; NE, not-evaluable; NR, not-reached; OS, overall survival; PFS, progression-free survival; Pl, placebo; Teff-high, high expression of effector T-cell gene signature in tumor defined as expression of PD-L1, CXCL9, and IFN-γ messenger RNA; WT, wild-type genotype, without *EGFR* or *ALK*.

carboplatin/nab-paclitaxel followed by maintenance atezolizumab (OS 18.6 months vs 13.9 months with chemotherapy; HR, 0.79; 95% CI, 0.64–0.98; $P = 0.033$) compared with carboplatin/nab-paclitaxel with the option to be followed by maintenance pemetrexed in IMpower130.[43] When stratified by PD-L1 expression, a trend toward OS benefit was observed within each cohort (OS 17.3 months vs 16.9 months with chemotherapy; HR, 0.84; 95% CI, 0.51–1.39 in PD-L1 high; OS 23.7 months vs. 15.9 months with chemotherapy; HR, 0.70; 95% CI, 0.45–1.08 in PD-L1 low; OS 15.2 months vs 12.0 months with chemotherapy; HR, 0.81; 95% CI, 0.61–1.08 in PD-L1 negative), in which PD-L1 high was defined as PD-L1 greater than or equal to 50% of tumor cells or greater than or equal to 10% of tumor-infiltrating immune cells, PD-L1 low as PD-L1 greater than or equal to 1% to 49% of tumor cells or greater than or equal to 1% and less than 10% of tumor-infiltrating immune cells, and PD-L1 negative as PD-L1 less than 1% of tumor cells and less than 1% of tumor-infiltrating immune cells.[43] In the squamous histology, PFS benefit with atezolizumab/carboplatin/nab-paclitaxel relative to carboplatin/nab-paclitaxel alone did not translate into OS benefit in IMpower131.[44] Atezolizumab is thus an option with chemotherapy with or without bevacizumab in driver-negative advanced NSCLC with nonsquamous histology. Most recently, cemiplimab has also been approved in combination with chemotherapy in November 2022 based on positive OS outcomes compared with chemotherapy alone in driver-negative advanced NSCLC in the phase 3 EMPOWER-Lung 3 (21.9 months vs 13.0 months with chemotherapy; HR, 0.71; 95% CI, 0.53–0.93), with OS benefit observed in the PD-L1 1% to 49%, but not in the less than 1% subgroup.[45]

Multiple complementary mechanisms including costimulatory or coinhibitory receptors play a role in antitumor immunity, of which PD-1/PD-L1 inhibitor is only one example of a coinhibitory immune receptor, and combination nonchemotherapy-based options have been explored.[46] CheckMate 227 evaluated combination immunotherapy, with nivolumab (anti-PD-1) and ipilimumab (anti-CTLA-4) as first-line treatment in advanced NSCLC.[47] Patients with PD-L1 greater than or equal to 1% (IHC 28–8) were randomized 1:1:1 to nivolumab/ipilimumab, chemotherapy, or nivolumab and patients with PD-L1 less than 1% were randomized to nivolumab/ipilimumab, chemotherapy, or nivolumab-chemotherapy. The primary end point of OS in PD-L1 greater than or equal to 1% was met with nivolumab/ipilimumab relative to chemotherapy (17.1 months vs 14.9 months with chemotherapy; HR, 0.79; 95% CI, 0.65–0.96; $P = 0.007$).[47] Improved OS with combination ICI was also demonstrated in the PD-L1 less than 1% cohort (17.2 months vs 12.2 months with chemotherapy; HR, 0.62; 95% CI, 0.49–0.79) on exploratory analysis.[47] Although combination nivolumab/ipilimumab was FDA-approved in May 2020 for first-line therapy for driver-negative advanced NSCLC only in the PD-L1 greater than or equal to 1% setting, nivolumab/ipilimumab is a reasonable chemotherapy-free first-line therapy for patients with advanced NSCLC with PD-L1 less than 1% with prior smoking history as per National Comprehensive Cancer Network guidelines. At more than 4 years of follow-up, improved OS with nivolumab/ipilimumab compared with chemotherapy was sustained in PD-L1 greater than or equal to 1% (17.1 months vs 14.9 months with chemotherapy; HR, 0.76; 95% CI, 0.65–0.90) and PD-L1 less than 1% populations (17.2 months vs 12.2 months with chemotherapy; HR, 0.64; 95% CI, 0.51–0.81).[48]

Following CheckMate 227, CheckMate 9LA also demonstrated superior OS relative to chemotherapy with combination nivolumab/ipilimumab with two cycles of doublet chemotherapy for induction and goal of rapid disease control in the initial phase of immunotherapy.[49] Improved OS was observed in all PD-L1 subpopulations (15.6 months vs 10.9 months with chemotherapy; HR, 0.66; 95% CI, 0.55–0.80) at

3.5 months longer follow-up than preplanned interim analysis, including in the PD-L1 less than 1% (16.8 months vs 9.8 months with chemotherapy; HR, 0.62; 95% CI, 0.45–0.85), leading to the FDA approval of nivolumab/ipilimumab with 2 cycles of doublet chemotherapy in May 2020 for any PD-L1. In the updated 3-year OS follow-up, sustained improvement in OS was observed (15.8 months vs 11.0 months with chemotherapy; HR, 0.74; 95% CI, 0.62–0.87) in all patients independent of PD-L1 and also specifically in the PD-L1 less than 1% (17.7 months vs 9.8 months with chemotherapy; HR, 0.67; 95% CI, 0.51–0.88).[50] Patients with squamous cell histology, who may have been associated with inferior outcomes compared with nonsquamous histology in prior chemoimmunotherapy trials,[31,32] demonstrated a comparable median OS benefit compared with adenocarcinoma histology in CheckMate 9LA (HR, 0.62; 95% CI, 0.45–0.86 in squamous; HR, 0.69; 95% CI, 0.55–0.87 in nonsquamous)[49] and thus, ipilimumab/nivolumab with 2 cycles of induction chemotherapy may be a reasonable first-line treatment choice for driver-negative advanced squamous cell NSCLC with PD-L1 less than 50%.

NEVER-SMOKERS

Never-smokers remain a subpopulation of interest given their lower responses to immunotherapy, attributed to reduced neoantigen presentation. In KEYNOTE-024 and KEYNOTE-042, no survival benefit was observed with pembrolizumab monotherapy compared with chemotherapy in never-smokers even within the subgroup of patients with PD-L1 greater than or equal to 50% (OS HR, 0.90; 95% CI, 0.11–7.59 at a median follow-up of 2 years in KEYNOTE-024[51]; OS HR, 1.10; 95% CI, 0.69–1.75 at a median follow-up of 1 year in KEYNOTE-042[19]). In CheckMate 227, never-smokers were in fact observed to have a trend toward improved survival with chemotherapy than with ipilimumab/nivolumab (15.2 months vs 19.6 months with chemotherapy; OS HR, 1.23; 95% CI, 0.76–1.98).[47] Based on these prior studies, never-smokers (≤100 life-time cigarettes) were ineligible to participate in the EMPOWER-Lung01 study[21] and thus, ICI monotherapy is not a suitable treatment choice for nonsmokers. A large retrospective analysis of two real-world multicenter cohorts (cohort 1 metastatic patients with PD-L1 ≥50% who received first-line pembrolizumab; cohort 2, metastatic patients with *EGFR/ALK* WT who received first-line platinum-doublet chemotherapy) was conducted to evaluate the correlation of smoking status to response to pembrolizumab.[52] In the 424 patients who were matched by multiple baseline characteristics including smoking status, never-smokers were observed to have a shorter PFS compared with current or former smokers within the matched pembrolizumab cohort (4.7 months vs 8.0 months current/former smokers; HR, 1.68; 95% CI, 1.17–2.40; $P = 0.0045$), and a longer PFS (7.4 months vs 6.0 months current/former smokers; HR, 0.68; 95% CI, 0.49–0.95; $P = 0.0255$) and OS (20.1 months vs 15.8 months current/former smokers; HR, 0.66; 95% CI, 0.45–0.97; $P = 0.0356$) compared with current or former smokers within the matched chemotherapy cohort.[52] Thus, chemotherapy-based regimens remain a preferred treatment option over ICI monotherapy in never-smokers with high PD-L1 expression.

In the combination chemoimmunotherapy trials, mixed results have been observed in never-smokers. Relative OS benefit with chemoimmunotherapy compared with chemotherapy-placebo was observed in KEYNOTE-189 (OS HR, 0.23; 95% CI, 0.10–0.54),[31] but not in EMPOWER-Lung3, in which a trend toward improved OS was in fact observed within the chemotherapy cohort relative to cemiplimab-chemotherapy (OS HR, 1.28; 95% CI, 0.53–3.08)[45] in the never-smoker subpopulation. The addition of bevacizumab demonstrated a nonsignificant trend toward improved OS in the ABCP cohort compared with BCP in *EGFR/ALK* WT treatment-naive patients with advanced NSCLC in the 3-year OS follow-up of IMpower150 in never-smokers (22.3 months vs 18.2 months with BCP; HR, 0.75; 95% CI, 0.49–1.14).[53] In contrast, in CheckMate 9LA, chemotherapy alone had a nonsignificant trend toward OS benefit compared with the addition of two cycles of chemotherapy with nivolumab/ipilimumab (14.1 months vs 17.8 months with chemotherapy; HR, 1.14; 95% CI, 0.66–1.97)[49] in the never-smoker subpopulation. Because the number of nonsmokers were small in these trials and observations are based on subgroup analyses and thus not sufficiently powered to detect meaningful differences between the chemotherapy or chemoimmunotherapy groups, the magnitude of potential benefit of chemoimmunotherapy in never-smokers remains inconclusive and combination chemoimmunotherapy with four cycles of induction chemotherapy with or without maintenance bevacizumab remains a reasonable first-line treatment option in never-smokers (**Fig. 1**).

DURATION OF IMMUNOTHERAPY

The National Comprehensive Cancer Network guidelines recommend a duration of 2 years of immunotherapy in treatment-naive patients with advanced NSCLC; however, the optimal duration of therapy is unknown. The phase 3 noninferiority DICIPLE study aimed to assess whether a shorter duration of immunotherapy was as effective as the arbitrary 2-year treatment.[54] In this trial, patients with advanced NSCLC who received first-line ipilimumab/nivolumab and had disease control at 6 months were randomized to observation alone with reintroduction of doublet immunotherapy on progression ("stop and go" strategy) versus continuation of doublet immunotherapy for up to 2 years. The trial was prematurely discontinued because the application for ipilimumab/nivolumab was withdrawn in Europe in January 2020,[55] but its preliminary data demonstrated that in the 71 patients who achieved disease control and were included in the analysis, no difference in PFS (HR, 0.65; 95% CI, 0.29–1.49; $P = 0.31$) or OS (reported data were immature; HR, 0.52; 95% CI, 0.13–2.12; $P = 0.36$) was observed between the two groups at a median follow-up of 21 months,

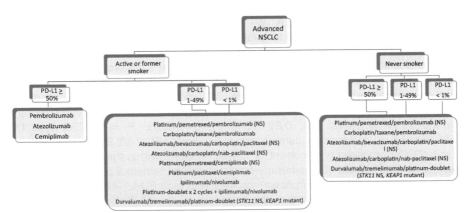

Fig. 1. Example of algorithm of treatment options for driver-negative advanced NSCLC by smoking status. In the regimens including atezolizumab, was defined to also include PD-L1 expression in tumor-infiltrating immune cells (IC): PD-L1 ≥50% of tumor cells (TC) or ≥10% of IC in high PD-L1 (noted as PD-L1 ≥50%), PD-L1 ≥1% of TC or IC and <50% of TC or <10% of IC in intermediate PD-L1 (noted as PD-L1 1-49%), and PD-L1 <1% of TC and IC in negative PD-L1 (noted as PD-L1 <1). NS, nonsquamous histology.

with no difference in grade 3 or higher immune-related side effects.[54] Although the trial was underpowered because of its early discontinuation, the study is hypothesis-generating and triggers an important question of whether a shorter, finite duration of therapy in advanced NSCLC is possible and remains to be further validated. With limited data in the first-line setting, in the second-line and beyond setting, continuous nivolumab was observed to have a superior PFS (24.7 months vs 9.4 months with fixed-duration nivolumab; HR, 0.56; 95% CI, 0.37–0.84) and OS (not reached vs 32.5 months with fixed-duration nivolumab; HR, 0.61; 95% CI, 0.37–0.99) compared with fixed-duration of nivolumab for 1 year in an exploratory analysis of Check-Mate153, a phase III/IV safety trial of nivolumab.[56] Until prospective trials are completed, optimal immunotherapy duration in advanced NSCLC in the first-line setting remains a shared clinical decision between the clinician and the patient.

IMMUNOTHERAPY SENSITIVITY, RESISTANCE, AND EXPLORATORY BIOMARKERS

Despite significant improvements in OS with ICI monotherapy and combination chemo-ICI, with up to one-third of patients alive in KEYNOTE-024[57] with pembrolizumab monotherapy and 20% alive in KEYNOTE-189[34] with chemoimmunotherapy at 5 years, response rates have only been reported to be about 50%. Thus, roughly 50% of patients not selected by PDL1 will experience primary resistance to chemoimmunotherapy, and 50% of those with PDL1 greater than or equal to 50% will experience primary resistance to PD1 axis inhibitor therapy alone. Although PD-L1 is currently the most reliable predictive biomarker for Immunotherapy response in advanced NSCLC, it remains imperfect because it lacks predictive potential in never-smokers and patients with driver mutations and often leads to variable testing results because of tumor heterogeneity. In addition, in the 5-year updated OS analysis of KEYNOTE-189, higher PD-L1 continued to demonstrate improved PFS with chemoimmunotherapy, but not for OS and biomarkers that may better predict long-term survival are still needed.[34]

Alternative biomarkers including tumor mutational burden (TMB) and its noninvasive counterpart, blood-based TMB (bTMB), have been explored. In the phase 3 CheckMate-026 study, which randomized treatment-naive advanced NSCLC without *EGFR* or *ALK* driver mutations to nivolumab or chemotherapy, the study did not meet its primary end point of PFS in the prespecific cohort of PD-L1 greater than or equal to 5%; however, patients with high TMB ($\geq$243 mutations/exome) were observed to have a superior PFS relative to chemotherapy compared with patients with low/medium TMB (low, 0–99 mutations/exome; medium, 100–242 mutations/exome).[25] In contrast, in the CheckMate 227 trial, no difference in median OS benefit was observed with TMB greater than or equal to 10 or TMB less than 10 with nivolumab/ipilimumab compared with chemotherapy.[58] Discordant results have also been observed with bTMB. Optimal PFS benefit was observed with atezolizumab relative to chemotherapy with bTMB greater than or equal to 16 (HR, 0.55; 95% CI, 0.33–0.92) in IMpower110,[20] and optimal OS benefit with durvalumab and tremelimumab relative to chemotherapy with bTMB greater than or equal to 20 in the MYSTIC trial,[26] both in exploratory analyses. However, in the BFAST trial cohort c analysis, the first phase 3 trial evaluating bTMB as a potential biomarker with ICI, no difference in PFS (HR, 0.77; 95% CI, 0.59–1.00) was demonstrated with atezolizumab monotherapy compared with chemotherapy in bTMB greater than or equal to 16.[59] Exploratory analysis of the BFAST (cohort c) trial demonstrated improved PFS with increased bTMB thresholds,[59] and whether bTMB may be a potential biomarker at higher bTMB thresholds remains inconclusive.

In addition to TMB, other biomarkers, such as *STK11* mutation associated with reduced PD-L1 expression[60] and *KEAP1* mutation associated with an immunosuppressive microenvironment,[61] identified in approximately 30% of lung adenocarcinomas,[62] have also been associated with reduced outcomes with immunotherapy, but only so far demonstrated in the *KRAS* mutant subgroup.[63] In the recently published POSEIDON trial,[64] which led to the FDA approval of combination durvalumab/tremelimumab/platinum-doublet chemotherapy in first-line *EGFR/ALK* WT NSCLC in November 2022, however, post hoc analysis demonstrated a trend toward OS benefit with the addition of durvalumab/tremelimumab to chemotherapy even within the *STK-11* mutant nonsquamous (HR, 0.56; 95% CI, 0.30–1.03) and *KEAP-1* mutant (HR, 0.43; 95% CI, 0.16–1.25) subgroups.[65] Although the analysis is only exploratory, durvalumab/tremelimumab/platinum-doublet chemotherapy may be a reasonable first-line option in *KRAS*-mutant patients with *STK-11* or *KEAP-1* mutations.

Multiple resistance mechanisms including alterations in T-cell signaling, alternate check-points (ie, TIGIT, LAG3), and microbiome, are being explored to improve immunotherapy clinical outcomes in advanced NSCLC.[66] Several clinical trials that use a biomarker directed treatment, such as KEYNOTE-495, which evaluates TMB and an immunogenic gene expression profile ($Tcell_{inf}GEP$) as predictive biomarkers, which has demonstrated preliminary clinical benefit within high TMB/high $Tcell_{inf}GEP$,[67] and INSIGNA (NCT03793179), which uses tumor informed signatures to evaluate differences in immunotherapy and chemotherapy sequencing are some examples of eagerly awaited trials to better identify patients who may derive greater benefit with immunotherapy-based regimens.

SUMMARY

PD-L1 continues to be the most reliable biomarker for the selection of treatment options in patients with advanced NSCLC with prior smoking history. Pembrolizumab, atezolizumab, and cemiplimab are all reasonable first-line immunotherapy options for PD-L1 greater than or equal to 50% in current or former smokers. For never-smokers with any PD-L1 and all patients with PD-L1 less than 50%, combination chemoimmunotherapy continues to be the favored treatment. In patients with PD-L1 less than 50% with prior smoking history, combination immunotherapy with short course induction chemotherapy or combination immunotherapy with ipilimumab/nivolumab are also reasonable first-line options in patients who may prefer "chemotherapy free" or short-term chemotherapy alternatives. Despite significant improvements in survival with the introduction of immunotherapy, only a minority of patients will achieve a sustained survival benefit, and a multibiomarker assay that may best predict immunotherapy response remains an active area of research.

CLINICS CARE POINTS

- Choice of first-line therapy for driver-negative metastatic NSCLC is dependent on multiple factors including PD-L1 TPS score, smoking history, disease burden, and performance status.
- PD-L1 is an established biomarker for immunotherapy monotherapy and chemoimmunotherapy in patients with prior smoking history.
- The significance of tumor PDL1 expression in advanced NSCLC in never smokers is uncertain.
- TMB and blood-TMB continue to be exploratory biomarkers in advanced NSCLC.

- Further research is needed to better selectively identify patients who may respond best to PD1 axis inhibitor therapy.

DISCLOSURES

Dr SY Kim has no disclosures. Dr S. Gettinger has received research funding for Yale University by BMS, NextCure, Genentech, Iovance, and Merck (drug only); serves on the safety board for BMS; and serves on the steering committee for the Iovance Clinical Trial.

REFERENCES

1. Schiller JH, Harrington D, Belani CP, et al. Comparison of four chemotherapy regimens for advanced non–small-cell lung cancer. N Engl J Med 2002;346:92–8.
2. Kelly K, Crowley J, Bunn PA Jr, et al. Randomized phase III trial of paclitaxel plus carboplatin versus vinorelbine plus cisplatin in the treatment of patients with advanced non–small-cell lung cancer: a southwest oncology group trial. J Clin Oncol 2001;19:3210–8.
3. Scagliotti GV, De Marinis F, Rinaldi M, et al. Phase III randomized trial comparing three platinum-based doublets in advanced non-small-cell lung cancer. J Clin Oncol 2002;20:4285 91.
4. Scagliotti GV, Parikh P, von Pawel J, et al. Phase III study comparing cisplatin plus gemcitabine with cisplatin plus pemetrexed in chemotherapy-naive patients with advanced-stage non-small-cell lung cancer. J Clin OncolJ Clin Oncol 2008;26: 3543–51.
5. Takezawa K, Okamoto I, Okamoto W, et al. Thymidylate synthase as a determinant of pemetrexed sensitivity in non-small cell lung cancer. Br J Cancer 2011; 104:1594–601.
6. Reck M, von Pawel J, Zatloukal P, et al. Phase III trial of cisplatin plus gemcitabine with either placebo or bevacizumab as first-line therapy for nonsquamous non-small-cell lung cancer: AVAiL. J Clin Oncol 2009;27:1227–34.
7. Reck M, von Pawel J, Zatloukal P, et al. Overall survival with cisplatin-gemcitabine and bevacizumab or placebo as first-line therapy for nonsquamous non-small-cell lung cancer: results from a randomised phase III trial (AVAiL). Ann Oncol 2010;21:1804–9.
8. Johnson DH, Fehrenbacher L, Novotny WF, et al. Randomized phase II trial comparing bevacizumab plus carboplatin and paclitaxel with carboplatin and paclitaxel alone in previously untreated locally advanced or metastatic non-small-cell lung cancer. J Clin Oncol 2004;22:2184–91.
9. Sandler A, Gray R, Perry MC, et al. Paclitaxel-carboplatin alone or with bevacizumab for non-small-cell lung cancer. N Engl J Med 2006;355:2542–50.
10. Jain RK. Normalizing tumor vasculature with anti-angiogenic therapy: a new paradigm for combination therapy. Nat Med 2001;7:987–9.
11. Willett CG, Boucher Y, di Tomaso E, et al. Direct evidence that the VEGF-specific antibody bevacizumab has antivascular effects in human rectal cancer. Nat Med 2004;10:145–7.
12. Boulanger J, Boursiquot JN, Cournoyer G, et al. Management of hypersensitivity to platinum- and taxane-based chemotherapy: cepo review and clinical recommendations. Curr Oncol 2014;21:e630–41.

13. Desai N, Trieu V, Yao Z, et al. Increased antitumor activity, intratumor paclitaxel concentrations, and endothelial cell transport of cremophor-free, albumin-bound paclitaxel, ABI-007, compared with cremophor-based paclitaxel. Clin Cancer Res 2006;12:1317–24.

14. Socinski MA, Bondarenko I, Karaseva NA, et al. Weekly nab-paclitaxel in combination with carboplatin versus solvent-based paclitaxel plus carboplatin as first-line therapy in patients with advanced non–small-cell lung cancer: final results of a phase III trial. J Clin Oncol 2012;30:2055–62.

15. Ishida Y, Agata Y, Shibahara K, et al. Induced expression of PD-1, a novel member of the immunoglobulin gene superfamily, upon programmed cell death. EMBO J 1992;11:3887–95.

16. Dong H, Strome SE, Salomao DR, et al. Tumor-associated B7-H1 promotes T-cell apoptosis: a potential mechanism of immune evasion. Nat Med 2002;8:793–800.

17. Curiel TJ, Wei S, Dong H, et al. Blockade of B7-H1 improves myeloid dendritic cell–mediated antitumor immunity. Nat Med 2003;9:562–7.

18. Reck M, Rodríguez-Abreu D, Robinson AG, et al. Pembrolizumab versus chemotherapy for PD-L1–positive non–small-cell lung cancer. N Engl J Med 2016;375: 1823–33.

19. Mok TSK, Wu YL, Kudaba I, et al. Pembrolizumab versus chemotherapy for previously untreated, PD-L1-expressing, locally advanced or metastatic non-small-cell lung cancer (KEYNOTE-042): a randomised, open-label, controlled, phase 3 trial. Lancet 2019;393:1819–30.

20. Herbst RS, Giaccone G, de Marinis F, et al. Atezolizumab for first-line treatment of PD-L1-selected patients with NSCLC. N Engl J Med 2020;383:1328–39.

21. Sezer A, Kilickap S, Gümüş M, et al. Cemiplimab monotherapy for first-line treatment of advanced non-small-cell lung cancer with PD-L1 of at least 50%: a multicentre, open-label, global, phase 3, randomised, controlled trial. Lancet 2021; 397:592–604.

22. Aguilar EJ, Ricciuti B, Gainor JF, et al. Outcomes to first-line pembrolizumab in patients with non-small-cell lung cancer and very high PD-L1 expression. Ann Oncol 2019;30:1653–9.

23. Ricciuti B, Elkrief A, Alessi JVM, et al. Three-year outcomes and correlative analyses in patients with non–small cell lung cancer (NSCLC) and a very high PD-L1 tumor proportion score (TPS) $\geq$ 90% treated with first-line pembrolizumab. J Clin Oncol 2022;40:9043.

24. Majem M.M., Cobo M., Isla D., et al., PD-(L)1 inhibitors as monotherapy for the first-line treatment of non-small-cell lung cancer patients with high PD-L1 expression: a network meta-analysis, J Clin Med, 10, 2021, doi:10.3390/jcm10071365.

25. Carbone DP, Reck M, Paz-Ares L, et al. First-line nivolumab in stage IV or recurrent non–small-cell lung cancer. N Engl J Med 2017;376:2415–26.

26. Rizvi NA, Cho BC, Reinmuth N, et al. Durvalumab with or without tremelimumab vs standard chemotherapy in first-line treatment of metastatic non–small cell lung cancer: the MYSTIC phase 3 randomized clinical trial. JAMA Oncol 2020;6: 661–74.

27. Middleton G, Brock K, Savage J, et al. Pembrolizumab in patients with non-small-cell lung cancer of performance status 2 (PePS2): a single arm, phase 2 trial. Lancet Respir Med 2020;8:895–904.

28. Lee SM, SSchulz C, Prabhash K, et al. IPSOS: results from a phase III study of first-line (1L) atezolizumab (atezo) vs single-agent chemotherapy (chemo) in patients (pts) with NSCLC not eligible for a platinum-containing regimen. Ann Oncol 2022;33:S808–69.

29. Boyer M, Şendur MAN, Rodríguez-Abreu D, et al. Pembrolizumab plus ipilimumab or placebo for metastatic non-small-cell lung cancer with PD-L1 tumor proportion score ≥ 50%: randomized, double-blind phase III KEYNOTE-598 study. J Clin Oncol 2021;39:2327–38.

30. Akinboro O, Vallejo JJ, Nakajima EC, et al. Outcomes of anti–PD-(L)1 therapy with or without chemotherapy (chemo) for first-line (1L) treatment of advanced non–small cell lung cancer (NSCLC) with PD-L1 score ≥ 50%: FDA pooled analysis. J Clin Oncol 2022;40:9000.

31. Gandhi L, Rodríguez-Abreu D, Gadgeel S, et al. Pembrolizumab plus chemotherapy in metastatic non–small-cell lung cancer. N Engl J Med 2018;378:2078–92.

32. Paz-Ares L, Luft A, Vicente D, et al. Pembrolizumab plus chemotherapy for squamous non–small-cell lung cancer. N Engl J Med 2018;379:2040–51.

33. Socinski MA, Jotte RM, Cappuzzo F, et al. Atezolizumab for first-line treatment of metastatic nonsquamous NSCLC. N Engl J Med 2018;378:2288–301.

34. Garassino MC, Gadgeel SM, Speranza G, et al. KEYNOTE-189 5-year update: first-line pembrolizumab(pembro) + pemetrexed (pem) and platinum vs placebo (pbo) + pem and platinum for metastatic nonsquamous NSCLC. Ann Oncol 2022; 33:S448–554.

35. Novello S, Kowalski DM, Luft A, et al. 5-year update from KEYNOTE-407: pembrolizumab plus chemotherapy in squamous non-small cell lung cancer (NSCLC). Ann Oncol 2022;33:S448–554.

36. Garon EB, Rizvi NA, Hui R, et al. Pembrolizumab for the treatment of non–small-cell lung cancer. N Engl J Med 2015;372:2018–28.

37. Borghaei H, Paz-Ares L, Horn L, et al. Nivolumab versus docetaxel in advanced nonsquamous non–small-cell lung cancer. N Engl J Med 2015;373:1627–39.

38. Herbst RS, Baas P, Kim DW, et al. Pembrolizumab versus docetaxel for previously treated, PD-L1-positive, advanced non-small-cell lung cancer (KEYNOTE-010): a randomised controlled trial. Lancet 2016;387:1540–50.

39. Gainor JF, Shaw AT, Sequist LV, et al. EGFR mutations and ALK rearrangements are associated with low response rates to PD-1 pathway blockade in non-small cell lung cancer: a retrospective analysis. Clin Cancer Res 2016;22:4585–93.

40. Akbay EA, Koyama S, Carretero J, et al. Activation of the PD-1 pathway contributes to immune escape in EGFR-driven lung tumors. Cancer Discov 2013;3: 1355–63.

41. Zhang N, Zeng Y, Du W, et al. The EGFR pathway is involved in the regulation of PD-L1 expression via the IL-6/JAK/STAT3 signaling pathway in EGFR-mutated non-small cell lung cancer. Int J Oncol 2016;49:1360–8.

42. Ota K, Azuma K, Kawahara A, et al. Induction of PD-L1 expression by the EML4-ALK oncoprotein and downstream signaling pathways in non-small cell lung cancer. Clin Cancer Res 2015;21:4014–21.

43. West H, McCleod M, Hussein M, et al. Atezolizumab in combination with carboplatin plus nab-paclitaxel chemotherapy compared with chemotherapy alone as first-line treatment for metastatic non-squamous non-small-cell lung cancer (IMpower130): a multicentre, randomised, openlabel, phase 3 trial. Lancet Oncol 2019;20:924–37.

44. Jotte R, Cappuzzo F, Vynnychenko I, et al. Atezolizumab in combination with carboplatin and nab-paclitaxel in advanced squamous NSCLC (IMpower131): results from a randomized phase III trial. J Thorac Oncol 2020;15:1351–60.

45. Gogishvili M, Melkadze T, Makharadze T, et al. Cemiplimab plus chemotherapy versus chemotherapy alone in non-small cell lung cancer: a randomized,

controlled, double-blind phase 3 trial. Nat Med 2022. https://doi.org/10.1038/s41591-022-01977-y.

46. Kraehenbuehl L, Weng CH, Eghbali S, et al. Enhancing immunotherapy in cancer by targeting emerging immunomodulatory pathways. Nat Rev Clin Oncol 2022; 19:37–50.

47. Hellmann MD, Paz-Ares L, Caro RB, et al. Nivolumab plus ipilimumab in advanced non–small-cell lung cancer. N Engl J Med 2019;381:2020–31.

48. Paz-Ares LG, Ramalingam SS, Ciuleanu TE, et al. First-line nivolumab plus ipilimumab in advanced NSCLC: 4-year outcomes from the randomized, open-label, phase 3 CheckMate 227 Part 1 trial. J Thorac Oncol 2022;17:289–308.

49. Paz-Ares L, Ciuleanu TE, Cobo M, et al. First-line nivolumab plus ipilimumab combined with two cycles of chemotherapy in patients with nonsmall-cell lung cancer (CheckMate 9LA): an international, randomised, open-label, phase 3 trial. Lancet Oncol 2021;22:198–211.

50. Paz-Ares LG, Ciuleanu TE, Cobo-Dols M, et al. First-line (1L) nivolumab (NIVO) + ipilimumab (IPI) + 2 cycles of chemotherapy (chemo) versus chemo alone (4 cycles) in patients (pts) with metastatic non-small cell lung cancer (NSCLC): 3-year update from CheckMate 9LA. J Clin Oncol 2022;40:LBA9026.

51. Reck M, Rodríguez–Abreu D, Robinson AG, et al. Updated analysis of KEYNOTE-024: pembrolizumab versus platinum-based chemotherapy for advanced non–small-cell lung cancer with PD-L1 tumor proportion score of 50% or greater. J Clin Oncol 2019;37:537–46.

52. Cortellini A, De Giglio A, Cannita K, et al. Smoking status during first-line immunotherapy and chemotherapy in NSCLC patients: a case-control matched analysis from a large multicenter study. Thorac Cancer 2021;12:880–9.

53. Socinski MA, Nishio M, Jotte RM, et al. IMpower150 final overall survival analyses for atezolizumab plus bevacizumab and chemotherapy in first-line metastatic nonsquamous NSCLC. J Thorac Oncol 2021;16:1909–24.

54. Zalcman G, FFlandin AM, Molinier O, et al. Nivolumab (Nivo) plus ipilimumab (Ipi) 6-months treatment versus continuation in patients with advanced non-small cell lung cancer (aNSCLC): Results of the randomized IFCT-1701 phase III trial. Ann Oncol 2022;33:S448–554.

55. European Medicine Agency. Opdivo: Withdrawal of the application to change the marketing authorisation, Available at: https://www.ema.europa.eu/en/medicines/human/withdrawn-applications/opdivo-2. 2020. Accessed October 1, 2022.

56. Waterhouse DM, Garon EB, Chandler J, et al. Continuous versus 1-year fixed-duration nivolumab in previously treated advanced non–smallcell lung cancer: CheckMate 153. J Clin Oncol 2020;38:3863–73.

57. Reck M, Rodríguez-Abreu D, Robinson AG, et al. Five-year outcomes with pembrolizumab versus chemotherapy for metastatic non–small-cell lung cancer with PD-L1 tumor proportion, Score ≥ 50. J Clin Oncol 2021;39:2339–49.

58. Hellmann MD, Ciuleanu TE, Pluzanski A, et al. Nivolumab plus ipilimumab in lung cancer with a high tumor mutational burden. N Engl J Med 2018;378:2093–104.

59. Peters S, Dziadziuszko R, Morabito A, et al. Atezolizumab versus chemotherapy in advanced or metastatic NSCLC with high blood-based tumor mutational burden: primary analysis of BFAST cohort C randomized phase 3 trial. Nat Med 2022;28:1831–9.

60. Lamberti G, Spurr LF, Li Y, et al. Clinicopathological and genomic correlates of programmed cell death ligand 1 (PD-L1)expression in nonsquamous non-small-cell lung cancer. Ann Oncol 2020;31:807–14.

61. Best SA, De Souza DP, Kersbergen A, et al. Synergy between the KEAP1/NRF2 and PI3K pathways drives non-small-celllung cancer with an altered immune microenvironment. Cell Metabol 2018;27:935–43.e4.

62. Network CGAR. Comprehensive molecular profiling of lung adenocarcinoma. Nature 2014;511:543.

63. Ricciuti B, Arbour KC, Lin JJ, et al. Diminished efficacy of programmed death-(Ligand)1 inhibitionin STK11- and KEAP1-mutant lung adenocarcinoma is affected by KRAS mutation status. J Thorac Oncol 2022;17:399–410.

64. Johnson ML, Cho BC, Luft A, et al. Durvalumab With or without tremelimumab in combination with chemotherapy as first-line therapy for metastatic non–small-cell lung cancer: the phase III POSEIDON study. J Clin OncolJ Clin Oncol 2022; 22:975.

65. Peters S, Cho BC, Luft A, et al. OA15.04 Association bbetween KRAS/STK11/KEAP1 mutations and outcomes in POSEIDON: durvalumab ± tremelimumab + chemotherapy in mNSCLC. J Thorac Oncol 2022;17:S39–41.

66. Vesely MD, Zhang T, Chen L. Resistance mechanisms to anti-PD cancer immunotherapy. Annu Rev Immunol 2022;40:45–74.

67. Gutierrez M, Lam WS, Hellman M, et al. 457 KEYNOTE-495/KeyImPaCT: interim analysis of a randomized, biomarker-directed, phase 2 trial of pembrolizumab-based combination therapy for non–small cell lung cancer (NSCLC). Journal for ImmunoTherapy of Cancer 2021;9:A485.

Targeted Therapy for Non–Small Cell Lung Cancer
First Line and Beyond

Elliott Brea, MD PhD[a], Julia Rotow, MD[b],*

KEYWORDS

- Non–small cell lung cancer • Oncogenes • Targeted therapy • Resistance

KEY POINTS

- Comprehensive genomic profiling is necessary to guide optimal first-line treatment in advanced/metastatic lung adenocarcinoma.
- Limited biomarker testing to include EGFR is now indicated in patients with surgically resectable early-stage or locally advanced lung adenocarcinoma.
- First-line therapy for NSCLC with most EGFR, ALK, ROS1, RET, NTRK, BRAF, or ME-Tex14 oncogenic alterations is generally the preferred treatment option. For KRAS G12C, HER2, and EGFR exon 20 insertions targeted therapies are currently approved for second line or later.
- Repeat genomic profiling at acquired targeted therapy resistance may offer personalized sequential targeted therapy strategies.

INTRODUCTION

The discovery of oncogenic driver alterations and the rapid expansion of associated oncogene-targeted therapeutic options have transformed outcomes for patients with non–small cell lung cancer (NSCLC) (**Fig. 1**). Targeted therapeutics generally offer the dual advantages of improved efficacy and improved tolerability compared with alternative therapeutic strategies. Targeted therapeutics have become the established standard of care for NSCLC bearing an actionable driver mutation, and for patients with an actionable driver the receipt of guideline-concordant care with a targeted therapy improves survival.[1]

PREVALENCE AND IDENTIFICATION OF ACTIONABLE ONCOGENIC DRIVERS

Established actionable driver alterations in lung cancer may be found in EGFR, BRAF, MET, KRAS, HER2, ALK, ROS1, RET, and NTRK (**Table 1**). Appropriate comprehensive

[a] Department of Medical Oncology, Dana-Farber Cancer Institute, SM353, 450 Brookline Avenue, Boston, MA 02215, USA; [b] Dana-Farber Cancer Institute, 450 Brookline Avenue, DA1240, Boston, MA 02215, USA
* Corresponding author.
E-mail address: julia_rotow@dfci.harvard.edu

Hematol Oncol Clin N Am 37 (2023) 575–594
https://doi.org/10.1016/j.hoc.2023.02.009
0889-8588/23/© 2023 Elsevier Inc. All rights reserved.
hemonc.theclinics.com

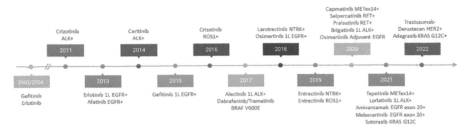

Fig. 1. Timeline of targeted therapy approvals for NSCLC. Key approvals of targeted thera-peutics in NSCLC, highlighting ongoing expansion in number of actionable oncogenic targets.

biomarker testing in patients with advanced NSCLC includes evaluation of all these tar-gets. Although this can be completed via single-gene panels, next-generation sequencing (NGS) offers an efficient comprehensive testing strategy. Actionable driver mutations are enriched in younger patients with minimal or no history of tobacco use and are most commonly identified in NSCLC with adenocarcinoma histology.[2] These alterations can be found at lower rates in other demographic groups and on rare occa-sions are found in squamous lung primaries.[3,4] For patients with lung adenocarcinoma aged less than 40 years the probability of an actionable driver alteration may be greater than 80%.[5] Of note, the recent approval of KRAS G12C-directed therapies has estab-lished a driver mutation that is enriched in older patients and those with a history of tobacco use.[2] Current practice guidelines call for completion of comprehensive genomic testing in advanced nonsquamous NSCLC and consideration for genomic testing in patients with squamous histology. Select biomarker testing is now also indi-cated in resectable NSCLC where PD-L1, EGFR, and in some circumstances ALK testing may guide recommendations around perioperative systemic therapy.

Modern hybrid capture-based DNA sequencing NGS assays have reduced sensi-tivity for detection of certain more-difficult-to-capture genomic alterations, including for most of the actionable gene fusions in NSCLC. RNA-sequencing-based assays can add sensitivity for gene fusion detection and can now be sent as commercial as-says in routine clinical practice. In one series, among NGS-negative adenocarcinoma 14% of tumors were positive for an oncogenic gene fusion or rearrangement by RNA sequencing.[6]

Plasma-based, cell-free DNA (cfDNA) sequencing assays offer a complementary strategy for biomarker testing. The more rapid turnaround times and the noninvasive nature of this assay may promote completion of biomarker testing before the initiation of first-line therapy.[7] The sensitivity of cfDNA for biomarker detection is impacted by the extent of systemic tumor DNA shed, and therefore a negative cfDNA assay cannot be used to reliably rule out the presence of an actionable driver. Patients with inade-quate tissue samples to permit full biomarker testing may require repeat tissue biopsy.

THE FUSION DRIVERS: ALK, ROS1, RET, AND NTRK
ALK Fusions

EML4-ALK fusions are identified in ~4% of lung adenocarcinomas,[8] and can be iden-tified via immunohistochemistry (IHC), fluorescence in situ hybridization (FISH), or NGS testing.[9]

The first ALK inhibitor, crizotinib, was approved by the US Food and Drug Adminis-tration (FDA) in 2011 and subsequently approved for first-line treatment following the PROFILE 1014 study, which demonstrated superiority to first-line platinum doublet

Table 1
Clinical efficacy of oncogene-targeted therapies in biomarker-selected advanced/metastatic non-small cell lung cancer

Oncogene/TKI	ORR (%)	PFS	OS	Trial/Reference
ALK				
Crizotinib 1L (vs chemo)	74% (vs 45%)	10.9 mo (vs 7.0 mo)	56.6% at 4 y (vs 49.1%)	PROFILE 1014[10,112]
Ceritinib 1L (vs chemo)	72.5% (vs 26.7%)	16.6 mo (vs 8.1 mo)	NR	ASCEND-4[13]
Brigatinib 1L (vs crizotinib)	71% (vs 60%)	24.0 mo (vs 11.1 mo)	71% at 3 y (vs 68%)	ALTA-1L[14,113]
Alectinib 1L (vs crizotinib)	82.9% (vs 75.5%)	34.8 mo (vs 10.9 mo)	62.5% at 5 y (vs 45.5%)	ALEX[11,12]
Lorlatinib 1L (vs crizotinib)	76% (vs 58%)	64% at 3 y (vs 19%)	NR	CROWN[15,16]
ROS1				
Crizotinib	72%	19.3 mo	51.4 mo	PROFILE 1001[21]
Entrectinib	68%	15.7 mo	47.8 mo	[23]
Lorlatinib (2L)	35%	DoR 13.8 mo	NR	[25]
RET				
Selpercatinib	84%	22 mo	NR	LIBRETTO-001[30]
Pralsetinib	72%	13 mo[a]	NR	ARROW[32]
NTRK				
Larotrectinib[b]	79%	28.5 mo	44.4 mo	[37]
Entrectinib[b]	57%	11 mo	21 mo	[38]
EGFR, common				
Osimertinib 1L (vs first-generation TKI)	80% (vs 76%)	18.9 mo (vs 10.2 mo)	38.6 mo (vs 31.8 mo)	FLAURA[44,45]
Erlotinib 1L (vs chemo)	83% (vs 36%)	13.1 mo (vs 4.6 mo)	22.8 mo (vs 27.2 mo)	OPTIMAL[114]
Afatinib (vs chemo)	56% (vs 23%)	11.1 mo (vs 6.9 mo)	28.2 mo (vs 28.2 mo)	LUX-Lung 3[115,116]
EGFR, uncommon				
Afatinib	71.1%	10.7 mo	19.4 mo	LUX-Lung 2,3,6[117]
Osimertinib	50%	8.2 mo	NR	[56]
EGFR exon 20ins				

(continued on next page)

Table 1
(continued)

Oncogene/TKI	ORR (%)	PFS	OS	Trial/Reference
Amivantamab 2L+	40%	8.3 mo	22.8 mo	CHRYSALIS[58]
Mobocertinib 2L+	25%–28%	7.3 mo	24 mo	EXCLAIM/PPP[59]
HER2 mutations				
T-DXd 2L+	55%	8.2 mo	17.8 mo	DESTINY-Lung01[64]
BRAF				
Dabrafenib/trametinib 1L	1L 62.3%	1L 10.8 mo	1L 17.3 mo	[118]
METex14				
Capmatinib	1L 68%,	1L 12.4 mo	NR	GEOMETRY mono-1[119]
Tepotinib	1L 61.3%	1L 13.8 mo	1L 18.8 mo	VISION[77,120]
KRAS G12 C				
Sotorasib 2L + vs chemo	28.1% (vs 13.2%)	5.6 mo (vs 4.5 mo)	10.6 mo (vs 11.3 mo)	CodeBreak 200[81]
Adagrasib 2L+	42.9%	6.5 mo	12.6 mo	KRYSTAL-1[82]

Abbreviations: 1L, first-line; 2L, second-line; BIRC, blinded independent review committee; chemo, chemotherapy; DoR, duration of response; Inv, investigator assessed; NR, not reached/reported; ORR, overall response rate; OS, overall survival; PFS, progression free survival; TKI, tyrosine kinase inhibitor.
[a] Including preamendment chemo-ineligible patient population.
[b] Fusion-positive solid tumors.

chemotherapy (overall response rate [ORR] 74% vs 45%, progression-free survival [PFS] 10.9 vs 7 months).[10] Subsequently the second-generation ALK inhibitors ceritinib, alectinib, and brigatinib were developed, offering greater potency and selectivity, greater central nervous system (CNS) activity, and improved side effect profiles. The phase 3 ALEX trial compared first-line alectinib with crizotinib and demonstrated superior median PFS (34.8 vs 10.9 months), 5-year OS [62.5% vs 45.5%], and CNS control with alectinib therapy,[11,12] and has been a preferred first-line therapy for ALK-positive lung cancer since its FDA approval in 2017. Both ceritinib and brigatinib also carry first-line approvals for ALK-positive lung cancer based on the ASCEND-4 and ALTA-1L studies, respectively, although they are less frequently used in first-line clinical practice.[13,14] The third-generation ALK inhibitor lorlatinib, initially used to manage acquired ALK second-site resistance mutations, has now also demonstrated superiority to crizotinib in the first-line setting based on data from the CROWN study. Although data are less mature, the 36-month PFS (64%) and CNS response rate (82% CNS ORR, 71% CNS complete response rate) also compare favorably with historical controls.[15,16] Alectinib and lorlatinib have not been directly compared in a prospective clinical trial and, although differing in adverse effect profiles, both remain preferred first-line treatment strategies for ALK-positive lung cancer. The available ALK inhibitors share some overlapping adverse effects, such as risk of LFT abnormalities, as well as more drug-specific toxicities including myalgias on alectinib, pulmonary toxicity on brigatinib, and neurocognitive and metabolic toxicities on lorlatinib.[12,14,15]

Both "on-target" acquired ALK resistance mutations and bypass pathway activation are observed at ALK tyrosine kinase inhibitor (TKI) resistance, and the spectrum of acquired resistance mutations differs by the ALK inhibitor. For example, the second-generation ALK TKIs are active against the crizotinib-resistant L1196M gatekeeper mutations, and lorlatinib is active against the G1202R solvent front mutation, which produces resistance to all first- and second-generation TKIs.[17] Lorlatinib has demonstrated activity in patients with progression on prior ALK TKI therapy, with higher response rates in patients with detectable acquired ALK mutations.[18] In patients with ALK-independent resistance mechanisms, MET amplification has emerged as a possible resistance pathway actionable via addition of a MET TKI.[19] Sequential ALK TKI therapy may produce compound ALK resistance mutations resistant to all currently approved ALK TKIs. Next-generation ALKi inhibitors are in development, which may target these compound mutations.[20]

ROS1 Fusions

Oncogenic ROS1 fusions are seen in approximately 1% of NSCLC.[16] ROS1 has a variety of fusion partners, with CD74 as the most common, followed by EZR, SDC4, and others.[17] Crizotinib was the first ROS1 inhibitor shown to have activity in patients with a response rate of 72% and a PFS of 19.3 months in the PROFILE 1001 trial.[21] Entrectinib, a ROS1 and TRK inhibitor, is also approved for ROS1-positive NSCLC with comparable response rate (68%) and median PFS (15.7 months). Entrectinib is also active against CNS metastases with an 80% intracranial response rate.[22,23] Both agents are an appropriate first-line treatment choice for ROS1-positive lung cancer given similar systemic efficacy data; crizotinib carries reduced risk of the neurocognitive adverse effects, which may render this strategy a preferred option for many patients, whereas entrectinib offers improved CNS control and is the preferred option in patients with known CNS involvement.

ALK, ROS1, RET, and NTRK share homologous kinase domains, and analogous acquired resistance mutations are observed at TKI resistance.[24] The most frequent on-target resistance mutation to ROS1 inhibitors is the ROS1 G2032 R solvent front mutation, which confers resistance to crizotinib, entrectinib, and lorlatinib. However, a wide range of second-site ROS1 mutations or bypass pathway activating mutations can be identified at TKI resistance, and the predicted activity of individual ROS1 inhibitors against these acquired mutations varies.[24] In clinic practice, or absent acquired resistance genomic profiling, off-label lorlatinib has shown activity at crizotinib resistance with a response rate of 35%.[25] Next-generation ROS1 inhibitors with predicted activity against ROS1 G2032 are in clinical development.[26,27]

RET Fusions

Oncogenic RET fusions are similarly rare but seen in 1% to 2% lung adenocarcinomas. RET has several fusion partners that have been detected, with the most common being KIF5B followed by CCDC6 with many others described.[28,29] Two potent and selective RET inhibitors, selpercatinib and pralsetinib, have shown high degrees of activity in patients previously treated or treatment-naive patients with RET fusions. In the LIBRETTO-001 trial, selpercatinib demonstrated an ORR of 61% for patients previously treated with chemotherapy and 84% (PFS 22.0 months) for treatment-naive patients.[30] In the ARROW study, pralsetinib demonstrated similarly high ORR of 72% in treatment-naive patients. Interpretation of first-line pralsetinib PFS data is complicated by initial first-line treatment only of those patients medically not eligible for platinum doublet chemotherapy followed by amendment to broaden enrollment criteria, with the median PFS across both study periods being 13 months and median PFS postamendment pending data maturity.[31,32] Tolerability is similar; both agents may cause hepatotoxicity with a greater reported rate of hypertension on selpercatinib and of cytopenias on pralsetinib.

The most common acquired second-site RET mutations following potent RET inhibitor therapy are the RET G810X solvent front mutations.[33] Off-target mutations in the MAPK pathway have also been observed such as KRAS, BRAF, MET amplification, and others.[34] Next-generation RET inhibitors such as LOXO-260 have emerged that show preclinical activity against G810X.[35]

NTRK Fusions

Oncogenic NTRK fusions are found across a wide spectrum of solid tumors and are rare in NSCLC, with prevalence below 1%. These fusions involve NTRK1, NTRK2, or NTRK3 (encoding TrkA, TrkB, or TrkC, respectively) with a variety of upstream fusion partners (eg, TPM3, CD74, ETV6) containing dimerization domains.[36] The Trk-selective TKI larotrectinib has demonstrated high response rate in a pooled analysis of NTRK fusion-positive solid tumors with an objective response rate of 79%, and with comparable ORR of 75% within NTRK-positive NSCLC. Responses are durable with a median PFS of 28.5 months. Larotrectinib is CNS active with a CNS response rate of 75%.[37] Entrectinib, an NTRK and ROS1 inhibitor, is also FDA approved for NTRK-positive solid tumors based on the pan-cancer ALKA/STARTRK-1/STARTRK-2 studies, however, with a lower pooled response rate of 57% and a median PFS of 11 months.[38] The NTRK second-site resistance mutations are analogous to those seen in ALK and ROS1 fusion-positive lung cancer.[39] Next-generation NTRK inhibitors, such as repotrectinib, predicted to be active against acquired resistance mutations are in clinical trials.[40]

EGFR ACTIVATING MUTATIONS

Activating EGFR mutations comprise the most common of the actionable genomic driver mutations in lung adenocarcinoma and are found in ~15% of patients in North

American populations and in up to 40% in Asian populations.[41] The EGFR mutations can be divided into 3 categories: (1) the common EGFR L858R and exon 19 deletions, (2) the uncommon EGFR activating mutations (eg, G719X, L861Q, S768I), and (3) the EGFR exon 20 insertions.[42]

There are currently 5 EGFR inhibitors with FDA approval for EGFR exon 19 deletions/L858R (~85% of EGFR-mutant lung cancer): the first-generation inhibitors erlotinib and gefitinib, the second-generation inhibitors afatinib and dacomitinib, and the third-generation inhibitor osimertinib. First-line osimertinib, first developed to treat the acquired EGFR T790M gatekeeper resistance mutation, was shown to be superior to first-generation EGFR TKIs in the phase 3 FLAURA study with a median PFS of 18.9 versus 10.2 months, improved overall survival of 38.6 versus 31.8 months, and improved CNS control (CNS ORR 91% vs 68%).[43,44] The use of a third-generation inhibitor is additionally associated with a lower risk of treatment-related cutaneous toxicities.[45]

Acquired resistance to osimertinib is heterogeneous and may include EGFR second-site mutations (eg, EGFR C797X, which impacts the residue at which osimertinib covalently binds), MET amplification, alternative oncogenic driver alterations (BRAF, RET, ALK fusions), RAS pathway mutations, and histologic transformation, some of which may lend themselves to off-label targeted therapy strategies.[46] Among the identifiable genomic mechanisms of resistance, EGFR C797X (~7%) and MET amplification (~15% to 30%) are the most common.[47] Repeat NGS profiling at acquired osimertinib resistance, although not mandated by standard of care, may inform subsequent treatment decisions. For example, the addition of tepotinib to osimertinib for acquired MET amplification was associated with a 54.5% response rate.[48] Case series and individual case reports have similarly suggested activity of combination TKI therapies targeting acquired RET, ALK, and BRAF activating alterations.[49–51] Other strategies under investigation include EGFR TKI/EGFR-MET bispecific combination therapy with amivantamab/lazertinib,[52] C797X-active fourth-generation EGFR TKIs,[53] and antibody-drug conjugate therapy[54] at EGFR TKI resistance.

The uncommon EGFR mutations (~10% of EGFR mutations[42]) are heterogeneous and variable in their responsiveness to EGFR TKI therapy. Afatinib is FDA approved for the most common of these uncommon mutations (G719X, L861Q, S768I) based on pooled analysis of the LUX lung studies with a response rate of 71.1%.[55] Osimertinib may also be used off-label, with a response rate of 50% in a smaller single-arm study, with favorable toxicity profile and CNS activity.[56] Structural modeling may inform therapy selection for the uncommon mutations.[42]

The EGFR exon 20 insertions (~5%–10% of EGFR mutations) are distinct in their resistance to the first- through third-generation EGFR inhibitors.[57] There are now 2 approved treatments for EGFR exon 20 insertions, both approved in the second-line or later setting. Amivantamab, an EGFR-MET bispecific antibody, was active in the CHRYSALIS study with a response rate of 40% (clinical benefit rate 74%) and a PFS of 8.3 months. Common adverse effects on this intravenous agent include risk of infusion reactions during first doses of treatment.[58] The EGFR exon 20 insertion-active TKI mobocertinib is also approved for previously treated EGFR exon 20ins-positive NSCLC with response rates of 25% to 28% and a median PFS of 7.3 months. Diarrhea is common on mobocertinib, occurring in more than 90% of patients.[59] Novel EGFR exon 20 inhibitors intended to offer greater potency, selectivity, and/or CNS activity are in development (eg, BLU-451,[60] CLN-081,[61] DZD9008[62]).

Other treatment strategies under evaluation include the role of upfront combination therapy for EGFR-mutated lung cancer. Examples of upfront combination strategies in clinical trials include use of first-line osimertinib plus platinum doublet chemotherapy (FLAURA2, NCT04035486) or amivantamab/lazertinib (MARIPOSA, NCT04487080).

HER2 ACTIVATING MUTATIONS

HER2, like EGFR, is a member of the ERBB family, and the 2 proteins share high kinase domain homology.[63] HER2 activating mutations, rather than overexpression, are the actionable biomarker of greatest interest in NSCLC. Most activating HER2 mutations in NSCLC (2% of lung adenocarcinoma) are HER2 exon 20 insertion mutations, predominantly the HER2 A775_G776insYVMA mutation.[63] Additional activating HER2 point mutations make up the remainder and are also encompassed by current HER2-targeted drug approvals. The HER2-ADC trastuzumab-deruxtecan (T-DXd) is the first approved agent for HER2-mutant NSCLC, with approval based on the DESTINY-Lung01 and DESTINY-Lung02 studies. In DESTINY-Lung01 T-DXd was active in previously treated patients with a response rate of 55% and disease control rate of 92%.[64] The FDA-approved dose was ultimately a lower dose (5.4 mg/kg) than that evaluated in Lung01, which produced a reduced risk of treatment-related toxicity, most notably a reduced risk of interstitial lung disease.[65] There are no current first-line HER2-targeted therapies in lung cancer, and chemoimmunotherapy is commonly used first line for this patient population. Current areas of active investigation in HER2-mutant lung cancer include evaluation of T-DXd in the first-line setting[66] and development of HER2 exon 20 insertion-active TKIs. Both pyrotinib and poziotinib, which inhibit EGFR and HER2 exon 20ins, have shown clinical activity, however were complicated by toxicity.[67,68] Additional HER2 exon 20ins-targeted TKIs are in development (NCT05650879, NCT05315700).

BRAF MUTATIONS

Activating BRAF mutations are found in ~3% of lung adenocarcinomas, ~50% of which will be the class I BRAF V600E mutation for which oncogene-targeted treatment with dabrafenib/trametinib is currently approved in NSCLC.[69] The BRAF V600E mutation leads to RAS-dependent monomeric BRAF activation. The remaining BRAF mutations are classified as class II or III mutations, and lead to MEK/ERK pathway activation either through RAS-independent dimerization (class II) or via RAS-dependent heterodimer formation.[70] Unlike EGFR and the fusion oncogenes, BRAF V600E mutations are less strongly associated with absent history of tobacco use or young age.[69] Following initial positive outcomes to BRAF inhibitor monotherapy with dabrafenib, combination BRAF/MEK inhibition with dabrafenib and trametinib was found in a single-arm study to be more active than historical controls with an ORR of 64% and a median PFS of 10.8 months.[71,72] Common toxicities include pyrexia, which may require antipyretic prophylaxis or steroid therapy; hypertension; and hepatotoxicity. Acquired secondary MAPK pathway activating mutations have been reported at TKI resistance,[73] with subsequent treatment options including standard chemoimmunotherapy strategies or consideration for RAS-pathway-directed clinical trial enrollment, because novel RAS/RAF pathway inhibitors continue to be evaluated for both BRAF V600E and non-V600E mutations (NCT04620330).

MET EXON 14 SKIPPING MUTATIONS

MET exon 14 skipping mutations encompasses a wide range of genomic alterations impacting the splice sites flanking exon 14, which contains regulatory elements important to MET degradation. Found in ~3% of lung adenocarcinoma, this driver alteration is enriched in the less common pulmonary sarcomatoid carcinoma[74] and, as for BRAF V600 E mutations, is less strongly associated with young age and absent tobacco use history.[75] Initial MET TKI activity in this setting was seen with off-label use of crizotinib, a multikinase inhibitor that inhibits both ALK and MET.[76] Subsequently the more potent MET inhibitors tepotinib and capmatinib were developed. Outcomes are comparable, and these are now the preferred first-line treatment of METex14-positive NSCLC. Tepotinib was evaluated in the VISION study, and although lower first-line response rates of 46% were reported in an initial study analysis, subsequent confirmatory cohorts demonstrated a first-line response rate of 62.3%.[77] Capmatinib was evaluated in the GEOMETRY trial and demonstrated an ORR of 68% in treatment-naive patients with a median PFS of 12.4 months.[40] Both agents have demonstrated CNS activity, with CNS response rates of 67% and 54% for tepotinib and capmatinib, respectively. These agents share an adverse effect profile including edema, hypoalbuminemia, hepatotoxicity, and gastrointestinal (GI) toxicities. Although there are no approved second-line MET inhibitors for use at acquired MET TKI resistance, class switching from type I (tepotinib, capmatinib, crizotinib) to type II (cabozantinib) MET TKIs may overcome MET second-site resistance mutations affecting Y1230 and D1228 residues at the type I TKI binding site.[78] Future strategies for targeting MET resistance include EGFR/MET bispecific antibody therapy with amivantamab, with encouraging interim data in the CHRYSALIS study.[79]

KRAS G12C MUTATIONS

Activating KRAS mutations are found in nearly 25% of lung adenocarcinoma. Half are the KRAS G12C mutation, the most common of the KRAS mutations in lung cancer.[1] KRAS had been deemed undruggable for decades, but this has changed in recent years with the development of the allosteric KRAS G12C inhibitors.[80] Both sotorasib and adagrasib carry indications for previously treated KRAS G12C+ lung adenocarcinoma. In the randomized phase 3 CodeBreak 200 study sotorasib was superior to docetaxel after prior platinum doublet and checkpoint inhibitor with ORR 28.1% versus 13.2% and PFS 5.6 versus 4.5 months, respectively.[81] Adagrasib received accelerated approval based on the phase 1/2 KRYSTAL-1 study in pretreated KRAS G12C+ NSCLC, with a reported ORR of 42.9% and a median PFS of 6.5 months. In patients with stable CNS metastasis an intracranial ORR of 32% was observed.[82] Common adverse effects in both KRAS G12C inhibitors include GI toxicities and aspartate aminotransferase/alanine aminotransferase level elevation. Diverse resistance mechanisms including secondary KRAS mutations, RAS/MAPK pathway activation, and alternative activating oncogenic driver alterations have been described.[83] The role of KRAS-targeted therapies first line and in combination with checkpoint inhibitor immunotherapy is the subject of ongoing clinical trials.[84] Strategies for targeting non-G12C KRAS-mutant NSCLC are also emerging with G12X RAS(ON) inhibitors, as well as targeting other components of the MAPK pathway.[85,86]

EMERGING ONCOGENIC DRIVERS AS THERAPEUTIC TARGETS

Several oncogene-activating genomic alterations are emerging therapeutic targets in NSCLC, with favorable clinical trial data. These alterations include MET amplification, HER2 overexpression, and the NRG1 fusions. High-level MET amplification is the best established of these potential therapeutic targets. Both MET TKIs capmatinib and tepotinib have been evaluated for MET amplification. In the GEOMETRY mono-1 study capmatinib had activity in patients with a gene copy number of at least 10 (ORR 40% in first-line setting), but more modest activity at lower gene copy numbers.[87] Tepotinib, in the VISION Cohort B, has also shown activity for MET gene amplification defined as a copy number of at least 2.5 by liquid biopsy, with a response rate of 42% and a response rate of 71% reported in a small cohort of 7 patients receiving first-line therapy.[88] The optimal strategy to identify and define MET gene amplification continues to be explored. Similarly, trastuzumab-deruxtecan has shown modest activity against HER2-overexpressing NSCLC, as defined by HER2 IHC score of 2+ or 3+, with a response rate of 24.5% in the DESTINY-Lung01 study.[89]

NRG1 fusions are a novel emerging fusion oncogene in solid tumors, a rare but potentially actionable target with a prevalence of approximately 0.2%. NRG1 is the ligand to HER3, and NRG1 fusions may increase local NRG1 concentrations at the cell membrane via fusion to transmembrane domains.[90] The HER2/HER3 and HER3-targeted antibodies zenocutuzumab and seribantumab have demonstrated early signs of clinical activity with response rates of ~30% in initial cohorts.[91,92]

IMMUNOTHERAPY IN ONCOGENE-DRIVEN LUNG CANCER

The finding of an oncogenic driver mutation has implications beyond the selection of a targeted therapy and impacts decision making around incorporation of immunotherapy into patient care (**Box 1**). In retrospective series low response rates are observed to checkpoint inhibitor monotherapy for the driver mutations often associated with limited tobacco use history (eg, EGFR, ALK, ROS1, RET, HER2).[93,94] In a prospective study of first-line pembrolizumab for EGFR-mutated NSCLC the response rate in EGFR-mutated disease was 0%.[95] Similarly subgroup analysis of early studies of nivolumab or pembrolizumab in the second-line setting showed lack of benefit in patients with EGFR-mutated NSCLC.[96,97] Conversely, the IMpower150 study continued to demonstrate survival benefit with addition of checkpoint inhibitor therapy to platinum/taxane/bevacizumab in a subgroup analysis of patients with EGFR-positive disease.[98] This study is unusual in permitting enrollment of patients with EGFR- or ALK-positive disease, a population excluded from most current immunotherapy combination studies. Of note these concerns regarding immunotherapy response do not extend in an established fashion to other driver mutations, and particularly do not extend to KRAS-mutant disease in which immunotherapy-containing regimens are standard first-line therapy.

Combination therapy with oncogene-targeted therapies and immunotherapy has demonstrated excess risk of toxicity for many, although not all, TKIs in NSCLC. For example, an ILD rate of 35% was reported on the combination of osimertinib plus

---

Box 1
Immunotherapy in oncogene-driven non–small cell lung cancer

Low response rates to checkpoint inhibitor monotherapy have been reported in oncogene-driven lung cancers (eg, EGFR, ALK, ROS1, RET, HER2).

Excess toxicity occurs with many TKI-plus immunotherapy combination regimens, which extends to risk when TKI therapy is used in the months following immunotherapy exposure.

Appropriate genomic biomarker testing should be completed before immunotherapy exposure if clinically feasible.

Optimal incorporation of perioperative and chemoimmunotherapy regimens into the management of oncogene-driven lung cancer remains an area of evolving clinical practice.

TKI, tyrosine kinase inhibitor.

durvalumab in the TATTON study,[99] and combination crizotinib plus nivolumab produced excess rates of hepatitis.[100] The effect of immunotherapy on toxicity risk may persist for many months after exposure, and increased risks of immune-related toxicity have been reported in patients who receive a TKI in the initial months after immunotherapy exposure. For example, higher rates of ILD occur in patients who receive osimertinib in the first 3 months after immunotherapy exposure, and elevated hepatotoxicity is seen in patients who receive crizotinib following immunotherapy.[101,102] A similar risk is not present with treatment in the opposite sequence, from TKI to immunotherapy, given the short half-lives of TKIs. These findings support the importance of completing genomic biomarker testing before immunotherapy exposure, and ongoing study is needed to clarify the optimal strategy to incorporate immunotherapy strategies into the management of oncogene-driven lung cancer.

Concerns regarding safety and efficacy in the metastatic setting may extend to the locally advanced setting, and avoidance of perioperative immunotherapy for patients with oncogenic drivers like EGFR and ALK may be reasonable in clinical practice. A retrospective review of EGFR-mutated NSCLC treated with consolidation durvalumab following chemoradiation as per the PACIFC regimen[103] demonstrated poor outcomes.[104] This remains an evolving area of study, and the extent to which these concerns apply to other driver alterations (RET, ROS1, HER2) remains an area of variable clinical practice absent prospective data.

PERIOPERATIVE USE OF TARGETED THERAPY

Adjuvant EGFR TKI therapy with osimertinib is indicated for resected NSCLC with an EGFR exon 19 deletion or L858 R mutation. This is the only currently approved perioperative targeted therapy regimen in NSCLC, with approval based on improved disease-free survival with 3 years adjuvant osimertinib in the ADAURA study, with overall survival outcomes pending data maturity.[105] Prior studies of earlier-generation EGFR TKIs not only demonstrated more modest disease-free survival advantages but also failed to demonstrate improvements in overall survival.[106] Both neoadjuvant and adjuvant use of oncogene targeted therapies are being evaluated in prospective studies (NCT04302025, NCT04351555).

DISCUSSION

The use of personalized therapeutic strategies in NSCLC has improved patient outcomes, with better quality of life on therapy and extended survival.[107] These improved outcomes are driven in large part by the availability of high-potency and selective targeted therapeutics with potential for prolonged duration of response, better-tolerated side effect profiles, and in many cases high activity for control of CNS disease. Shared patterns of resistance via second-site resistance mutations, MET amplification, and other bypass pathway activation may lend themselves to sequential targeted therapies strategies, further extending the duration of benefit (**Fig. 2**).

Current clinical practice has lagged behind guideline-recommended testing standards, with as few as 50% of patients with advanced lung adenocarcinoma receiving optimal biomarker testing before first-line therapy.[108] Completion of comprehensive genomic testing improves patient survival, and the use of concurrent tissue- and plasma-based assays increases the probability of comprehensive testing before the first cycle of systemic therapy. In one series, comprehensive testing was associated with near doubling of overall survival (22.1 vs 11.6 months).[7,109] Disparities in access to optimal testing may further impact access to optimal care and its associated survival advantages.[110]

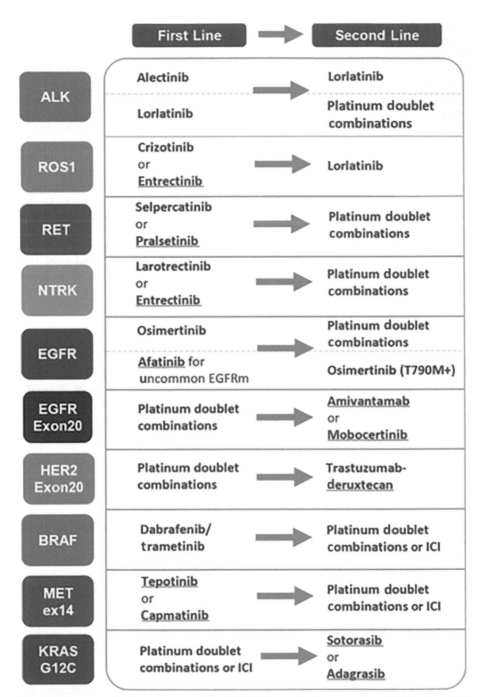

Fig. 2. TKI sequencing in oncogene-driven NSCLC. Suggested sequencing of TKI and non-TKI strategies in oncogene-driven subsets of NSCLC, highlighting settings in which sequential TKI therapy is feasible. NGS profiling at acquired TKI resistance may offer additional targeted therapy options either via clinical trial enrollment or via off-label drug access. ICI, immune checkpoint inhibitor; TKI, tyrosine kinase inhibitor.

With perioperative approvals of EGFR-targeted therapy and checkpoint inhibitor immunotherapies, personalized treatment strategies have begun to move toward the management of earlier-stage NSCLC. The role of perioperative use of agents targeting the full spectrum of oncogenic driver mutations is under clinical investigation,[111] predicting for a future where comprehensive genomic testing will be indicated in early-stage disease as it is now in advanced disease. These advances bring hope for improved outcomes related to personalized medicine across the continuum of lung cancer management.

CLINICS CARE POINTS

- All patients with advanced/metastatic nonsquamous NSCLC require genomic testing to include at minimum testing for actionable alterations in EGFR, ALK, ROS1, RET, NTRK, BRAF, METex14, HER2, and KRAS. Selected patients with squamous histology may also benefit from genomic testing. NGS testing offers a comprehensive testing strategy if feasible.

- Repeat genomic testing at acquired TKI resistance, although not mandated by standard of care, may offer subsequent personalized treatment options.

- Patients with resectable NSCLC require EGFR and PD-L1 biomarker testing.

- Immunotherapy monotherapy should be avoided early in the course of EGFR, ASLK, ROS1, RET, and HER2-postitive NSCLC given limited reported treatment efficacy.

DISCLOSURE

Dr E. Brea reports no conflicts of interest. Dr J. Rotow reports consulting or honoraria from AstraZeneca, Genentech, Guardant Health, Janssen, Gritstone Oncology, Lilly, Takeda, BioAtla, Summit Therapeutics, and G1 Therapeutics, and grant support in the form of institutional clinical trial funding from AstraZeneca, United Kingdom, BioAtla, AbbVie, United States, Blueprint Medicines, RedCloud Bio, EpimAb, and Loxo Oncology, United States.

REFERENCES

1. Singal G, Miller PG, Agarwala V, et al. Association of Patient Characteristics and Tumor Genomics With Clinical Outcomes Among Patients With Non-Small Cell Lung Cancer Using a Clinicogenomic Database. JAMA 2019;321(14):1391–9.
2. Sequist LV, Heist RS, Shaw AT, et al. Implementing multiplexed genotyping of non-small-cell lung cancers into routine clinical practice. Ann Oncol 2011; 22(12):2616–24.
3. Heist RS, Sequist LV, Engelman JA. Genetic changes in squamous cell lung cancer: a review. J Thorac Oncol 2012;7(5):924–33.
4. Joshi A, Zanwar S, Noronha V, et al. EGFR mutation in squamous cell carcinoma of the lung: does it carry the same connotation as in adenocarcinomas? OncoTargets Ther 2017;10:1859–63.
5. Gitlitz BJ, Novello S, Vavalà T, et al. The Genomics of Young Lung Cancer: Comprehensive Tissue Genomic Analysis in Patients Under 40 With Lung Cancer. JTO Clin Res Rep 2021;2(7):100194.
6. Benayed R, Offin M, Mullaney K, et al. High Yield of RNA Sequencing for Targetable Kinase Fusions in Lung Adenocarcinomas with No Mitogenic Driver Alteration Detected by DNA Sequencing and Low Tumor Mutation Burden. Clin Cancer Res 2019;25(15):4712–22.

7. Aggarwal C, Marmarelis ME, Hwang W-T, et al. Association of comprehensive molecular genotyping and overall survival in patients with advanced non-squamous non-small cell lung cancer. J Clin Oncol 2022;40(16_suppl):9022.

8. Pikor LA, Ramnarine VR, Lam S, et al. Genetic alterations defining NSCLC sub-types and their therapeutic implications. Lung Cancer 2013;82(2):179–89.

9. Lin C, Shi X, Yang S, et al. Comparison of ALK detection by FISH, IHC and NGS to predict benefit from crizotinib in advanced non-small-cell lung cancer. Lung Cancer 2019;131:62–8.

10. Solomon BJ, Mok T, Kim DW, et al. First-line crizotinib versus chemotherapy in ALK-positive lung cancer. N Engl J Med 2014;371(23):2167–77.

11. Mok T, Camidge DR, Gadgeel SM, et al. Updated overall survival and final progression-free survival data for patients with treatment-naive advanced ALK-positive non-small-cell lung cancer in the ALEX study. Ann Oncol 2020; 31(8):1056–64.

12. Peters S, Camidge DR, Shaw AT, et al. Alectinib versus Crizotinib in Untreated ALK-Positive Non-Small-Cell Lung Cancer. N Engl J Med 2017;377(9):829–38.

13. Soria JC, Tan DS, Chiari R, et al. First-line ceritinib versus platinum-based chemo-therapy in advanced ALK-rearranged non-small-cell lung cancer (ASCEND-4): a randomised, open-label, phase 3 study. Lancet 2017;389(10072):917–29.

14. Camidge DR, Kim HR, Ahn MJ, et al. Brigatinib Versus Crizotinib in ALK Inhibitor-Naive Advanced ALK-Positive NSCLC: Final Results of Phase 3 ALTA-1L Trial. J Thorac Oncol 2021;16(12):2091–108.

15. Shaw AT, Bauer TM, de Marinis F, et al. First-Line Lorlatinib or Crizotinib in Advanced ALK-Positive Lung Cancer. N Engl J Med 2020;383(21):2018–29.

16. Solomon BJ, Bauer TM, Mok TSK, et al. Efficacy and safety of first-line lorlatinib versus crizotinib in patients with advanced, ALK-positive non-small-cell lung cancer: updated analysis of data from the phase 3, randomised, open-label CROWN study. Lancet Respir Med 2022;S2213-2600(22):437–44.

17. Gainor JF, Dardaei L, Yoda S, et al. Molecular Mechanisms of Resistance to First- and Second-Generation ALK Inhibitors in ALK-Rearranged Lung Cancer. Cancer Discov 2016;6(10):1118–33.

18. Shaw AT, Solomon BJ, Besse B, et al. ALK Resistance Mutations and Efficacy of Lorlatinib in Advanced Anaplastic Lymphoma Kinase-Positive Non-Small-Cell Lung Cancer. J Clin Oncol 2019;37(16):1370–9.

19. Dagogo-Jack I, Yoda S, Lennerz JK, et al. MET Alterations Are a Recurring and Actionable Resistance Mechanism in ALK-Positive Lung Cancer. Clin Cancer Res 2020;26(11):2535–45.

20. Fujino T, Nguyen L, Yoda S, et al. Preclinical activity of NVL-655 in patient-derived models of ALK cancers, including those with lorlatinib-resistant G1202R/L1196M compound mutation. European Journal of Cancer 2022;174:S78–9.

21. Shaw AT, Riely GJ, Bang YJ, et al. Crizotinib in ROS1-rearranged advanced non-small-cell lung cancer (NSCLC): updated results, including overall survival, from PROFILE 1001. Ann Oncol 2019;30(7):1121–6.

22. Dziadziuszko R, Krebs MG, De Braud F, et al. Updated Integrated Analysis of the Efficacy and Safety of Entrectinib in Locally Advanced or Metastatic ROS1 Fusion-Positive Non-Small-Cell Lung Cancer. J Clin Oncol 2021;39(11):1253–63.

23. Drilon A, Chiu C-H, Fan Y, et al. Long-Term Efficacy and Safety of Entrectinib in ROS-Fusion Positive NSCLC. JTO Clinical and Research Reports 2022;3(6): 100332.

24. Davare MA, Vellore NA, Wagner JP, et al. Structural insight into selectivity and resistance profiles of ROS1 tyrosine kinase inhibitors. Proceedings of the

National Academy of Sciences of the United States of America 2015;112(39): E5381–90.

25. Shaw AT, Solomon BJ, Chiari R, et al. Lorlatinib in advanced ROS1-positive non-small-cell lung cancer: a multicentre, open-label, single-arm, phase 1-2 trial. Lancet Oncol 2019;20(12):1691–701.

26. Yun MR, Kim DH, Kim SY, et al. Repotrectinib Exhibits Potent Antitumor Activity in Treatment-Naïve and Solvent-Front-Mutant ROS1-Rearranged Non-Small Cell Lung Cancer. Clin Cancer Res 2020;26(13):3287–95.

27. Zhou C, Fan H, Wang Y, et al. Taletrectinib (AB-106; DS-6051b) in metastatic non-small cell lung cancer (NSCLC) patients with ROS1 fusion: Preliminary results of TRUST. J Clin Oncol 2021;39(15_suppl):9066.

28. Kohno T, Ichikawa H, Totoki Y, et al. KIF5B-RET fusions in lung adenocarcinoma. Nat Med 2012;18(3):375–7.

29. Takeuchi K, Soda M, Togashi Y, et al. RET, ROS1 and ALK fusions in lung cancer. Nat Med 2012;18(3):378–81.

30. Drilon A, Subbiah V, Gautschi O, et al. Selpercatinib in Patients With RET Fusion–Positive Non–Small-Cell Lung Cancer: Updated Safety and Efficacy From the Registrational LIBRETTO-001 Phase I/II Trial. J Clin Oncol 2022;41(2):385–94.

31. Gainor JF, Curigliano G, Kim DW, et al. Pralsetinib for RET fusion-positive non-small-cell lung cancer (ARROW): a multi-cohort, open-label, phase 1/2 study. Lancet Oncol 2021;22(7):959–69.

32. Griesinger F, Curigliano G, Thomas M, et al. Safety and efficacy of pralsetinib in ROS-fusion positive non-small-cell lung cancer including as first-line therapy: update from the ARROW trial. Ann Oncol 2022;33(11):1168–78.

33. Lin JJ, Liu SV, McCoach CE, et al. Mechanisms of resistance to selective RET tyrosine kinase inhibitors in RET fusion-positive non-small-cell lung cancer. Ann Oncol 2020;31(12):1725–33.

34. Rosen EY, Won HH, Zheng Y, et al. The evolution of RET inhibitor resistance in RET-driven lung and thyroid cancers. Nat Commun 2022;13(1):1450.

35. Pennell NA, Wirth LJ, Gainor JF, et al. A first-in-human phase 1 study of the next-generation RET inhibitor, LOXO-260, in RET inhibitor refractory patients with RET-altered cancers (trial in progress). J Clin Oncol 2022;40(16_suppl): TPS8595.

36. Farago AF, Taylor MS, Doebele RC, et al. Clinicopathologic Features of Non-Small-Cell Lung Cancer Harboring an NTRK Gene Fusion. JCO Precis Oncol 2018;2018. PO.18.00037.

37. Hong DS, DuBois SG, Kummar S, et al. Larotrectinib in patients with TRK fusion-positive solid tumours: a pooled analysis of three phase 1/2 clinical trials. Lancet Oncol 2020;21(4):531–40.

38. Doebele RC, Drilon A, Paz-Ares L, et al. Entrectinib in patients with advanced or metastatic NTRK fusion-positive solid tumours: integrated analysis of three phase 1-2 trials. Lancet Oncol 2020;21(2):271–82.

39. Cocco E, Scaltriti M, Drilon A. NTRK fusion-positive cancers and TRK inhibitor therapy. Nat Rev Clin Oncol 2018;15(12):731–47.

40. Cho BC, Doebele RC, Lin J, et al. MA11.07 Phase 1/2 TRIDENT-1 Study of Repotrectinib in Patients with ROS1+ or NTRK+ Advanced Solid Tumors. J Thorac Oncol 2021;16(3):S174–5.

41. Midha A, Dearden S, McCormack R. EGFR mutation incidence in non-small-cell lung cancer of adenocarcinoma histology: a systematic review and global map by ethnicity (mutMapII). Am J Cancer Res 2015;5(9):2892–911.

42. Robichaux JP, Le X, Vijayan RSK, et al. Structure-based classification predicts drug response in EGFR-mutant NSCLC. Nature 2021;597(7878):732–7.
43. Reungwetwattana T, Nakagawa K, Cho BC, et al. CNS Response to Osimertinib Versus Standard Epidermal Growth Factor Receptor Tyrosine Kinase Inhibitors in Patients With Untreated EGFR-Mutated Advanced Non–Small-Cell Lung Cancer. J Clin Oncol 2018;36(33):3290–7.
44. Ramalingam SS, Vansteenkiste J, Planchard D, et al. Overall Survival with Osimertinib in Untreated, EGFR-Mutated Advanced NSCLC. N Engl J Med 2019; 382(1):41–50.
45. Soria JC, Ohe Y, Vansteenkiste J, et al. Osimertinib in Untreated EGFR-Mutated Advanced Non-Small-Cell Lung Cancer. N Engl J Med 2018;378(2):113–25.
46. Leonetti A, Sharma S, Minari R, et al. Resistance mechanisms to osimertinib in EGFR-mutated non-small cell lung cancer. Br J Cancer 2019;121(9):725–37.
47. Ramalingam SS, Zhang N, Yu J, et al. MA07.03 Real-world Landscape of EGFR C797X Mutation as a Resistance Mechanism to Osimertinib in Non-small Cell Lung Cancer. J Thorac Oncol 2022;17(9):S67–8.
48. Mazieres J, Kim T, Lim B, et al. LBA52 - Tepotinib + osimertinib for EGFRm NSCLC with MET amplification (METamp) after progression on first-line (1L) osimertinib: Initial results from the INSIGHT 2 study. Ann Oncol 2022;33(7): S808–69.
49. Schrock AB, Zhu VW, Hsieh W-S, et al. Receptor Tyrosine Kinase Fusions and BRAF Kinase Fusions are Rare but Actionable Resistance Mechanisms to EGFR Tyrosine Kinase Inhibitors. J Thorac Oncol 2018;13(9):1312–23.
50. Huang Y, Gan J, Guo K, et al. Acquired BRAF V600E Mutation Mediated Resistance to Osimertinib and Responded to Osimertinib, Dabrafenib, and Trametinib Combination Therapy. J Thorac Oncol 2019;14(10):e236–7.
51. Rotow J, Patel J, Hanley M, et al. FP14.07 Combination Osimertinib plus Selpercatinib for EGFR-mutant Non-Small Cell Lung Cancer (NSCLC) with Acquired RET fusions. J Thorac Oncol 2021;16(3):S230.
52. Shu C, Goto K, Ohe Y, et al. 1193MO - Amivantamab plus lazertinib in postosimertinib, post-platinum chemotherapy EGFR-mutant non-small cell lung cancer (NSCLC): Preliminary results from CHRYSALIS-2. Ann Oncol 2021;32(5): S949–1039.
53. Shum E, Elamin YY, Piotrowska Z, et al. A phase 1/2 study of BLU-945 in patients with common activating EGFR-mutant non–small cell lung cancer (NSCLC): SYMPHONY trial in progress. J Clin Oncol 2022;40(16_suppl):TPS9156.
54. Jänne PA, Baik C, Su WC, et al. Efficacy and Safety of Patritumab Deruxtecan (HER3-DXd) in EGFR Inhibitor-Resistant, EGFR-Mutated Non-Small Cell Lung Cancer. Cancer Discov 2022;12(1):74–89.
55. Yang JC, Schuler M, Popat S, et al. Afatinib for the Treatment of NSCLC Harboring Uncommon EGFR Mutations: A Database of 693 Cases. J Thorac Oncol 2020;15(5):803–15.
56. Cho JH, Lim SH, An HJ, et al. Osimertinib for Patients With Non-Small-Cell Lung Cancer Harboring Uncommon EGFR Mutations: A Multicenter, Open-Label, Phase II Trial (KCSG-LU15-09). J Clin Oncol 2020;38(5):488–95.
57. Vyse S, Huang PH. Targeting EGFR exon 20 insertion mutations in non-small cell lung cancer. Signal Transduct Targeted Ther 2019;4(1):5.
58. Park K, Haura EB, Leighl NB, et al. Amivantamab in EGFR Exon 20 Insertion-Mutated Non-Small-Cell Lung Cancer Progressing on Platinum Chemotherapy: Initial Results From the CHRYSALIS Phase I Study. J Clin Oncol 2021;39(30): 3391–402.

59. Zhou C, Ramalingam SS, Kim TM, et al. Treatment Outcomes and Safety of Mobocertinib in Platinum-Pretreated Patients With EGFR Exon 20 Insertion–Positive Metastatic Non–Small Cell Lung Cancer: A Phase 1/2 Open-label Nonrandomized Clinical Trial. JAMA Oncol 2021;7(12):e214761.

60. Spira AI, Yu HA, Sun L, et al. Phase 1/2 study of BLU-451, a central nervous system (CNS) penetrant, small molecule inhibitor of EGFR, in incurable advanced cancers with EGFR exon 20 insertion (ex20ins) mutations. J Clin Oncol 2022; 40(16_suppl):TPS9155.

61. Yu HA, Tan DS-W, Smit EF, et al. Phase (Ph) 1/2a study of CLN-081 in patients (pts) with NSCLC with EGFR exon 20 insertion mutations (Ins20). J Clin Oncol 2022;40(16_suppl):9007.

62. Yang JC-H, Wang M, Mitchell P, et al. Preliminary safety and efficacy results from phase 1 studies of DZD9008 in NSCLC patients with EGFR Exon20 insertion mutations. J Clin Oncol 2021;39(15_suppl):9008.

63. Friedlaender A, Subbiah V, Russo A, et al. EGFR and HER2 exon 20 insertions in solid tumours: from biology to treatment. Nat Rev Clin Oncol 2022;19(1):51–69.

64. Li BT, Smit EF, Goto Y, et al. Trastuzumab Deruxtecan in HER2-Mutant Non–Small-Cell Lung Cancer. N Engl J Med 2021;386(3):241–51.

65. Goto K, Sang-We K, Kubo T, et al. LBA55 - Trastuzumab deruxtecan (T-DXd) in patients (Pts) with HER2-mutant metastatic non-small cell lung cancer (NSCLC): Interim results from the phase 2 DESTINY-Lung02 trial. Ann Oncol 2022;33(7): S808–69.

66. Li BT, Ahn M-J, Goto K, et al. Open-label, randomized, multicenter, phase 3 study evaluating trastuzumab deruxtecan (T-DXd) as first-line treatment in patients with unresectable, locally advanced, or metastatic non–small cell lung cancer (NSCLC) harboring HER2 exon 19 or 20 mutations (DESTINY-Lung04). J Clin Oncol 2022;40(16_suppl):TPS9137.

67. Song Z, Li Y, Chen S, et al. Efficacy and safety of pyrotinib in advanced lung adenocarcinoma with HER2 mutations: a multicenter, single-arm, phase II trial. BMC Med 2022;20(1):42.

68. Elamin YY, Robichaux JP, Carter BW, et al. Poziotinib for Patients With HER2 Exon 20 Mutant Non-Small-Cell Lung Cancer: Results From a Phase II Trial. J Clin Oncol 2022;40(7):702–9.

69. Dagogo-Jack I, Martinez P, Yeap BY, et al. Impact of BRAF Mutation Class on Disease Characteristics and Clinical Outcomes in BRAF-mutant Lung Cancer. Clin Cancer Res 2019;25(1):158–65.

70. Fontana E, Valeri N. Class(y) Dissection of BRAF Heterogeneity: Beyond Non-V600. Clin Cancer Res 2019;25(23):6896–8.

71. Planchard D, Besse B, Groen HJ, et al. Dabrafenib plus trametinib in patients with previously treated BRAF(V600E)-mutant metastatic non-small cell lung cancer: an open-label, multicentre phase 2 trial. Lancet Oncol 2016;17(7):984–93.

72. Planchard D, Smit EF, Groen HJM, et al. Dabrafenib plus trametinib in patients with previously untreated BRAF(V600E)-mutant metastatic non-small-cell lung cancer: an open-label, phase 2 trial. Lancet Oncol 2017;18(10):1307–16.

73. Facchinetti F, Lacroix L, Mezquita L, et al. Molecular mechanisms of resistance to BRAF and MEK inhibitors in BRAF(V600E) non-small cell lung cancer. Eur J Cancer 2020;132:211–23.

74. Liu X, Jia Y, Stoopler MB, et al. Next-Generation Sequencing of Pulmonary Sarcomatoid Carcinoma Reveals High Frequency of Actionable MET Gene Mutations. J Clin Oncol 2016;34(8):794–802.

75. Le X, Hong L, Hensel C, et al. Landscape and Clonal Dominance of Co-occurring Genomic Alterations in Non-Small-Cell Lung Cancer Harboring MET Exon 14 Skipping. JCO Precis Oncol 2021;5. PO.21.00135.
76. Drilon A, Clark JW, Weiss J, et al. Antitumor activity of crizotinib in lung cancers harboring a MET exon 14 alteration. Nature Med 2020;26(1):47–51.
77. Thomas M, Garassino M, Felip E, et al. OA03.05 Tepotinib in Patients with MET Exon 14 (METex14) Skipping NSCLC: Primary Analysis of the Confirmatory VISION Cohort C. J Thorac Oncol 2022;17(9):S9–10.
78. Recondo G, Bahcall M, Spurr LF, et al. Molecular Mechanisms of Acquired Resistance to MET Tyrosine Kinase Inhibitors in Patients with MET Exon 14-Mutant NSCLC. Clin Cancer Res 2020;26(11):2615–25.
79. Krebs M, Spira AI, Cho BC, et al. Amivantamab in patients with NSCLC with MET exon 14 skipping mutation: Updated results from the CHRYSALIS study. J Clin Oncol 2022;40(16_suppl):9008.
80. Huang L, Guo Z, Wang F, et al. KRAS mutation: from undruggable to druggable in cancer. Signal Transduct Targeted Ther 2021;6(1):386.
81. Johnson M, De Langen J, Waterhouse D, et al. LBA10 - Sotorasib versus docetaxel for previously treated non-small cell lung cancer with KRAS G12C mutation: CodeBreaK 200 phase III study. Ann Oncol 2022;33(7):S808–69.
82. Jänne PA, Riely GJ, Gadgeel SM, et al. Adagrasib in Non–Small-Cell Lung Cancer Harboring a KRASG12C Mutation. N Engl J Med 2022;387(2):120–31.
83. Awad MM, Liu S, Rybkin II, et al. Acquired Resistance to KRASG12C Inhibition in Cancer. N Engl J Med 2021;384(25):2382 93.
84. Jänne PA, Smit EF, de Marinis F, et al. LBA4 Preliminary safety and efficacy of adagrasib with pembrolizumab in treatment-naive patients with advanced non-small cell lung cancer (NSCLC) harboring a KRAS G12C mutation. Annals of Oncology 2022;16:100104.
85. Jacobs F, Cani M, Malapelle U, et al. Targeting KRAS in NSCLC: Old Failures and New Options for "Non-G12C" Patients. Cancers 2021;13(24):6332.
86. Koltun ES, Rice MA, Gustafson WC, et al. Abstract 3597: Direct targeting of KRASG12X mutant cancers with RMC-6236, a first-in-class, RAS-selective, orally bioavailable, tri-complex RASMULTI(ON) inhibitor. Cancer Res 2022; 82(12_Supplement):3597.
87. Wolf J, Seto T, Han JY, et al. Capmatinib in MET Exon 14-Mutated or MET-Amplified Non-Small-Cell Lung Cancer. N Engl J Med 2020;383(10):944–57.
88. Le X, Paz-Ares LG, Van Meerbeeck J, et al. Tepotinib in patients (pts) with advanced non-small cell lung cancer (NSCLC) with MET amplification (METamp). J Clin Oncol 2021;39(15_suppl):9021.
89. Nakagawa K, Nagasaka M, Felip E, et al. OA04.05 Trastuzumab Deruxtecan in HER2-Overexpressing Metastatic Non-Small Cell Lung Cancer: Interim Results of DESTINY-Lung01. J Thorac Oncol 2021;16(3):S109–10.
90. Nagasaka M, Ou S-HI. NRG1 and NRG2 fusion positive solid tumor malignancies: a paradigm of ligand-fusion oncogenesis. Trends in cancer 2022; 8(3):242–58.
91. Schram AM, O'Reilly EM, O'Kane GM, et al. Efficacy and safety of zenocutuzumab in advanced pancreas cancer and other solid tumors harboring NRG1 fusions. J Clin Oncol 2021;39(15_suppl):3003.
92. Carrizosa DR, Burkard ME, Elamin YY, et al. CRESTONE: Initial efficacy and safety of seribantumab in solid tumors harboring NRG1 fusions. J Clin Oncol 2022;40(16_suppl):3006.

93. Mazieres J, Drilon A, Lusque A, et al. Immune checkpoint inhibitors for patients with advanced lung cancer and oncogenic driver alterations: results from the IMMUNOTARGET registry. Ann Oncol 2019;30(8):1321–8.

94. Negrao MV, Skoulidis F, Montesion M, et al. Oncogene-specific differences in tumor mutational burden, PD-L1 expression, and outcomes from immunotherapy in non-small cell lung cancer. Journal for immunotherapy of cancer 2021;9(8): e002891.

95. Lisberg A, Cummings A, Goldman JW, et al. A Phase II Study of Pembrolizumab in EGFR-Mutant, PD-L1+, Tyrosine Kinase Inhibitor Naïve Patients With Advanced NSCLC. J Thorac Oncol 2018;13(8):1138–45.

96. Borghaei H, Paz-Ares L, Horn L, et al. Nivolumab versus docetaxel in advanced nonsquamous non-small-cell lung cancer. N Engl J Med 2015;373:1627–39.

97. Herbst RS, Baas P, Kim DW, et al. Pembrolizumab versus docetaxel for previously treated, PD-L1-positive, advanced non-small-cell lung cancer (KEYNOTE-010): a randomised controlled trial. Lancet 2016;387(10027):1540–50.

98. Nogami N, Barlesi F, Socinski MA, et al. IMpower150 Final Exploratory Analyses for Atezolizumab Plus Bevacizumab and Chemotherapy in Key NSCLC Patient Subgroups With EGFR Mutations or Metastases in the Liver or Brain. J Thorac Oncol 2022;17(2):309–23.

99. Ahn MJ, Cho BC, Ou X, et al. Osimertinib Plus Durvalumab in Patients With EGFR-Mutated, Advanced NSCLC: A Phase 1b, Open-Label, Multicenter Trial. J Thorac Oncol 2022;17(5):718–23.

100. Spigel DR, Reynolds C, Waterhouse D, et al. Phase 1/2 Study of the Safety and Tolerability of Nivolumab Plus Crizotinib for the First-Line Treatment of Anaplastic Lymphoma Kinase Translocation — Positive Advanced Non–Small Cell Lung Cancer (CheckMate 370). J Thorac Oncol 2018;13(5):682–8.

101. Schoenfeld AJ, Arbour KC, Rizvi H, et al. Severe immune-related adverse events are common with sequential PD-(L)1 blockade and osimertinib. Ann Oncol 2019;30(5):839–44.

102. Lin JJ, Chin E, Yeap BY, et al. Increased Hepatotoxicity Associated with Sequential Immune Checkpoint Inhibitor and Crizotinib Therapy in Patients with Non–Small Cell Lung Cancer. J Thorac Oncol 2019;14(1):135–40.

103. Antonia SJ, Villegas A, Daniel D, et al. Overall Survival with Durvalumab after Chemoradiotherapy in Stage III NSCLC. N Engl J Med 2018;379(24):2342–50.

104. Aredo JV, Mambetsariev I, Hellyer JA, et al. Durvalumab for Stage III EGFR-Mutated NSCLC After Definitive Chemoradiotherapy. J Thorac Oncol 2021; 16(6):1030–41.

105. Wu Y-L, Tsuboi M, He J, et al. Osimertinib in Resected EGFR-Mutated Non–Small-Cell Lung Cancer. N Engl J Med 2020;383(18):1711–23.

106. Wu Y-L, Zhong W, Wang Q, et al. CTONG1104: Adjuvant gefitinib versus chemotherapy for resected N1-N2 NSCLC with EGFR mutation—Final overall survival analysis of the randomized phase III trial 1 analysis of the randomized phase III trial. J Clin Oncol 2020;38(15_suppl):9005.

107. Kris MG, Johnson BE, Berry LD, et al. Using multiplexed assays of oncogenic drivers in lung cancers to select targeted drugs. JAMA 2014;311(19):1998–2006.

108. Robert NJ, Espirito JL, Chen L, et al. Biomarker testing and tissue journey among patients with metastatic non-small cell lung cancer receiving first-line therapy in The US Oncology Network. Lung Cancer 2022;166:197–204.

109. Presley CJ, Tang D, Soulos PR, et al. Association of Broad-Based Genomic Sequencing With Survival Among Patients With Advanced Non–Small Cell Lung Cancer in the Community Oncology Setting. JAMA 2018;320(5):469–77.

110. Bruno DS, Hess LM, Li X, et al. Disparities in Biomarker Testing and Clinical Trial Enrollment Among Patients With Lung, Breast, or Colorectal Cancers in the United States. JCO Precision Oncology 2022;6:e2100427.
111. Sepesi B, Jones DR, Meyers BF, et al. LCMC LEADER neoadjuvant screening trial: LCMC4 evaluation of actionable drivers in early-stage lung cancers. J Clin Oncol 2022;40(16_suppl):TPS8596.
112. Solomon BJ, Kim DW, Wu YL, et al. Final Overall Survival Analysis From a Study Comparing First-Line Crizotinib Versus Chemotherapy in ALK-Mutation-Positive Non-Small-Cell Lung Cancer. J Clin Oncol 2018;36(22):2251–8.
113. Camidge DR, Kim HR, Ahn M-J, et al. Brigatinib versus Crizotinib in ALK-Positive Non–Small-Cell Lung Cancer. N Engl J Med 2018;379(21):2027–39.
114. Zhou C, Wu YL, Chen G, et al. Erlotinib versus chemotherapy as first-line treatment for patients with advanced EGFR mutation-positive non-small-cell lung cancer (OPTIMAL, CTONG-0802): a multicentre, open-label, randomised, phase 3 study. Lancet Oncol 2011;12(8):735–42.
115. Sequist LV, Yang JC, Yamamoto N, et al. Phase III study of afatinib or cisplatin plus pemetrexed in patients with metastatic lung adenocarcinoma with EGFR mutations. J Clin Oncol 2013;31(27):3327–34.
116. Yang JC-H, Wu Y-L, Schuler M, et al. Afatinib versus cisplatin-based chemotherapy for EGFR mutation-positive lung adenocarcinoma (LUX-Lung 3 and LUX-Lung 6): analysis of overall survival data from two randomised, phase 3 trials. Lancet Oncol 2015;16(2):141–51.
117. Yang JC, Sequist LV, Geater SL, et al. Clinical activity of afatinib in patients with advanced non-small-cell lung cancer harbouring uncommon EGFR mutations: a combined post-hoc analysis of LUX-Lung 2, LUX-Lung 3, and LUX-Lung 6. Lancet Oncol 2015;16(7):830–8.
118. Planchard D, Besse B, Groen HJM, et al. Phase 2 Study of Dabrafenib Plus Trametinib in Patients With BRAF V600E-Mutant Metastatic NSCLC: Updated 5-Year Survival Rates and Genomic Analysis. J Thorac Oncol 2022;17(1):103–15.
119. Wolf J, Garon EB, Groen HJM, et al. Capmatinib in MET exon 14-mutated, advanced NSCLC: Updated results from the GEOMETRY mono-1 study. J Clin Oncol 2021;39(15_suppl):9020.
120. Paik PK, Veillon R, Cortot A, et al. Phase II study of tepotinib in NSCLC patients with METex14 mutations. J Clin Oncol 2019;37(suppl):abstr 9005.

What Is New in Small Cell Lung Cancer

Robert Matera, MD[a],*, Anne Chiang, MD, PhD[a]

KEYWORDS

- Drug • Immunotherapy • Radiation • Small cell lung cancer

KEY POINTS

- SCLC is a rare yet aggressive subtype of lung cancer with a poor prognosis.
- Addition of immunotherapy in the front-line setting is now standard of care for extensive stage SCLC patients though clinical benefit remains modest.
- Lurbinectedin is the second FDA approved therapy for use in relapsed/refractory SCLC.
- Stratification of SCLC tumors based on expression of transcription factors rather than genetic alterations is promising though clinical utility has not yet been proven.
- Clinical trials examining role of checkpoint inhibition, oncogenic transcription, epigenetic regulation, and DNA repair are currently underway with a variety of drugs of different classes.

INTRODUCTION

Small cell lung cancer (SCLC) is a rare yet aggressive lung cancer subtype with an extremely poor prognosis of around 1 year. SCLC accounts for 15% of all newly diagnosed lung cancers and is characterized by rapid growth with high potential for metastatic spread and treatment resistance.[1]

Although traditional TMN lung cancer staging is prognostic, SCLC is classically divided into limited stage (LS) and extensive stage (ES) disease. Limited disease accounts for 25% of newly diagnosed cases and defines disease that can be treated in a single radiation field.[2] This previously included only tumors that were restricted to a single hemithorax; however, due to advances in radiation techniques, select patients with contralateral disease may still be categorized as LS disease. Definitive platinum-based chemotherapy with concurrent radiation is standard of care for these patients. Surgical resection is considered in rare circumstances of early-stage disease, especially node negative or N1 disease.

Most of the patients, 75% to 80%, are categorized as ES at the time of diagnosis. Treatment of ES-SCLC has traditionally consisted of a platinum-containing agent in

[a] Department of Hematology and Oncology, Yale New Haven Hospital, 20 York Street, New Haven, CT, USA
* Corresponding author. 20 York Street, New Haven, CT 06510.
E-mail address: robert.matera@yale.edu

Hematol Oncol Clin N Am 37 (2023) 595–607
https://doi.org/10.1016/j.hoc.2023.02.010
0889-8588/23/© 2023 Elsevier Inc. All rights reserved.

combination with etoposide, a regimen that was established in 1992.[3] Recently, the addition of immunotherapy has been shown to improve outcomes. Although significant, the gains from immunotherapy are modest, improving median survival by 2 to 3 months. Much effort has been placed on further improving these outcomes. In the article the authors review some of the most notable of these efforts, including trials of novel immunotherapy agents, novel disease targets, and multiple drug combinations.

In addition, the understanding of SCLC biology is undergoing a paradigm shift. The emergence of discrete molecular subtypes has stratified a disease previously thought to be genomically more homogenous and offers new insights that will guide drug development and clinical trial design.

Extensive Stage Disease

Since the 1990s, the combination of a platinum agent with etoposide was the most widely used standard-of-care regimen for ES disease.[3] Irinotecan was initially shown to be superior to etoposide in one phase III trial.[4] However, 2 subsequent studies[5,6] failed to replicate this finding. Platinum/etoposide has remained the standard of care for more than 30 years until recently when a survival benefit was found with the addition of immune checkpoint inhibitors (ICIs) to traditional chemotherapy.

Programmed cell death ligand 1 inhibitors

Impower133,[7] a double-blinded phase III clinical trial randomized 403 patients to receive carboplatin and etoposide with or without atezolizumab, a monoclonal antibody inhibitor of antiprogrammed cell death ligand 1 (PD-L1). After 4 cycles, patients randomized to the atezolizumab arm continued on atezolizumab maintenance every 3 weeks until disease progression or intolerable toxicity. Median progression-free survival (PFS) in the atezolizumab group was 5.2 months versus 4.3 months in the chemotherapy-only arm (hazard ratio [HR] 0.77, p = 0.02). Median overall survival (OS) was also significantly increased in the immunotherapy arm to 12.3 months compared with 10.3 months in the chemotherapy group (HR = 0.70, p = 0.007). Based on these data, in March 2019 the Food and Drug Administration (FDA) approved atezolizumab in combination with carboplatin and etoposide for the first-line treatment of ES-SCLC.

Approximately 1 year later, the FDA granted approval to a second PD-L1 inhibitor, durvalumab, for the same indication based on the results of the CASPIAN trial.

The CASPIAN trial was an open-label, international phase III clinical trial[8]; 805 patients were randomized 1:1:1 to receive platinum-etoposide alone or in combination with either durvalumab or durvalumab plus tremelimumab, an anticytotoxic T-lymphocyte antigen 4 (CTLA4) antibody. After 4 to 6 cycles, patients in durvalumab and durvalumab plus tremelimumab arms continued on maintenance durvalumab or durvalumab plus tremelimumab, respectively, until disease progression or intolerable side effects. Median OS was significantly increased in the durvalumab plus chemotherapy arm at 13.0 months compared with 10.3 months in the chemotherapy-only arm (HR = 0.73, p = 0.0047). Two-year OS rate was 22.2% versus 14.4% in chemotherapy alone, and an updated analysis showed that at 3 years, patients receiving durvalumab were 3 times more likely to be alive than those receiving chemotherapy alone (3-year survival rate of 17.6% vs 5.8%).[9] After more than 30 years without new treatment options, PD-L1 inhibitors offered 2 new FDA-approved treatment options, and chemoimmunotherapy has become the new standard of care in the first-line setting for ES disease; this has prompted further investigations in 2 categories: identifying more effective immunotherapy agents or adding agents to the established chemoimmunotherapy backbone.

Novel programmed cell death protein 1 inhibitors

Serplulimab, a novel antiprogrammed cell death protein 1 (PD-1) monoclonal antibody was shown to improve median OS and median PFS when added to a chemotherapy backbone compared with chemotherapy alone in patients with SCLC. In a randomized, phase III trial 585 patients with ES-SCLC were randomized 2:1 to receive serplulimab plus carboplatin and etoposide versus carboplatin and etoposide alone.[10] The median OS was increased to 15.4 months in the serplulimab arm versus 10.9 months in the chemotherapy-alone arm (HR = 0.63, p < 0.001). The overall side-effect profile was similar to that of other PD-1 inhibitors without new toxicities identified. At 2 years, 43% of patients in the serplulimab arm were alive compared with 7.9% of controls.

Although cross-trial comparisons should be interpreted with caution, serplulimab is associated with the longest improvement in survival. However, serplulimab is not yet FDA approved and is similar to the approved PDL-1 agents. It will be interesting to see if this increased survival benefit is enough to sway clinical practice.

Adding to chemoimmunotherapy

Two large trials found no benefit to adding an additional immunomodulatory agent to an established chemoimmunotherapy backbone.

Tremelimumab, a humanized, monoclonal antibody that inhibits anticytotoxic CTLA4 was shown in preclinical models and other solid tumors to synergistically enhance T-cell activation when used in combination with a PD-L1 inhibitor.[11,12]

In the CASPIAN trial, tremelimumab did not significantly improve OS when added to durvalumab, platinum, and etoposide compared with platinum and etoposide alone (median OS 10.4 months vs 10.5 months). Although not directly compared, the durvalumab and durvalumab plus tremelimumab arms had similar 2-year (22.9 months vs 22.9 months) and 3-year median OS rates (17.6 months durvalumab and 15.3 months durvalumab plus tremelimumab), suggesting tremelimumab did not enhance durvalumab maintenance.

T-cell immunoreceptor with immunoglobulin and immunoreceptor tyrosine–based inhibitory motif domains (TIGIT) is a negative immune checkpoint expressed on T cell and natural killer cells, which dampens immune response by completing with CD226, a stimulating molecule.[13] Preclinical models showed that suppression of TIGIT had a synergistic effect on immune activation and tumor rejection when combined with PD-L1 blockade.[13] SKYSCRAPER-02[14] evaluated the addition of tiragolumab, an anti-TIGIT monoclonal antibody, to a standard frontline chemoimmunotherapy regimen.

Four hundred ninety patients were randomized to receive atezolizumab, carboplatin, and etoposide with or without tiragolumab followed by maintenance with either atezolizumab or atezolizumab plus tiragolumab. No benefit was seen with the addition of tiragolumab in either median PFS or median OS. Median PFS was 5.4 months in the tiragolumab arm versus 5.6 months (HR = 1.1, p = 0.35). Median OS was 13.6 months in both arms (p = 0.8).

It is unclear why combined checkpoint blockade has not proved effective in SCLC in the front-line setting (there have been signals of benefit in relapsed disease as demonstrated by Checkmate 032; discussed later). However, the inefficacy may be due to a lack of established biomarkers to select the appropriate patient populations. Unlike in non–SCLC (NSCLC), PD-L1 expression has not been shown to be predictive of immunotherapy response in SCLC.[15,16]

Reducing adverse events

Trilaciclib, a selective CDK4/6 inhibitor and first-in-class myelopreservation agent, was evaluated in a placebo-controlled, randomized, phase II trial.[17] One hundred seven patients were randomized to receive stand-of-care carboplatin and etoposide with or without trilaciclib given on days 1, 2, and 3 of each cycle (for up to 4 cycles). Patients treated with trilaciclib had fewer total grade 3 and higher adverse events (62% vs 87%) as well as significantly less grade 4 neutropenia (49% vs 2%, p < 0.0001) and dose reductions per 100 cycles (8.5 vs 2.1, p = 0.0195). Patients also tended to require less red blood cell transfusions and granulocyte colony-stimulation factor (GCSF) administration, although these did not reach statistical significance. Another phase II study showed similar benefits when trilaciclib was given in relapsed/refractory patients.[18] Trilaciclib significantly reduced the duration of severe neutropenia with cycle 1 (2 days vs 7 days, p < 0.0001) and occurrence of severe neutropenia (40.6 vs 75.9%, p = 0.016). Based on these studies, trilaciclib was FDA approved to decrease the incidence of chemotherapy-induced myelosuppression in patients with ES-SCLC receiving platinum/etoposide-containing or topotecan-containing regimens. In contrast to the more traditionally used GCSF, which acts only on granulocyte precursors, trilaciclib is not lineage-specific and preserves precursors of all cell lines through chemotherapy.

Limited Stage Disease

Currently, the standard of care for LS disease consists of concurrent chemoradiotherapy (CCRT) with a platinum agent in addition to etoposide followed by prophylactic cranial irradiation in responders.[19] The recent benefit of immunotherapy therapy in the ES setting has sparked several investigations in the use of ICIs in LS disease.

It has been proposed that the local damage caused by radiation increases the presence of neoantigens and thus primes the systemic immune system against all sites of the tumor. Immunotherapy can potentially augment this response,[20] providing a rationale for concurrent immunotherapy with radiation. In addition, there may be an additional benefit, whereby local radiation can cause regression of distant tumors, a phenomenon termed the abscopal effect.[21]

Although several studies are ongoing, 2 have published data to date. In a 2020 phase I/II study, 40 patients were treated with CCRT plus pembrolizumab followed by pembrolizumab consolidation for up to 16 cycles.[22] At a median follow-up of 23.1 months, median PFS was 19.7 months and median OS was 39.5 months; this was compared favorably against an accepted median OS of 30 months with standard-of-care CCRT alone established by the CONVERT trial.[23] There were initial concerns about synergistic toxicity with concurrent immunotherapy and radiation therapy; however, the toxicity profile in this study was manageable with no grade 5 events and rare grade 4 toxicities (neutropenia and respiratory failure in 2 and 1 patients, respectively).

The STIMULI trial was a phase II study investigating the role of dual ICI consolidation. One hundred fifty-three patients were randomized to nivolumab plus ipilimumab or observation following CCRT.[24] Neither median PFS nor median OS was significantly different at a median follow-up of 22.4 months. The median time to treatment discontinuation was 1.7 months largely due to the high prevalence of treatment-related toxicities in the experimental arm; 62% and 25% of patients experienced grade 3 or grade 4 toxicities, respectively.

Given the promising results of concurrent and consolidative pembrolizumab, several studies are underway examining the role of immunotherapy agents in various aspects of LS disease treatment. ACHILIES and ADRIATIC will explore the role of ICI consolidation. The phase II ACHILIES study (NCT03540420) will randomize patients to atezolizumab consolidation if up to 12 months versus observation following CCRT. The larger, phase III ADRIATIC study[25] investigates the role of combined ICI randomizing patients to durvalumab, durvalumab plus tremelimumab, or placebo following concurrent CCRT. Studies in which ICI is given concurrently with CCRT and then followed by ICI consolidation are also underway for both atezolizumab (NRG-LU005, NCT03811002) and durvalumab (DOLPHIN, NCT04602533) as are investigations of ICI in combination with other agents such as TIGIT (NCT04308785) and poly(adenosine diphosphate-ribose) polymerase (PARP) inhibitors (KEYLYNK-013, NCT046 24204). The tole of sequential therapy/ICI induction is also under active investigation (NCT05034133).

Relapsed/Refractory Disease

Despite high initial response rates approaching 60% to 80%, most patients with SCLC will eventually have disease progression. Alternative second-line options are currently limited. Since 1997, topotecan, a topoisomerase I inhibitor, remained the only FDA-approved option in the second-line setting[26] with an overall response rate (ORR) of 6.4% and 38% in patients who relapsed less than or greater than 3 months from chemotherapy, respectively. The median OS was approximately 5 months in both groups. In 2020, lurbinectedin, a selective inhibitor of oncogenic transcription, was FDA approved for relapsed/refractory disease based on the results of a phase II study showing an ORR of 35%, and median duration of response was 5.3 months.[27] Several other therapies have been trialed in this space with varying results.

Antiprogrammed cell death ligand 1 agents

In 2018, nivolumab was granted accelerated FDA approval based on results of the phase I/II CheckMate-032 trial showing efficacy in the third-line setting. Of note, in this study, the combination nivolumab plus ipilimumab had numerically higher 1-year OS compared with nivolumab monotherapy (43% vs 33%), although these differences were not statistically significant. However, approval was withdrawn after confirmatory studies CheckMate 451[28] and CheckMate 331[29] failed to demonstrate an improvement in OS. Similarly, in 2019, accelerated approval was granted for pembrolizumab in the third-line setting based on the results of KEYNOTE-158[30] and KEYNOTE-028.[31] However, the sponsor withdrew the application for approval after the confirmatory phase III trial, KEYNOTE-604[32] failed to show improvement in OS with the addition of pembrolizumab to chemotherapy in the first-line setting. The failure of pembrolizumab and nivolumab despite effectiveness of other immunotherapy agents was surprising. Study investigators suggest that KEYNOTE 604 may have enrolled sicker patients, as this study included a higher proportion of patients with more than 3 metastases and larger tumor size. It is possible that a subpopulation would have benefit from these therapies; however, predictive and prognostic biomarkers do not currently exist to identify these patients.

Delta-like protein 3

Delta-like protein 3 (DLL3) is an inhibitory Notch ligand. It is present in more than 80% of SCLC tumors yet not expressed in detectable levels in normal tissue, making it an attractive agent for tumor selectivity.[33] Several agents of different drug classes have been developed using this selective target.

Rovalpituzumab tesirine. Rovalpituzumab tesirine (Rova-T) is an antibody drug conjugate composed of an immunoglobulin G monoclonal antibody directed against DLL3 linked to pyrrolobenzodiazepine, a potent DNA crosslinking agent.[34]

In a phase II single-arm study of Rova-T after 2 or more lines of treatment (TRINITY), Rova-T showed an ORR of 12% and disease control rate of 70% with slightly higher response rates seen in tumors with greater than 75% DLL3 positivity.[35] This prompted 2 subsequent phase III trials examining the role of Rova-T in earlier treatment. The phase III, open-label TAHOE trial evaluated the efficacy of Rova-T in the second-line setting and enrolsment was discontinued after median OS was found to be higher in the topotecan arm.[36] Rova-T was also briefly evaluated in the first-line setting in the phase III MERU study,[37] which was stopped early after a futility analysis showed shorter OS in the Rova-T arm. After two phase III trials failed to show efficacy, manufacturing of Rova-T was discontinued.

AMG 757. AMG757 is a half-life extended, bispecific T-cell engager (BiTE) with affinity for DLL3 on SCLC tumor cells and CD3 on T-lymphocytes. An updated analysis of an ongoing phase I study of AMG757 monotherapy following at least one line of platinum-based chemotherapy showed an acceptable safety profile at 10 escalating dose levels. Unconfirmed partial response was seen in 63% (5 of 8) of patients, suggesting promising antitumor activity, and further studies are ongoing.[38]

DNA damage/repair
Thomas and colleagues[39,40] postulated that high levels of replication stress is a hallmark of SCLC tumors and may be vulnerable to drugs that inhibit the replication stress response, specifically ataxia telangiectasia mutated and rad3 related (ATR). In a phase II trial of berzosertib, a first-in-class ATR inhibitor combined with topotecan showed an overall response rate of 36% (9 of 25 patients). At a median follow-up of 20.7 months, median PFS was 4.8 months and median OS was 8.5 months. Unfortunately, this trail was discontinued after an interim analysis found it was unlikely to meet endpoints. Further phase I/II studies are ongoing with berzosertib in combination with sacituzumab govitecan (NCT04826341).

Epigenetic regulation
Inhibitors of lysine-specific histone demethylase 1A (LSD1) have shown antitumor effects in preclinical models.[41] When 6 ASCL1-positive patient-derived xenografts were treated with an ORY-1001, a novel LSD1 inhibitor, 5 of 6 tumors tumors showed significant growth inhibiton.[42] It was shown that tumor suppression was mediated through suppression of ASCl1, a neuroendocrine transcription factor. Futhermore, transcription factor suppression was due to activation of NOTCH, an endogenous activator of ASCL1. Consistent with this, mouse models lacking ASCL1 did not respond to ORY-1001 therapy.[42] It has also been demonstrated that LSD1 inhibition may augment immunotherapy in refractory SCLC models through upregulation of antigen presentation machinery.[43] A phase I/II study of bomedemstat, an oral LSD1 inhibitor, in combination with maintenance immunotherapy, is currently ongoing (NCT05191797). Targeting transcription factor expression through alternative mechanisms is also currently under investigation, including with inhibitors of enhancer-of-zeste-2-polycomb-repressive-complex-2-subunit and histone deacetylase.

Combination therapy
Immunotherapy plus tyrosine kinase inhibitors. Sintilimab, an anti-PD1 monoclonal antibody, was tested in combination with anlotinib, an antiangiogenic tyrosine kinase inhibitor in the second-line setting in a single-arm objective performance trial of 42 patients.[44] The combination of sintilimab and anlotinib showed an ORR of 49% with disease control rate of 80%. Median PFS and median OS were 6 and 16 months, respectively. Ninety-five percent of patients experienced at least one treatment-related adverse event, with hypothyroidism and hypoproteinemia being the most common. Of note, in this study 43% of patients were nonsmokers, which may limit comparisons to the general population; this may be due to genetic differences in the sample population that was limited to Chinese patients or an enriched proportion of SCLC

transdifferentiated from adenocarcinoma.[45] Anlotinib is currently undergoing evaluation in the first-line setting with chemotherapy and durvalumab (NCT04660097) as well as in maintenance after first-line chemotherapy (NCT03780283) and in combination with other checkpoint inhibitors (NCT04165330, NCT04731909, NCT04620837).

Poly(adenosine diphosphate-ribose) polymerase inhibitor plus temozolomide. Talazoparib, a PARP inhibitor was tested in combination with TMZ, an oral alkylating agent in the relapsed/refractory setting following first-line platinum-based chemotherapy.[46] A phase II, open-label, single-arm study showed daily talazoparib plus low-dose TMZ yielded a median PFS of 4.5 months and median OS 11.9 months. Serial analysis of cell-free DNA showed appearance of treatment-related mutations and was associated with superior disease control. Adverse events were mainly hematologic, with thrombocytopenia, anemia, and neutropenia being the most common. Prior early studies have also shown benefit to TMZ in combination with other PARP-inhibitors, such as olaparib[47] and veliparib[48]; however, both trials used TMZ at significantly higher doses, indicating a lower dose may be sufficient. The efficacy of TMZ, in combination with PARP and checkpoint inhibition, is currently undergoing investigation (NCT03830918).

Molecular Subtypes

Until recently, SCLC has been considered a relatively homogenous disease, and all patients with extensive disease are treated with a similar chemoimmunotherapy drug regimen. Unlike in NSCLC where genomic testing yielded the identification of targetable "driver mutations," genomic analysis of SCLC did not lead to clinically meaningful disease stratification. One exception is transdifferentiation of NSCLC adenocarcinomas to SCLC as a mechanism of estimated glomerular filtration rate resistance, which are generally thought to be genetically distinct from de novo disease.[45]

Initial genomic studies of SCLC showed a near universal loss of RB1 and TP53 as well as very high tumor mutation burden at 6 to 8 protein changing mutations per million base pairs.[49] Mutations in genes that encode histone modifiers (CREBBP, EP300, and MLL) and amplification of SOX2 were also noted[49,50] in addition to loss of function of Notch family proteins gene.[51] However, a multifaceted genomic analysis of 110 SCLC tumors identified known oncogenic driver mutations in less than 5% of samples; these included mutations in BRAF, KIT, and PIK3CA.

More recently it was shown that SCLC can be stratified into subgroups characterized by expression of specific transcription factors.[52–54] The classifications SCLC-A, SCLC-N, and SCLC-P were proposed to identify tumors that maximally express transcription factors achaete-scute homologue 1 (ASCL1), neurogenic differentiation factor 1 (NeuroD1), or POU class 2 homeobox 3 (POU2F3), respectively. A fourth subgroup, SCLC-Y, defined by expression of yes-associated protein 1 (YAP1), was initially suggested but immunohistochemistry studies do not reliably demonstrate expression of YAP1 as a unique category.[55] Using nonnegative matrix factorization, SCLC-A, -N, and -P subgroups were confirmed and an alternative fourth subtype, SCLC-inflammatory (SCLC-I), was proposed.[56] SCLC-I is characterized by low expression of ASCL1, NeuroD1, and POU2F3 and does not have a unique transcriptional signature. However, SCLC-I tumors have significantly higher expression of many immune checkpoint proteins and human leukocyte antigens.

There is emerging evidence that SCLC subgroups are clinically distinct and may have differential response to therapy. Gay and colleagues retrospectively stratified IMpower133 patients into SCLC-A, -N, -P, and -I subgroups and compared the outcomes of each group. SCLC-I patients seemed to derive the most benefit from atezolizumab with median OS of 18 months compared with 10 months for patients with SCLC-I who received only chemotherapy. Patients with SCLC-P had the worst outcomes, with median OS of 6 months in the placebo group (compared with a median of 10 months in A, N, and I), suggesting that POU2F3 may be a marker of poor prognosis. IMpower133 was not powered for subgroup analysis, and these differences in OS across SCLC subcategories were not statically significant. However, they speak to the notion that subgroup classification is clinically relevant and may be predictive of response to both novel and established therapies.

Complicating the picture, a single molecular subgroup designation may not be representative or remain constant throughout the course of disease. Several studies have demonstrated different subtype populations within a single tumor, suggesting the existence of intertumoral heterogenicity.[56,57] In addition, studies using genetically engineered mouse models of SCLC have shown that tumors may undergo transition from one subtype to another throughout the course of disease.[58]

SUMMARY

The last several years have seen more advancement in the treatment in SCLC than any other time in history. The addition of immunotherapy to traditional chemotherapy was the first regimen to significantly improve outcomes in more than 3 decades. There are now 2 FDA agents, atezolizumab and durvalumab, in the first-line setting for ES disease. Although this represents a tremendous achievement, the absolute benefit of immunotherapy remains modest, typically adding 2 to 5 months to median OS.[8,7,10] Unfortunately, attempts to augment this regimen with synergistic agents such at anti-CTLA or anti-TIGIT have failed to prolong survival in the first-line setting.

CCRT remains the standard of care for LS disease; however, there have been promising results with the addition of pembrolizumab to this regimen.[22] The incorporation of immunotherapy in the LS-SCLC setting is now an area of intense research. Multiple immunotherapy agents, including novel drugs and drug combinations, are under investigation in various stages of treatment including induction, concurrent with CCRT and as consolidation.

In relapsed disease, lurbinectedin became the second FDA-approved agent in this disease space, alongside topotecan.[27] Of note, the phase III Atlantis trial failed to show a difference in median OS between lurbinectedin plus doxorubicin vs physician's choice (topotecan or cyclophosphamide plus doxorubicin plus vincristine) in patients with SCLC who relapsed after platinum-based chemotherapy.[59] However, the dose of lurbinectedin was 35% lower than the typical 3.2 mg/m^2 dosing used in Trigo and colleagues that led to the drugs approval. More importantly, only 6% of patients were previously treated with immunotherapy, and this small group of patients seemed to have numerically longer median PFS than the physician's choice group (6.9 months vs 4.2 months). Now that immunotherapy is standard of care in the first line, it is possible this regimen may be more effective in the current treatment landscape. In addition, there is an going trial evaluating the role of lurbinectedin in combination with atezolizumab as maintenance in the front-line setting (NCT05091567).

FDA approval was withdrawn for 2 anti-PD1 agents, pembrolizumab and nivolumab, after confirmatory phase III studies failed to show benefit. In addition, trials of monoclonal DLL3 inhibitors did not prolong survival. However, AMG757, a BiTE with affinity for DLL3 and CD3, shows promising results in earl trials, suggesting that DLL3 may still be a beneficial target. Multiple drug combinations have also shown early signs of benefit in this space, specifically sintilimab and anlotinib. The combination with anlotinib with other immunotherapy agents is currently being studied in multiple different lines of treatment as are combination of PARP inhibitors and TMZ.

Finally, the identification of molecular subtypes based on transcription factor expression has been a paradigm shifting discovery. Once thought to be a genomically homogenous disease, SCLC can now be stratified into clinically meaningful subgroups. Retrospective studies have shown that distinct groups derive differential benefit from a given treatment. For example, in IMpower133, SCLC-I had a larger improvement in OS with atezolizumab than any other subgroup; this offers insight into the failures of previous drugs that may have only benefited a limited number of subgroups. More importantly, it informs study design going forward and allows the exploitation of unique vulnerabilities of each individual subtype.

CLINICS CARE POINTS

- Durvalumab and atezolizumab significantly improve survival when added to a chemotherapy in the extensive disease setting.
- The addition of immunotherapy in the limited disease setting is a topic of intense study; however, chemotherapy and radiation remain the standard of care.
- SCLC is heterogenous and can be divided into at least 4 distinct subtypes (SCLC-A, SCLC-N, SCLC-P, and SCLC-I) based on the expression profile of transcription factors. For now, subtype designation does not alter treatment; however, this is under investigation.

REFERENCES

1. Gazdar AF, Bunn PA, Minna JD. Small-cell lung cancer: what we know, what we need to know and the path forward. Nat Rev Cancer 2017;17:725–37.
2. Amini A, Byers LA, Welsh JW, et al. Progress in the management of limited-stage small cell lung cancer. Cancer 2014;120:790–8.
3. Roth BJ, Johnson DH, Einhorn LH, et al. Randomized study of cyclophosphamide, doxorubicin, and vincristine versus etoposide and cisplatin versus alternation of these two regimens in extensive small-cell lung cancer: a phase III trial of the Southeastern Cancer Study Group. J Clin Oncol 1992;10:282–91.
4. Noda K, Nishiwaki Y, Kawahara M, et al. Irinotecan plus cisplatin compared with etoposide plus cisplatin for extensive small-cell lung cancer. N Engl J Med 2002; 346:85–91.
5. Hanna N, Bunn PA Jr, Langer C, Einhorn L, et al. Randomized phase III trial comparing irinotecan/cisplatin with etoposide/cisplatin in patients with previously untreated extensive-stage disease small-cell lung cancer. J Clin Oncol 2006;24: 2038–43.
6. Lara PN Jr, Natale R, Crowley J, et al. Phase III trial of irinotecan/cisplatin compared with etoposide/cisplatin in extensive-stage small-cell lung cancer: clinical and pharmacogenomic results from SWOG S0124. J Clin Oncol 2009;27:2530.
7. Horn L, Mansfield AS, Szczęsna A, et al. First-line atezolizumab plus chemotherapy in extensive-stage small-cell lung cancer. N Engl J Med 2018;379: 2220–9.
8. Paz-Ares L, Dvorkin M, Chen Y, et al. Durvalumab plus platinum–etoposide versus platinum–etoposide in first-line treatment of extensive-stage small-cell lung cancer (CASPIAN): a randomised, controlled, open-label, phase 3 trial. Lancet 2019;394:1929–39.

9. Paz-Ares L, Chen Y, Reinmuth N, et al. Durvalumab, with or without tremelimumab, plus platinum-etoposide in first-line treatment of extensive-stage small-cell lung cancer: 3-year overall survival update from CASPIAN. ESMO Open 2022;7:100408.

10. Cheng Y, Han L, Wu L, et al. Serplulimab, a novel anti-PD-1 antibody, plus chemotherapy versus chemotherapy alone as first-line treatment for extensive-stage small-cell lung cancer: An international randomized phase 3 study. J Clin Oncol 2022;40:8505.

11. Eroglu Z, Kim DW, Wang X, et al. Long term survival with cytotoxic T lymphocyte-associated antigen 4 blockade using tremelimumab. Eur J Cancer 2015;51:2689–97.

12. Tarhini AA, Kirkwood JM. Tremelimumab (CP-675,206): a fully human anticytotoxic T lymphocyte-associated antigen 4 monoclonal antibody for treatment of patients with advanced cancers. Expet Opin Biol Ther 2008;8:1583–93.

13. Johnston RJ, Comps-Agrar L, Hackney J, et al. The immunoreceptor TIGIT Regulates Antitumor and Antiviral CD8+ T Cell Effector Function. Cancer Cell 2014;26:923–37.

14. Rudin CM, Liu SV, Lu S, et al. SKYSCRAPER-02: Primary results of a phase III, randomized, double-blind, placebo-controlled study of atezolizumab (atezo) + carboplatin + etoposide (CE) with or without tiragolumab (tira) in patients (pts) with untreated extensive-stage small cell lung cancer (ES-SCLC). J Clin Oncol 2022;40:LBA8507.

15. Frese KK, Simpson KL, Dive C. Small cell lung cancer enters the era of precision medicine. Cancer Cell 2021;39:297–9.

16. Schultheis AM, Scheel AH, Ozretić L, et al. PD-L1 expression in small cell neuroendocrine carcinomas. Eur J Cancer 2015;51:421–6.

17. Daniel D, Kuchava V, Bondarenko I, et al. 1742PD - Trilaciclib (T) decreases myelosuppression in extensive-stage small cell lung cancer (ES-SCLC) patients receiving first-line chemotherapy plus atezolizumab. Ann Oncol 2019;30:v713.

18. Hart LL, Ferrarotto R, Andric ZG, et al. Myelopreservation with trilaciclib in patients receiving topotecan for small cell lung cancer: results from a randomized, double-blind, placebo-controlled phase II study. Adv Ther 2021;38:350–65.

19. Simone CB II, Bogart JA, Cabrera AR, et al. Radiation therapy for small cell lung cancer: an ASTRO clinical practice guideline. Practical Radiation Oncology 2020;10:158–73.

20. Kodet O, Němejcova K, Strnadová K, et al. The Abscopal Effect in the Era of checkpoint inhibitors. Int J Mol Sci 2021;22:7204.

21. Mole R. Whole body irradiation—radiobiology or medicine? Br J Radiol 1953;26:234–41.

22. Welsh JW, Heymach JV, Guo C, et al. Phase 1/2 trial of pembrolizumab and concurrent chemoradiation therapy for limited-stage SCLC. J Thorac Oncol 2020;15:1919–27.

23. Faivre-Finn C, Snee M, Ashcroft L, et al. Concurrent once-daily versus twice-daily chemoradiotherapy in patients with limited-stage small-cell lung cancer (CONVERT): an open-label, phase 3, randomised, superiority trial. Lancet Oncol 2017;18:1116–25.

24. Peters S, Pujol J-L, Dafni U, et al. Consolidation nivolumab and ipilimumab versus observation in limited-disease small-cell lung cancer after chemo-radiotherapy—results from the randomised phase II ETOP/IFCT 4-12 STIMULI trial. Ann Oncol 2022;33:67–79.

25. Senan S, Okamoto I, Lee G-w, et al. Design and rationale for a phase III, randomized, placebo-controlled trial of durvalumab with or without tremelimumab after concurrent chemoradiotherapy for patients with limited-stage small-cell lung cancer: the ADRIATIC study. Clin Lung Cancer 2020;21:e84–8.

26. Ardizzoni A, Hansen H, Dombernowsky P, et al. Topotecan, a new active drug in the second-line treatment of small-cell lung cancer: a phase II study in patients with refractory and sensitive disease. The European Organization for Research and Treatment of Cancer Early Clinical Studies Group and New Drug Development Office, and the Lung Cancer Cooperative Group. J Clin Oncol 1997;15: 2090–6.

27. Trigo J, Subbiah V, Besse B, et al. Lurbinectedin as second-line treatment for patients with small-cell lung cancer: a single-arm, open-label, phase 2 basket trial. Lancet Oncol 2020;21:645–54.

28. Owonikoko TK, Park K, Govindan R, et al. Nivolumab and Ipilimumab as maintenance therapy in extensive-disease small-cell lung cancer: CheckMate 451. J Clin Oncol 2021;39:1349–59.

29. Spigel D, Vicente D, Ciuleanu T, et al. Second-line nivolumab in relapsed small-cell lung cancer: CheckMate 331. Ann Oncol 2021;32:631–41.

30. Marabelle A, Le DT, Ascierto PA, et al. Efficacy of pembrolizumab in patients with noncolorectal high microsatellite instability/mismatch repair–deficient cancer: results from the phase II KEYNOTE-158 study. J Clin Oncol 2020;38:1.

31. Ott PA, Elez E, Hiret S, et al. Pembrolizumab in patients with extensive-stage small-cell lung cancer: results from the phase Ib KEYNOTE-028 study. J Clin Oncol 2017;35:3823–9.

32. Rudin CM, Awad MM, Navarro A, et al. Pembrolizumab or Placebo plus etoposide and platinum as first-line therapy for extensive-stage small-cell lung cancer: randomized, double-blind, phase III KEYNOTE-604 study. J Clin Oncol 2020;38: 2369–79.

33. Saunders LR, Bankovich AJ, Anderson WC, et al. A DLL3-targeted antibody-drug conjugate eradicates high-grade pulmonary neuroendocrine tumor-initiating cells in vivo. Sci Transl Med 2015;7:302ra136.

34. Rudin CM, Pietanza MC, Bauer TM, et al. Rovalpituzumab tesirine, a DLL3-targeted antibody-drug conjugate, in recurrent small-cell lung cancer: a first-in-human, first-in-class, open-label, phase 1 study. Lancet Oncol 2017;18:42–51.

35. Morgensztern D, Besse B, Greillier L, et al. Efficacy and safety of rovalpituzumab tesirine in third-line and beyond patients with DLL3-expressing, relapsed/refractory small-cell lung cancer: results from the phase II TRINITY StudyPhase II study results of rova-T in DLL3-expressing SCLC. Clin Cancer Res 2019;25:6958–66.

36. Blackhall F, Jao K, Greillier L, et al. Efficacy and safety of rovalpituzumab tesirine compared with topotecan as second-line therapy in DLL3-high SCLC: results from the phase 3 TAHOE study. J Thorac Oncol 2021;16:1547–58.

37. Johnson ML, Zvirbule Z, Laktionov K, et al. Rovalpituzumab tesirine as a maintenance therapy after first-line platinum-based chemotherapy in patients with extensive-stage–SCLC: results from the phase 3 MERU study. J Thorac Oncol 2021;16:1570–81.

38. Owonikoko TK, Champiat S, Johnson ML, et al. Updated results from a phase 1 study of AMG 757, a half-life extended bispecific T-cell engager (BiTE) immuno-oncology therapy against delta-like ligand 3 (DLL3), in small cell lung cancer (SCLC). J Clin Oncol 2021;39:8510.

39. Thomas A., Takahashi N., Rajapakse V.N., et al., Therapeutic targeting of ATR yields durable regressions in small cell lung cancers with high replication stress, Cancer Cell, 39, 2021, 566–579.e567.

40. Blackford AN, Jackson SP, ATM ATR. the trinity at the heart of the DNA damage RESPONSE. Mol Cell 2017;66:801–17.

41. Borromeo MD, Savage TK, Kollipara RK, et al. ASCL1 and NEUROD1 reveal heterogeneity in pulmonary neuroendocrine tumors and regulate distinct genetic programs. Cell Rep 2016;16:1259–72.

42. Augert A, Eastwood E, Ibrahim AH, et al. Targeting NOTCH activation in small cell lung cancer through LSD1 inhibition. Sci Signal 2019;12:eaau2922.

43. Nguyen EM, Taniguchi H, Chan JM, et al. Targeting lysine-specific demethylase 1 rescues major histocompatibility complex class I antigen presentation and overcomes programmed death-ligand 1 blockade resistance in SCLC. J Thorac Oncol 2022;17:1014–31.

44. Ma S, He Z, Wang L, et al. Sintilimab plus anlotinib as second or further-line therapy for small cell lung cancer: An objective performance trial. J Clin Oncol 2022; 40:8516.

45. Yu HA, Arcila ME, Rekhtman N, et al. Analysis of tumor specimens at the time of acquired resistance to EGFR-TKI Therapy in 155 patients with EGFR-mutant lung cancersmechanisms of acquired resistance to EGFR-TKI therapy. Clin Cancer Res 2013;19:2240–7.

46. Goldman J, Cummings A, Mendenhall M, et al. OA12. 03 phase 2 study analysis of talazoparib (TALA) plus temozolomide (TMZ) for extensive-stage small cell lung cancer (ES-SCLC). J Thorac Oncol 2022;17:S32.

47. Farago AF, Yeap BY, Stanzione M, et al. Combination olaparib and temozolomide in relapsed small-cell lung cancerolaparib and temozolomide in SCLC. Cancer Discov 2019;9:1372–87.

48. Pietanza MC, Waqar SN, Krug LM, et al. Randomized, double-blind, phase II study of temozolomide in combination with either veliparib or placebo in patients with relapsed-sensitive or refractory small-cell lung cancer. J Clin Oncol 2018;36: 2386.

49. Peifer M, Fernández-Cuesta L, Sos ML, et al. Integrative genome analyses identify key somatic driver mutations of small-cell lung cancer. Nat Genet 2012;44: 1104–10.

50. Rudin CM, Durinck S, Stawiski EW, et al. Comprehensive genomic analysis identifies SOX2 as a frequently amplified gene in small-cell lung cancer. Nat Genet 2012;44:1111–6.

51. George J, Lim JS, Jang SJ, et al. Comprehensive genomic profiles of small cell lung cancer. Nature 2015;524:47–53.

52. Huang YH, Klingbeil O, He XY, et al. POU2F3 is a master regulator of a tuft cell-like variant of small cell lung cancer. Genes Dev 2018;32:915–28.

53. Rudin CM, Poirier JT, Byers LA, et al. Molecular subtypes of small cell lung cancer: a synthesis of human and mouse model data. Nat Rev Cancer 2019;19: 289–97.

54. Zhang W, Girard L, Zhang YA, et al. Small cell lung cancer tumors and preclinical models display heterogeneity of neuroendocrine phenotypes. Transl Lung Cancer Res 2018;7:32–49.

55. Baine MK, Hsieh M-S, Lai WV, et al. SCLC subtypes defined by ASCL1, NEUROD1, POU2F3, and YAP1: a comprehensive immunohistochemical and histopathologic characterization. J Thorac Oncol 2020;15:1823–35.

56. Gay CM, Stewart CA, Park EM, et al. Patterns of transcription factor programs and immune pathway activation define four major subtypes of SCLC with distinct therapeutic vulnerabilities. Cancer Cell 2021;39:346–360 e347.
57. Simpson KL, Stoney R, Frese KK, et al. A biobank of small cell lung cancer CDX models elucidates inter- and intratumoral phenotypic heterogeneity. Nat Can 2020;1:437–51.
58. Ireland AS, Micinski AM, Kastner DW, et al. MYC drives temporal evolution of small cell lung cancer subtypes by reprogramming neuroendocrine fate. Cancer Cell 2020;38:60–78.e12.
59. Aix SP, Ciuleanu TE, Navarro A, et al. Combination lurbinectedin and doxorubicin versus physician's choice of chemotherapy in patients with relapsed small-cell lung cancer (ATLANTIS): a multicentre, randomised, open-label, phase 3 trial. Lancet Respir Med 2023;11:74–86.

Lung Cancer Supportive Care and Symptom Management

Johnathan Yao, MD[a], Madison Novosel, BA[b], Shreya Bellampalli, BS[c], Jennifer Kapo, MD[d], Julia Joseph, MD[a], Elizabeth Prsic, MD[e,*]

KEYWORDS

- Advanced lung cancer • Palliative care • Symptom management • Cancer pain

KEY POINTS

- Cancer-associated symptoms related to the underlying malignancy or cancer-directed therapy negatively impact quality of life. Among patients with lung cancer, pain and dyspnea are prevalent.
- Pain is a common adverse event experienced by patients with advanced lung cancer. Appropriate analgesia is essential to improve patient quality of life, morbidity, and mortality.
- Oncological emergencies (e.g. hypercalcemia, SIADH and spinal cord compression) may be life-threatening complications of advanced lung cancer and warrant prompt diagnosis and management.
- Patients with advanced lung cancer often experience significant psychosocial stressors (e.g. fatigue, anxiety, financial toxicity) which may decrease their quality of life, complicate the receipt of cancer-directed therapy, and increase risk of morbidity and mortality.

INTRODUCTION

Despite significant advances in therapy and diagnosis, lung cancer remains the leading cause of cancer-related death among men and women globally.[1] Given the

[a] Yale Internal Medicine-Traditional Residency Program, Department of Internal Medicine, Yale School of Medicine, Yale University, 333 Cedar Street, PO Box 208030, New Haven, CT 06520-8030, USA; [b] Chronic Disease Epidemiology, Yale School of Public Health, Yale University, 60 College Street, New Haven, CT 06510, USA; [c] Medical Scientist Training Program, Mayo Clinic Alix School of Medicine, Mayo Clinic, 200 First Street Southwest, Rochester, MN 55905, USA; [d] Department of General Internal Medicine, Yale School of Medicine, Yale University, 333 Cedar Street, PO Box 208025, New Haven, CT 06520, USA; [e] Section of Medical Oncology, Department of Medicine, Yale School of Medicine, Yale University, 333 Cedar Street, PO Box 208028, New Haven, CT 06520, USA
* Corresponding author. Section of Medical Oncology, Palliative Care Program, Yale School of Medicine, Yale University, 333 Cedar Street, PO Box 208028, New Haven, CT 06520-8028, USA.
E-mail address: elizabeth.prsic@yale.edu
Twitter: @ElizabethPrsic (E.P.)

Hematol Oncol Clin N Am 37 (2023) 609–622
https://doi.org/10.1016/j.hoc.2023.02.011
0889-8588/23/© 2023 Elsevier Inc. All rights reserved.

significant mortality, morbidity, and treatment-related adverse events, supportive care is an essential element in the care of patients with lung cancer.

BACKGROUND

Despite advances in the diagnosis and management of lung cancer, lung cancer remains the leading cause of cancer death.[1] Of primary risk factors, tobacco smoking remains the predominant risk factor. Other risk factors include occupational and environmental exposures and chronic lung disease.[2] This review focuses on supportive care and symptom management among patients with lung cancer.

MORTALITY

Lung cancer remains the leading cause of cancer-associated deaths for both men and women globally despite significant advances in the diagnosis and management of disease.[3,4] Overall, lung cancer causes more deaths than breast, prostate, colorectal, and brain cancers combined.[4] In fact, lung cancer accounts for nearly 20% of cancer-associated deaths worldwide.[3] With increased industrialization and access to tobacco worldwide, the worldwide incidence of lung cancer continues to increase.[5] In 2018, more than 2,000,000 individuals were diagnosed with lung cancer with more than 1,700,000 deaths estimated in 2018.[3]

Immunotherapy and targeted agents have dramatically changed management of lung cancers in both the curative and the palliative settings. Management options may include surgical resection, radiation therapy, chemotherapy, targeted therapies, and/or immunotherapy. Furthermore, with development and implementation of lung cancer screening, cancers may be detected earlier and improve morbidity and mortality associated with the disease.[6] Despite advances, lung cancer mortality and morbidity remain significant, underlining the importance of supportive care and symptom management in this patient population.

MORBIDITY

Lung cancer-associated morbidity and symptom burden remain major challenges for the millions of individuals diagnosed with lung cancer annually. With increasing survival and time on treatment, patients may face increasingly complex toxicities related to cancer-directed therapies. This is particularly relevant in the setting of immunotherapy-related adverse events, which may contribute to long-term or permanent medical complications (eg, hypothyroidism, diabetes mellitus, and hypopituitarism).[7]

PROGNOSTIC UNCERTAINTY

With advances in lung cancer management have come improvements in early detection and disease-specific survival. However, patients and families are faced with increasingly complex treatment-related decisions in the setting of serious illness, as well as prognostic uncertainty. Patients with advanced cancer who do not receive prognostic information may overestimate their life expectancy. Furthermore, these patients may be more likely to receive aggressive care at the end of life (EOL) that may not be aligned with their goals of care.[8] Aggressive medical care at the EOL for patients with advanced cancer may be associated with poor quality of care.[9,10] Early palliative care may help patients to improve understanding of their prognosis over time and to choose care that is more consistent with their goals of care near the EOL.[8]

ONCOLOGIC EMERGENCIES

Within lung cancer, there are several oncologic emergencies clinicians may encounter commonly.

Hypercalcemia

Hypercalcemia of malignancy may present with nausea, vomiting, constipation, and altered mental status. Symptoms are most common with calcium levels greater than 14 mg/dL; however, symptoms may also present more acutely with a rapid increase in levels. Hypercalcemia is a common complication of malignancies, occurring in up to a third of patients with advanced cancer. It is more common among patients with squamous cell cancer of the lung. Historically, hypercalcemia has been associated with a poor prognosis; recent data suggest an in-hospital mortality greater than 5%.[11,12] Hydration and administration of bisphosphonates are the primary methods of hypercalcemia treatment. Calcitonin causes a rapid decline in calcium but is short-acting and associated with tachyphylaxis owing to downregulation of calcitonin receptors.[13] Bisphosphonates, such as zoledronate, decreases calcium in 4 to 10 days, with a therapeutic duration of 4 to 6 weeks.[14] Denosumab, an RANK-ligand inhibitor, can also lower serum calcium by reducing bone resorption, but at significantly increased cost relative to bisphosphonates.[15]

Syndrome of Inappropriate Secretion of Antidiuretic Hormone

Syndrome of Inappropriate secretion of antidiuretic hormone (SIADH), commonly seen in small cell lung cancer (SCLC), may present as nausea, myalgias, headache, and neurologic symptoms (eg, seizures, comas), when sodium levels are less than 135 mEq/L, decreased serum osmolarity less than 280 mmol/L, and concentrated urine greater than 100 mOsm/L. SCLC can ectopically secrete excess antidiuretic hormone. Fluid restriction (limit of 500–1000 mL) will usually correct SIADH over the course of several days. A goal correction of 4 to 8 mmol/L per day is necessary to avoid central pontine myelinolysis. Oral salt tablets can also be used, or in patients with severe symptoms, hypertonic saline may be required.[16]

Superior Vena Cava Syndrome

Superior vena cava syndrome (SVCS) may present as cough, dyspnea, dysphagia, and swelling or discoloration of the neck, face, and upper extremities. More severely, patients may have life-threatening vascular involvement. SVCS is due to compression of the superior vena cava (SVC), which leads to edema and retrograde flow. Thrombi may be associated with the presence of SVCS. Specifically, the SVC extends to the right atrium and is enveloped by lymph nodes that drain from the right thoracic cavity. As such, around 80% of SVCS cases are due to direct extension from a centrally located right-sided tumor. Treatment may include radiation and chemotherapy to reduce tumor burden or stenting of obstructed vasculature. Steroids may be helpful adjuncts in select situations (eg, lymphoma). Combination chemotherapy is effective and may be preferable in the appropriate clinical setting because it can avoid a large radiation field and treat distant metastases. Relief of SVCS is usually observed after 7 to 10 days with appropriate treatment.[17]

Spinal Cord Compression

Spinal cord compression (SCC) is a dangerous complication of lung cancer, which can lead to permanent neurologic impairment, including incontinence, loss of sensory function, and paraplegia. SCC should be on the differential diagnosis for any patient with cancer who complains of new or changed back pain. Pain may be exacerbated by sneezing, coughing, or lying down. Up to 20% of patients with lung cancer may present with SCC at the time of diagnosis.[16] Diagnostic imaging should include MR imaging of the total spine. Corticosteroids should be administered promptly (ideally within 12 hours of diagnosis) to reduce vasogenic edema. Dosing typically begins with dexamethasone 10 mg once, followed by 4 mg every 6 hours.[18] Neurosurgery should be consulted to evaluate for possible surgical intervention. Finally, radiation oncology should also be consulted for symptom palliation.[19]

Malignant Pericardial Effusion

Lung cancer constitutes over half of pericardial involvement documented among patients with cancer.[20] Malignant pericardial effusions can present with dyspnea, orthopnea, fatigue, palpitations, and dizziness. For patients with suspected cardiac tamponade, physical examination findings may include pulsus paradoxus, tachycardia, distended neck veins, narrow pulse pressure, and distant heart sounds. With a high clinical suspicion from the history and physical examination, pericardial effusions can be diagnosed with echocardiogram and treated with pericardiocentesis. Among patients who present with large pericardial effusions, the elderly and those with lung cancer have worse survival.[21]

Increased Intracranial Pressure

A new, changed, or persistent headache in a patient with cancer should always raise concern for increased intracranial pressure (ICP) related to central nervous system metastases. Headaches associated with increased ICP are often worse at night or in the morning upon waking owing to decreased venous drainage in the supine position. Headaches may be associated with nausea and vomiting and typically improve rapidly with steroids. Notably, ICP-related headaches may be resistant to nonopioid analgesics (eg, acetaminophen or ibuprofen). For patients with signs or symptoms associated with ICP, immediate consultation of radiation oncology and neurosurgery is appropriate.

More advanced sequelae of increased ICP may include changes in breathing, hypertension, and bradycardia (ie, symptoms related to the Cushing reflex). Leptomeningeal metastases may present with symptoms consistent with increased ICP, or with neurologic complications (eg, altered mental status, seizures). Leptomeningeal disease is most commonly diagnosed by lumbar puncture, but can also be identified by subarachnoid masses, diffuse contrast enhancement of the meninges, or hydrocephalus without a mass lesion on imaging.[22]

Initial management involves initiation of systemic steroids. Dexamethasone is the preferred agent typically beginning with 10 mg once, followed by 4 mg every 6 hours for patients with moderate to severe associated symptoms.[23] Of note, intravenous (IV) dosing and oral steroid dosing are equivalent assuming the oral route is safe and effective.[23] Side effects of steroids are dose-dependent; steroid taper should be initiated rapidly, but titrated as clinically tolerated.[23]

Whole brain radiation therapy (WBRT) is often used to treat brain metastases and may be associated with several adverse side effects, including memory loss, fatigue, radiation-induced alopecia, and neurocognitive dysfunction. Stereotactic radiosurgery (SRS) may be used for patients with a limited number of central nervous system metastases. SRS has been shown to be highly effective in the local control of brain metastases and offers several advantages.[24] This includes fewer overall systemic side effects, single-session delivery of high-dose radiation, and allowing for the maintenance of systemic chemotherapy and/or immunotherapy without interruption.

Several studies have demonstrated that patients treated with SRS alone were less likely to have cognitive decline when compared with patients treated with SRS + WBRT, and importantly, no significant differences in overall survival have been demonstrated.[24–26]

SYMPTOMS
Dyspnea

Dyspnea, defined as the sensation of breathlessness, is a common and debilitating symptom in patients with advanced cancer. Among patients with lung cancer, dyspnea may be caused by malignant pleural effusions, direct invasion into the airway or pulmonary vasculature, and pulmonary lymphangitic carcinomatosis. Further, pulmonary embolism, post-obstructive pneumonia, and pericardial effusion may present with dyspnea. Pneumonitis may be a treatment-related cause of dyspnea. Consequences of dyspnea include fatigue, anxiety, drowsiness, and decreased performance status. National Comprehensive Cancer Network (NCCN) guidelines recommend the use of both pharmacologic and nonpharmacologic interventions for managing dyspnea.[27] Nonpharmacologic interventions include fans, bilevel ventilation, cooler temperatures, stress management, and relaxation therapy.[28] Of the nonpharmacologic interventions, fans and bilevel ventilation were found to be more effective, whereas behavioral therapy and relaxation were not associated with improving dyspnea.[28] Positioning may also improve dyspnea, where clinically appropriate. Supervised exercise-based pulmonary rehabilitation has also been found to improve cardiorespiratory fitness and functional capacity in patients with lung cancer and compromised lung function.[29] Among pharmacologic approaches, opioids are the standard of care for pharmacologic management of dyspnea resistant to nonpharmacologic therapy.[30] Benzodiazepines may also be a helpful adjunct if dyspnea is associated with anxiety, although evidence supporting its use in this setting is limited. Importantly, their concurrent use with opioids may increase the risk of respiratory depression.

Cancer Pain

Pain is a common complication of patients with advanced cancer and is associated with increased readmission, morbidity, and mortality.[16,31] Poor pain control may be associated with increased risk of falls, delirium, decreased performance status, increased depression, anxiety, and decreased quality of life (QOL).

Most of the pain syndromes in patients with lung cancer result from direct metastatic involvement. With bone involvement, the combination of direct nerve injury, release of inflammatory factors, and bone fractures may contribute to pain.[32] In addition to nociceptive cancer pain, neuropathic pain may arise from malignancy itself (eg, direct nerve injury or plexopathy) or from cytotoxic therapy (eg, taxanes, platinums).[16]

Opioids are commonly used as first-line therapy for moderate to severe cancer-associated pain (**Fig. 1**). Generally, higher-potency opioids, such as morphine, hydromorphone, or oxycodone, are used first line.[33] Lower-potency opioids, such as tramadol and codeine, have more variable pharmacokinetics and may be less efficacious in certain individuals.[33] Short-acting opioids should be given every 3 to 4 hours as needed, with longer intervals only where appropriate in the setting of renal or hepatic dysfunction.[33] If more frequent (eg, 4–5 doses per 24 hours) short-acting opioid dosing is required, patients may benefit from long-acting formulations to support chronic, cancer-associated pain.[33] If a short-acting dose is

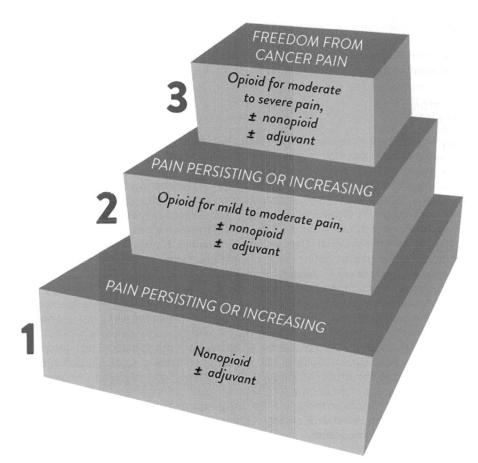

Fig. 1. The 3-step analgesic ladder. (*From* WHO Guidelines for the Pharmacological and Radiotherapeutic Management of Cancer Pain in Adults and Adolescents. Geneva: World Health Organization; 2018. Figure A1.1, The three-step analgesic ladder. Available from: https://www.ncbi.nlm.nih.gov/books/NBK537489/figure/appannex1.fig1/; with permission. (Figure A1.1 in original).[34])

ineffective, increase dose by 50% for moderately controlled pain, or 100% for severe, poorly controlled pain. Transdermal fentanyl may be helpful for chronic, stable pain in patients with difficulty maintaining oral administration (eg, severe nausea, recurrent small bowel obstructions).[33] Patient-controlled analgesia may be helpful in selected patients who have severe pain, requiring IV route of administration and rapid titration.[33]

Although opioids are used frequently to manage moderate to severe cancer-associated pain, opioid-sparing agents, such as acetaminophen or nonsteroidal anti-inflammatory drugs, may be helpful. Opioid-sparing adjuncts are particularly important in the management of neuropathic pain.

Neuropathic Pain

Neuropathic pain is characterized by paresthesia, hyperalgesia, and allodynia (pain related to a stimulus that usually does not provoke pain) and can result in decreased performance status and cognitive and social functioning.[35,36] The majority of patients with cancer presenting with neuropathic pain experience symptoms related to malignancy, owing to either direct nerve damage or secondary to chemotherapy, radiation, or surgery.[36] Neuropathic pain responds variably to opioids, although methadone may have improved efficacy owing to its N-methyl-D-aspartate receptor antagonist effect.[37] However, data supporting the use of methadone for adults with neuropathic pain are mixed.[38] Medications, such as pregabalin, duloxetine, gabapentin, and glucocorticoids, are often prescribed to treat neuropathic pain symptoms, but many patients remain refractory posttreatment.[39–41] Current research for effective neuropathic pain management remains largely in preclinical stages with surgical, viral, and chemotherapy-induced animal models, although some therapies have moved beyond to clinical trials.[35,42,43]

Nonpharmacologic therapies may also be effective in the management of cancer pain. Radiation oncology is a particularly effective modality for palliation, particularly for bone metastases.[24] Palliative radiation may also help support symptomatic relief.[24] Finally, acupuncture and massage therapy may be effective in managing cancer pain and neuropathy.[33,44,45]

Nausea

Nausea and vomiting are among the most debilitating side effects of cancer treatments. Antiemetic medications are most effective when given prophylactically in the setting of chemotherapy-induced nausea and vomiting (CINV).[46] The American Society of Clinical Oncology (ASCO) has guidelines based on systematic review of medical literature that stratify treatment based on emetogenicity of cancer-directed therapy. In general, patients receiving highly emetogenic agents should receive neurokinin 11 (NK1) receptor antagonist, serotonin (5-HT3) receptor antagonist, and dexamethasone and olanzapine for prophylaxis. Platinum-based therapies are more likely to cause delayed and/or persistent CINV and require focused supportive care. Patients treated with moderate-emetic-risk regimens should be offered a 2-drug combination of 5-HT3 receptor antagonist and dexamethasone. Finally, patients receiving low-emetic-risk cancer-directed therapies should be offered a 5-HT3 receptor antagonist or dexamethasone before treatment. Patients treated with minimal-emetic-risk cancer-directed therapies should not be offered routine antiemetic prophylaxis.

Breakthrough nausea can be managed with olanzapine, which can achieve control in up to 70% patients with refractory CINV.[47] Alternatively, ASCO 2020 guidelines suggest using an NK1 antagonist, a 5-HT3 antagonist, a dopaminergic antagonist (prochlorperazine, haloperidol), or a benzodiazepine (eg, lorazepam, alprazolam).[48]

Numerous causes may contribute to nausea and vomiting in patients with lung cancer, in addition to CINV. Increased ICP can also present with nausea and vomiting. Management of ICP is covered separately in this review. Nausea may also present in the setting of increased abdominal distention related to bowel obstruction, liver capsule distension, or constipation. Vestibular dysfunction related to vertigo or middle ear causes may also present with nausea. Vestibular causes of nausea may respond well to meclizine, scopolamine, or other agents with anticholinergic effects.

A risk factor of poorly controlled symptoms is anticipatory nausea and vomiting (ANV), or conditioned nausea and vomiting, which can occur in up to a third of patients.[49] Risk factors include poor nausea control with cancer-directed therapy, age less than 50 years, female gender, motion sickness, and history of pregnancy-associated nausea. Behavioral or psychological therapy is first-line therapy for ANV. Other approaches include scheduled antiemetics, benzodiazepines, and potentially, cannabinoids. However, evidence for the use of cannabinoids latter remains insufficient for guideline-based recommended antiemetic therapy.

Side-effect profile, adverse effects, and patient comorbidities should be considered when selecting an antiemetic. For instance, metoclopramide may be helpful in patients with a history of diabetic gastropathy, decreased motility, or constipation given its pro-motility effects. In patients with prolonged QT, caution should be taken when prescribing QT-prolonging agents, such as ondansetron and other 5HT-3 antagonists. In patients with insomnia and weight loss, olanzapine may help support nausea and has mild sedating effects along with increased appetite. For patients with cancer-associated fatigue or liver capsule distention as well as nausea, low-dose steroids (eg, dexamethasone 2–4 mg daily) may serve as a helpful adjunct for multiple symptoms. Although cannabinoids and acupuncture may be helpful adjuncts for antiemetics, data remain insufficient for guideline-based recommendations supporting their use.[50]

Psychosocial Needs

Patients who have cancer experience significant psychosocial distress. The NCCN defines distress as an unpleasant, multidimensional experience of a social, psychological, and/or spiritual nature that may interfere with a patient's emotions, actions, and ability to cope with symptoms and treatment.[51] Distress can negatively affect a patient's morbidity, functional impairment, and QOL.[52] Studies show that up to 45% of patients routinely report significant psychosocial distress, yet fewer than 10% are referred for psychosocial care.[53] Among the most common causes of patient distress include fatigue, pain, fears, worry, nervousness, and sadness.[54] These symptoms can be supported by integrated palliative care.[55] In addition, social workers may also be equipped to benefit patients with psychosocial needs owing to their training in counseling, care coordination, and other patient-centered skills.[56] Financial toxicity is common in patients with lung cancer; approximately half of patients with cancer or cancer survivors report personal economic burdens related to care.[57] It is important to support patients facing financial toxicity and advocate for equitable access to affordable cancer care.

PALLIATIVE CARE

Palliative care is an interdisciplinary approach focusing on improving QOL for patients living with serious illness and their families.[58] Given the significant morbidity and mortality associated with lung cancer, early integration of palliative care is an essential element of cancer care. In fact, early integration may improve survival as well as QOL for patients with non–small cell lung cancer (NSCLC) and is recommended by the NCCN for all patients diagnosed with NSCLC and select patients with SCLC.[59–61]

Palliative care provides additional support for patients with serious comorbid physical conditions, complex symptom management, psychosocial needs, spiritual or existential distress, poor prognosis, and those requiring communication support or advance care planning.[27]

Although early integration of palliative care is recommended for patients with advanced NSCLC and concurrently with cancer-directed therapy, there is significant variability in terms of available specialty support nationally.[61,62] Although the vast majority of large, urban hospitals in the United States have palliative care services, less than a quarter of smaller rural hospitals have similar support.[63]

Despite guideline recommendations and clinical benefits, only a quarter of patients with metastatic lung cancer in the United States received palliative care.[64,65] Among patients with advanced NSCLC, patients from minority groups are less likely to access palliative care support.[65] In fact, of patients with advanced NSCLC cancer, only 20% of black patients and 15.9% of Hispanic patients received palliative care.[66]

Goals of Care

Communication between clinicians and patients is essential to ensure that care provided is consistent with patient goals. A major focus of goals of care conversations is discussion of medically intensive care at the EOL. Most patients in the United States prefer to die in nonhospital settings.[67] However, patients with often experience high emergency room utilization and hospital admission, which may not be consistent with previously stated goals.[54] Patients who receive chemotherapy near the EOL are more likely to experience emergency department (ED) visits, inpatient admissions, and death in the hospital compared with those who do not receive chemotherapy the last 30 days of life.[68] Palliative care has demonstrated significant improvement in the quality of care at the EOL for patients with advanced cancer, as well as significant health care cost savings.[69,70] Among patients with lung cancer, early palliative care referral is associated with lower risk of late chemotherapy.[9,65] There are well-documented disparities in terms of palliative care among patients with advanced cancer, and health care utilization at the EOL, with racial-ethnic minorities having decreased access to palliative care, increased health care utilization, and medically aggressive care at the EOL.[10,71]

Hospice Utilization

Hospice care focuses on caring for patients with serious illness who are approaching the EOL. Patients with a serious medical illness and a prognosis of 6 months or less are eligible for the Medicare hospice benefit. Hospice care aims to address symptoms and to support patients and their caregivers, rather than cure the underlying disease.

Patients with advanced lung cancer enrolled in hospice in the last 30 days of life experienced lower rates of hospitalization, ED visits, and chemotherapy and radiation at the EOL.[72] These measures may be associated with poorer quality of care at the EOL. Furthermore, decreased health care utilization was associated with decreased health care spending in the last 30 days of life.[72]

LUNG CANCER SURVIVORSHIP

NCCN guidelines identify individuals as cancer survivors as those living with cancer and those free of cancer.[73] There are more than 380,000 estimated lung cancer survivors in the United States as of 2019.[74] This number is increasing every year as a result of screening, early detection, and advances in treatment. Challenges to lung cancer survivorship include high recurrence rates, most often within the first 2 years of completely resected early-stage cancer. Long-term complications of disease and treatment may include pain, neuropathy, hearing loss, cognitive decline, and psychological distress. Persistent tobacco use and medical comorbidities related to past use also contribute to the complex care needs of this patient population.

SUMMARY

Advances in lung cancer care have improved understanding of the disease, as well as treatment, supportive care, and survival.[75] Supportive care and symptom management are key components of the care of patients with lung cancer. Every clinician should understand the diagnosis and management of oncology emergencies associated with advanced lung cancer and be able to expertly manage cancer-associated pain and identify and support psychosocial needs. For patients with advanced disease, early integration of palliative care improves QOL and may improve survival. Finally, for patients nearing the EOL, hospice care offers more comprehensive, supportive care for patients and families.

DISCLOSURE

The authors have no financial interests or relationships to disclose.

REFERENCES

1. Romaszko AM, Doboszyńska A. Multiple primary lung cancer: A literature review. Adv Clin Exp Med 2018;27(5):725–30.
2. Bade BC, Dela Cruz CS. Lung Cancer 2020: Epidemiology, Etiology, and Prevention. Clin Chest Med 2020;41(1):1–24.
3. Thandra KC, Barsouk A, Saginala K, et al. Epidemiology of lung cancer. Contemp Oncol 2021;25(1):45–52.
4. American Cancer Society. Cancer Facts & Figures. American Cancer Society. Available at: https://www.cancer.org/content/dam/cancer-org/research/cancer-facts-and-statistics/annual-cancer-facts-and-figures/2022/2022-cancer-facts-and-figures.pdf. Accessed September 30, 2022.
5. Barta JA, Powell CA, Wisnivesky JP. Global Epidemiology of Lung Cancer. Ann Glob Health 2019;85(1). https://doi.org/10.5334/aogh.2419.
6. Meza R, Jeon J, Toumazis I, et al. Evaluation of the Benefits and Harms of Lung Cancer Screening With Low-Dose Computed Tomography: Modeling Study for the US Preventive Services Task Force. JAMA 2021;325(10):988–97.
7. Martins F, Sofiya L, Sykiotis GP, et al. Adverse effects of immune-checkpoint inhibitors: epidemiology, management and surveillance. Nat Rev Clin Oncol 2019;16(9):563–80.
8. Enzinger AC, Zhang B, Schrag D, et al. Outcomes of Prognostic Disclosure: Associations With Prognostic Understanding, Distress, and Relationship With Physician Among Patients With Advanced Cancer. J Clin Oncol 2015;33(32):3809–16.
9. Woldie I, Elfiki T, Kulkarni S, et al. Chemotherapy during the last 30 days of life and the role of palliative care referral, a single center experience. BMC Palliat Care 2022;21(1):20.
10. Johnson LA, Ellis C. Chemotherapy in the Last 30 Days and 14 Days of Life in African Americans With Lung Cancer. Am J Hosp Palliat Care 2021;38(8):927–31.
11. Ralston SH, Gallacher SJ, Patel U, et al. Cancer-associated hypercalcemia: morbidity and mortality. Clinical experience in 126 treated patients. Ann Intern Med 1990;112(7):499–504.
12. Wright JD, Tergas AI, Ananth CV, et al. Quality and Outcomes of Treatment of Hypercalcemia of Malignancy. Cancer Invest 2015;33(8):331–9.
13. Goldner W. Cancer-Related Hypercalcemia. J Oncol Pract 2016;12(5):426–32.
14. Fojo AT. Chapter 122: 'Metabolic emergencies. In: Hellman and Rosenberg's cancer: Principles and Practice of oncology. Philadelphia, PA: Wolters Kluwer Health; 2015. p. 1822–31.
15. Hu MI, Glezerman IG, Leboulleux S, et al. Denosumab for treatment of hypercalcemia of malignancy. J Clin Endocrinol Metab 2014;99(9):3144–52.
16. Gould Rothberg BE, Quest TE, Yeung SJ, et al. Oncologic emergencies and urgencies: A comprehensive review. CA Cancer J Clin 2022;72(6):570–93.
17. Zimmerman S, Davis M. Rapid Fire: Superior Vena Cava Syndrome. Emerg Med Clin North Am 2018;36(3):577–84.

18. Kumar A, Weber MH, Gokaslan Z, et al. Metastatic Spinal Cord Compression and Steroid Treatment: A Systematic Review. Clin Spine Surg 2017;30(4):156–63.

19. Becker K.P. and Baehring J.M., Chapter 121: spinal cord compression, In: DeVita V.T. Lawrence T.S., Rosenberg S.A., DeVita, Hellman and Rosenberg's cancer: Principles and Practice of oncology, 2015, Wolters Kluwer Health, Philadelphia, PA, 1810-1815.

20. Strobbe A, Adriaenssens T, Bennett J, et al. Etiology and Long-Term Outcome of Patients Undergoing Pericardiocentesis. J Am Heart Assoc 2017;6(12). https://doi.org/10.1161/jaha.117.007598.

21. Ahmed T, Mouhayar E, Song J, et al. Predictors of Recurrence and Survival in Cancer Patients With Pericardial Effusion Requiring Pericardiocentesis. Front Cardiovasc Med 2022;9:916325.

22. Grossman SA, Krabak MJ. Leptomeningeal carcinomatosis. Cancer Treat Rev 1999;25(2):103–19.

23. Chang SM, Messersmith H, Ahluwalia M, et al. Anticonvulsant prophylaxis and steroid use in adults with metastatic brain tumors: summary of SNO and ASCO endorsement of the Congress of Neurological Surgeons guidelines. Neuro Oncol 2019;21(4):424–7.

24. Yaeh A, Nanda T, Jani A, et al. Control of brain metastases from radioresistant tumors treated by stereotactic radiosurgery. J Neuro Oncol 2015;124(3):507–14.

25. Lutz S, Balboni T, Jones J, et al. Palliative radiation therapy for bone metastases: Update of an ASTRO Evidence-Based Guideline. Pract Radiat Oncol 2017; 7(1):4–12.

26. Aoyama H, Tago M, Kato N, et al. Neurocognitive function of patients with brain metastasis who received either whole brain radiotherapy plus stereotactic radiosurgery or radiosurgery alone. Int J Radiat Oncol Biol Phys 2007;68(5):1388–95.

27. National Comprehensive Cancer Network. Palliative Care (Version 1.2022). Available at: https://www.nccn.org/professionals/physician_gls/pdf/palliative.pdf.

28. Gupta A, Sedhom R, Sharma R, et al. Nonpharmacological Interventions for Managing Breathlessness in Patients With Advanced Cancer: A Systematic Review. JAMA Oncol 2021;7(2):290–8.

29. Deng GE, Rausch SM, Jones LW, et al. Complementary therapies and integrative medicine in lung cancer: Diagnosis and management of lung cancer, 3rd ed: American College of Chest Physicians evidence-based clinical practice guidelines. Chest 2013;143(5 Suppl):e420S–36S.

30. Hui D, Bohlke K, Bao T, et al. Management of Dyspnea in Advanced Cancer: ASCO Guideline. J Clin Oncol 2021;39(12):1389–411.

31. Coyne CJ, Reyes-Gibby CC, Durham DD, et al. Cancer pain management in the emergency department: a multicenter prospective observational trial of the Comprehensive Oncologic Emergencies Research Network (CONCERN). Support Care Cancer 2021;29(8):4543–53.

32. Mantyh PW. Bone cancer pain: from mechanism to therapy. Curr Opin Support Palliat Care 2014;8(2):83–90.

33. National Comprehensive Cancer Network. Adult Cancer Pain (Version 2.2022). Available at: https://www.nccn.org/professionals/physician_gls/pdf/pain.pdf.

34. WHO guidelines for the pharmacological and radiotherapeutic management of cancer pain in adults and Adolescents. Figure A1.1, the three-step analgesic ladder. Geneva: World Health Organization; 2018.

35. Cavalli E, Mammana S, Nicoletti F, et al. The neuropathic pain: An overview of the current treatment and future therapeutic approaches. Int J Immunopathol

Pharmacol 2019;33. https://doi.org/10.1177/2058738419838383. 20587384 19838383.

36. Edwards HL, Mulvey MR, Bennett MI. Cancer-Related Neuropathic Pain. Cancers 2019;11(3). https://doi.org/10.3390/cancers11030373.

37. McPherson ML. Methadone: a complex and challenging analgesic, but it's worth it!. In: Demystifying opioid conversion calculators. American Society of Health System Pharmacists 2018;2nd edition:180.

38. McNicol ED, Ferguson MC, Schumann R. Methadone for neuropathic pain in adults. Cochrane Database Syst Rev 2017;5(5):Cd012499.

39. De Santis S, Borghesi C, Ricciardi S, et al. Analgesic effectiveness and tolerability of oral oxycodone/naloxone and pregabalin in patients with lung cancer and neuropathic pain: an observational analysis. OncoTargets Ther 2016;9: 4043–52.

40. Gül Ş K, Tepetam H, Gül HL. Duloxetine and pregabalin in neuropathic pain of lung cancer patients. Brain Behav 2020;10(3):e01527.

41. Chow R, Novosel M, So OW, et al. Duloxetine for prevention and treatment of chemotherapy-induced peripheral neuropathy (CIPN): systematic review and meta-analysis. BMJ Support Palliat Care 2022. https://doi.org/10.1136/spcare-2022-003815.

42. Alles SRA, Smith PA. Peripheral Voltage-Gated Cation Channels in Neuropathic Pain and Their Potential as Therapeutic Targets. Front Pain Res (Lausanne) 2021;2:750583.

43. Khanna R, Yu J, Yang X, et al. Targeting the CaVα-CaVβ interaction yields an antagonist of the N-type CaV2.2 channel with broad antinociceptive efficacy. Pain 2019;160(7):1644–61.

44. Ge L, Wang Q, He Y, et al. Acupuncture for cancer pain: an evidence-based clinical practice guideline. Chin Med 2022;17(1):8.

45. Boyd C, Crawford C, Paat CF, et al. The Impact of Massage Therapy on Function in Pain Populations-A Systematic Review and Meta-Analysis of Randomized Controlled Trials: Part II, Cancer Pain Populations. Pain Med 2016;17(8):1553–68.

46. Roila F, Molassiotis A, Herrstedt J, et al. 2016 MASCC and ESMO guideline update for the prevention of chemotherapy- and radiotherapy-induced nausea and vomiting and of nausea and vomiting in advanced cancer patients. Ann Oncol 2016;27(suppl 5):v119–33.

47. Vig S, Seibert L, Green MR. Olanzapine is effective for refractory chemotherapy-induced nausea and vomiting irrespective of chemotherapy emetogenicity. J Cancer Res Clin Oncol 2014;140(1):77–82.

48. Hesketh PJ, Kris MG, Basch E, et al. Antiemetics: ASCO Guideline Update. J Clin Oncol 2020;38(24):2782–97.

49. Kamen C, Tejani MA, Chandwani K, et al. Anticipatory nausea and vomiting due to chemotherapy. Eur J Pharmacol 2014;722:172–9.

50. Hesketh PJ, Kris MG, Basch E, et al. Antiemetics: American Society of Clinical Oncology Clinical Practice Guideline Update. J Clin Oncol 2017;35(28):3240–61.

51. Riba MB, Donovan KA, Andersen B, et al. Distress Management, Version 3.2019, NCCN Clinical Practice Guidelines in Oncology. J Natl Compr Canc Netw 2019; 17(10):1229–49.

52. Butt Z, Wagner LI, Beaumont JL, et al. Longitudinal screening and management of fatigue, pain, and emotional distress associated with cancer therapy. Support Care Cancer 2008;16(2):151–9.

53. Carlson LE, Bultz BD. Cancer distress screening. Needs, models, and methods. J Psychosom Res 2003;55(5):403–9.

54. Hildenbrand JD, Park HS, Casarett DJ, et al. Patient-reported distress as an early warning sign of unmet palliative care needs and increased healthcare utilization in patients with advanced cancer. Support Care Cancer 2022;30(4):3419–27.

55. Fulton JJ, LeBlanc TW, Cutson TM, et al. Integrated outpatient palliative care for patients with advanced cancer: A systematic review and meta-analysis. Palliat Med 2019;33(2):123–34.

56. Meier DE, Beresford L. Social workers advocate for a seat at palliative care table. J Palliat Med 2008;11(1):10–4.

57. Smith GL, Banegas MP, Acquati C, et al. Navigating financial toxicity in patients with cancer: A multidisciplinary management approach. CA Cancer J Clin 2022; 72(5):437–53.

58. Aragon KN. Palliative Care in Lung Cancer. Clin Chest Med 2020;41(2):281–93.

59. Temel JS, Greer JA, Muzikansky A, et al. Early palliative care for patients with metastatic non-small-cell lung cancer. N Engl J Med 2010;363(8):733–42.

60. Maione P, Perrone F, Gallo C, et al. Pretreatment quality of life and functional status assessment significantly predict survival of elderly patients with advanced non-small-cell lung cancer receiving chemotherapy: a prognostic analysis of the multicenter Italian lung cancer in the elderly study. J Clin Oncol 2005; 23(28):6865–72.

61. National Comprehensive Cancer Network. Non-Small Cell Lung Cancer (Version 5.2022). Available at: https://www.nccn.org/professionals/physician_gls/pdf/nscl.pdf.

62. Ferrell BR, Temel JS, Temin S, et al. Integration of Palliative Care Into Standard Oncology Care: American Society of Clinical Oncology Clinical Practice Guideline Update. J Clin Oncol 2017;35(1):96–112.

63. Morrison RS, Meier DE. America's Care of Serious Illness: 2019 State-By-State Report Card on Access to Palliative Care in Our Nation's Hospitals. Center to Advance Palliative Care and the National Palliative Care Research Center. Available at: https://reportcard.capc.org/. Accessed September 30, 2022.

64. Ferrell B, Sun V, Hurria A, et al. Interdisciplinary Palliative Care for Patients With Lung Cancer. J Pain Symptom Manage 2015;50(6):758–67.

65. Cole AP, Nguyen DD, Meirkhanov A, et al. Association of Care at Minority-Serving vs Non-Minority-Serving Hospitals With Use of Palliative Care Among Racial/Ethnic Minorities With Metastatic Cancer in the United States. JAMA Netw Open 2019;2(2):e187633.

66. Stein JN, Rivera MP, Weiner A, et al. Sociodemographic disparities in the management of advanced lung cancer: a narrative review. J Thorac Dis 2021;13(6): 3772–800.

67. Hays JC, Galanos AN, Palmer TA, et al. Preference for place of death in a continuing care retirement community. Gerontol 2001;41(1):123–8.

68. Bao Y, Maciejewski RC, Garrido MM, et al. Chemotherapy Use, End-of-Life Care, and Costs of Care Among Patients Diagnosed With Stage IV Pancreatic Cancer. J Pain Symptom Manage 2018;55(4):1113–21.e3.

69. Sheridan PE, LeBrett WG, Triplett DP, et al. Cost Savings Associated With Palliative Care Among Older Adults With Advanced Cancer. Am J Hosp Palliat Care 2021;38(10):1250–7.

70. Vranas KC, Lapidus JA, Ganzini L, et al. Association of Palliative Care Use and Setting With Health-care Utilization and Quality of Care at the End of Life Among Patients With Advanced Lung Cancer. Chest 2020;158(6):2667–74.

71. Chen Y, Criss SD, Watson TR, et al. Cost and Utilization of Lung Cancer End-of-Life Care Among Racial-Ethnic Minority Groups in the United States. Oncol 2020; 25(1):e120–9.

72. Kalidindi Y, Segel J, Jung J. Impact of Hospice on Spending and Utilization Among Patients With Lung Cancer in Medicare. Am J Hosp Palliat Care 2020; 37(4):286–93.

73. National Comprehensive Cancer Network. Survivorship (Version 1.2022). Available at: https://www.nccn.org/professionals/physician_gls/pdf/survivorship.pdf.

74. Rajapakse P. An Update on Survivorship Issues in Lung Cancer Patients. World J Oncol 2021;12(2–3):45–9.

75. Thai AA, Solomon BJ, Sequist LV, et al. Lung cancer. Lancet 2021;398(10299): 535–54.

New Therapies on the Horizon

Alissa J. Cooper, MD*, Rebecca S. Heist, MD, MPH

KEYWORDS

- Immune checkpoints • Immunotherapy resistance • Antibody-drug conjugate
- Novel therapies • Lung cancer

KEY POINTS

- Although immune checkpoint inhibitors have transformed the prognosis and treatment of lung cancer patients, the field now grapples with the management of the disease that has progressed on standard programmed death ligand 1 blockade.
- Strategies include combination therapies, the incorporation of agents which target alternative immune checkpoint targets, and novel immunomodulatory therapies such as vaccines, adoptive T-cell therapies, and oncolytic viruses.
- A novel agent class combining features of targeted therapy and cytotoxic chemotherapy is the antibody-drug conjugates, which hold promise as potent options for treatment.

INTRODUCTION

The advent of checkpoint inhibitor immunotherapies in standard management of lung cancer has transformed the field over the past few years.[1–6] Though these advances have significantly improved outcomes for patients with lung cancer, there remains a high unmet need for new effective therapies for patients whose disease has progressed on currently available treatment. Ongoing research has focused on promising new avenues in lung cancer treatment; two areas of particular interest are antibody-drug conjugates (ADCs), which hold great potential as a treatment that combines the potency of cytotoxic chemotherapy with the precision of targeted therapy, and novel immunotherapies, both as monotherapies and in combination with standard of care programmed death receptor 1 (PD-1) and programmed death ligand 1 (PD-L1) immune checkpoint inhibitors (ICIs). This review aims to describe encouraging new developments with novel immune therapies and ADCs for the treatment of lung cancer.

Characterizing Immune Checkpoint Inhibitors Resistance

Despite a substantial proportion of patients with lung cancer deriving benefit from currently available PD-1 and PD-L1 inhibitors, inevitably some patients will develop

Massachusetts General Hospital Cancer Center, Harvard Medical School, 55 Fruit Street, Yawkey 7B, Boston, MA 02114, USA
* Corresponding author.
E-mail address: acooper@mgh.harvard.edu

Hematol Oncol Clin N Am 37 (2023) 623–658
https://doi.org/10.1016/j.hoc.2023.02.004
0889-8588/23/© 2023 Elsevier Inc. All rights reserved.

hemonc.theclinics.com

acquired resistance (disease progression on therapy following an initial clinical benefit of 6 months or greater) and others will demonstrate primary resistance (disease progression after at least 6 weeks but not more than 6 months on treatment).[7] Multiple factors contribute to the clinical phenotype of progression, chief among them the tumor microenvironment, which itself is influenced by germline and tumor genetics, prior treatment history, and clinical and demographic characteristics.[8–11] Patients with acquired resistance may benefit from combination therapies intended to restore sensitivity to immune modulation,[7] whereas those with primary resistance to PD-(L)1 inhibitors might require alternative novel modalities entirely. Although data are still emerging regarding these populations of patients, one study demonstrated that rapid progression, or progressive disease within 6 weeks of ICI initiation, in pretreated non-small cell lung cancer (NSCLC) patients comprised 8% of evaluable cases.[12]

STRATEGIES TO OVERCOME IMMUNE CHECKPOINT INHIBITORS RESISTANCE
Combination Therapies with Programmed Death Ligand 1 Inhibitors

Currently, the only approved combination therapy with PD-(L)1 inhibitors is the cytotoxic T-lymphocyte-associated protein 4 (CTLA-4) inhibitor ipilimumab, which can be used in *EGFR/ALK*-negative, PD-L1+ NSCLC in combination with PD-1 inhibitor nivolumab, or in combination with nivolumab and two cycles of chemotherapy.[13] Other novel combination therapies in development are listed in **Table 1** with select combination strategies detailed below.

DNA damage repair pathways

Preclinical and translational data have indicated that poly ADP ribose polymerase (PARP) inhibitors promote immune priming through multiple mechanisms related to DNA damage; additionally, their administration leads to the upregulation of PD-L1 expression.[14] In a first-line phase I study of veliparib and nivolumab in combination with platinum doublet chemotherapy, combination therapy was found to be tolerable and the confirmed objective response rate (ORR) was 40%.[15] A first-line phase II study of niraparib plus pembrolizumab showed differential efficacy by PD-L1 level: for patients with tumor proportion score (TPS) ≥ 50%, ORR was 56.3%, whereas for patients with TPS 1-49%, ORR was 20.0%.[16] The combination of ICI and PARP inhibitors is currently being tested in the ORION trial (maintenance durvalumab plus olaparib or durvalumab alone following treatment with platinum doublet and durvalumab; NCT03775486) and in the Javelin PARP Medley trial (avelumab plus talazoparib in ICI-pretreated or -naive patients; NCT03330405). The HUDSON trial (NCT03334617), enrolling patients whose disease progressed on PD-(L)1 blockade, tested the combination of olaparib and durvalumab in biomarker-matched and biomarker-unmatched patients without notable efficacy.[17]

Another potential target has emerged in the ataxia-telangiectasia-mutated kinase gene (ATM). Preclinical studies have shown that loss of ATM signaling drives dependence on ataxia telangiectasia and Rad3-related protein kinase (ATR).[18,19] The combination of durvalumab with the ATR inhibitor ceralasertib demonstrated median progression-free survival (PFS) 7.43 months (80% CI 3.45–9.46) and median overall survival (OS) 15.80 months (80% CI 11.01–NC) in NSCLC patients with ATM mutations.[17] A first-line phase Ib trial is investigating the combination of the ATR inhibitor berzosertib with chemoimmunotherapy in advanced squamous NSCLC (NCT04216316).

Anti-angiogenic agents

There is a strong preclinical rationale for the addition of anti-angiogenic agents to immunotherapy. The dysfunctional and abnormal vasculature generated by the tumor

Table 1
Selected clinical trials of combination therapies with programmed death ligand 1 inhibitors

Target	Agent	Strategy	NCT Identifier/Phase	Population
Small molecule inhibitors				
PARP-i	Olaparib	Maintenance durvalumab + olaparib or placebo after induction chemo + durva	NCT03775486 Phase II	Treatment-naive
		Durvalumab + olaparib	NCT03334617 Phase II	Prior PD-(L)1 inhibitor
		Maintenance pembrolizumab + olaparib vs pembro + pemetrexed after induction	NCT03976323 Phase III	Treatment-naive, non-sq
		Maintenance pembrolizumab + olaparib vs pembrolizumab + placebo after induction	NCT03976362 Phase III	Treatment-naive, sq
	Talazoparib	Avelumab + talazoparib	NCT04173507 Phase II	Prior PD-(L)1 inhibitor SLFN11+ SCLC
		Maintenance atezolizumab + talozaparib vs atezolizumab after induction	NCT04334941 Phase II	
	Niraparib	Dostarlimab + niraparib as 2L treatment	NCT04701307 Phase II	Stage III NSCLC; SCLC or neuroendocrine
		Niraparib ± pembrolizumab or dostarlimab	NCT03308942 Phase II	Treatment-naive; Prior PD-(L)1 inhibitor
	Fluzoparib	Maintenance camrelizumab + fluzoparib after 1L SCLC treatment	NCT04782089 Phase II	SCLC, not progressed
ATR-i	Berzosertib	Carboplatin/gemcitabine/ pembrolizumab + berzosertib	NCT04216316 Phase Ib/II	No PD-(L)1 inhibitor in prior 1 year, sq
AXL-i, MET-i	Glesatinib	Nivolumab + glesatinib	NCT02954991 Phase II	Prior PD-(L)1 inhibitor
AXL-i	Bemcentinib	Pembrolizumab + bemcentinib	NCT03184571 Phase II	ICI-naive; Prior PD-(L)1 inhibitor
PI3K-i	Copanlisib	Durvalumab + copanlisib as consolidation after CRT	NCT04895579 Phase Ib	Following CRT
		Nivolumab + copanlisib	NCT03735628 Phase Ib	If nivolumab indicated
	Idealisib	Pembrolizumab + idealisib	NCT03257722 Phase Ib/II	Prior PD-(L)1 inhibitor

(continued on next page)

Table 1
(continued)

Target	Agent	Strategy	NCT Identifier/Phase	Population
MET-i	Capmatinib	Pembroliuzmab + capmatinib	-	Treatment-naive, PD-L1 ≥ 50%
		Spartalizumab + capmatinib vs docetaxel	NCT03647488 Phase II	Prior PD-(L)1 inhibitor
MEK-i	Binimetinib	Pembrolizumab + binimetinib	NCT03991819 Phase I/Ib	ICI-naive, PD-L1 ≥ 50%
	Trametinib	Pembrolizumab + trametinib	NCT03299088 Phase I	KRAS-mut, prior chemo and targeted therapy
		Pembrolizumab + trametinib	NCT03225664 Phase Ib/II	Prior ICI
Anti-angiogenic agents	multi-TKI-i	Sitravatinib		
		Nivolumab + sitravatinib	NCT02954991 Phase II	Prior PD-(L)1 inhibitor
		Nivolumab + sitravatinib vs docetaxel	NCT03906071 Phase III	Prior PD-(L)1 inhibitor
		Tislelizumab + sitravatinib vs docetaxel	NCT04921358 Phase III	Prior PD-(L)1 inhibitor
		Pembrolizumab + sitravatinib	NCT04925986 Phase II	Treatment-naive, sq
	Cabozantininb	Nivolumab + cabozantinib vs cabo alone vs standard chemotherapy	NCT04310007 Phase II	Prior PD-(L)1 inhibitor
		Atezolizumab + cabozantinib vs docetaxel	NCT04471428 Phase III	Prior PD-(L)1 inhibitor
	Lenvatinib	Pembrolizumab + levatinib	NCT02501096 Phase I/II	Prior PD-(L)1 inhibitor
		Pembrolizumab + levatinib vs docetaxel	NCT03976375 Phase III	Prior PD-(L)1 inhibitor
		Pembrolizumab + levatinib vs placebo	NCT04676412 Phase III	Treatment-naive, PD-L1 ≥ 1%
	mAb	Bevacizumab		
		Atezolizumab + bevacizumab vs atezolizumab alone	NCT03896074 Phase II	Treatment-naive, PD-L1 ≥ 1%
	Ramucirumab	Pembrolizumab + ramucirumab + docetaxel	NCT04340882 Phase II	Prior PD-(L)1 inhibitor
		Atezolizumab + ramucirumab	NCT03689855 Phase II	Prior ICI

	Target	Agent	Regimen	NCT / Phase	Status
Inhibitory immune checkpoints	TIGIT	Vibostolimab	Pembrolizumab + vibostolimab or pembrolizumab + vibostolimab + docetaxel vs docetaxel	NCT04725188 Phase II	Prior PD-(L)1 inhibitor
		Ociperlimab	Tislelizumab + ociperlimab vs pembrolizumab vs tislelizumab	NCT04746924 Phase III	ICI-naive
		Tiragolumab	Atezolizumab + tiragolumab	NCT03563716 Phase II	Treatment-naive, PD-L1 ≥ 1%
		Domvanalimab	Zimberelimab + domvanalimab + etrumadenant (adenosine-i)	NCT04791839 Phase II	Prior PD-(L)1 inhibitor
		IBI939	Sintilimab + IBI939	NCT04672369 Phase I	ICI-naive
	LAG-3	Eftilagimod alpha	Pembrolizumab + eftilagimod alpha	NCT03625323 Phase II	ICI-naive; Prior ICI
		RO7247669	PD1-LAG3 bispecific antibody	NCT04140500 Phase I	Prior PD-(L)1 inhibitor, PD-L1 ≥ 1%
		LAG525	Spartalizumab + LAG525	NCT03365791 Phase I	ICI-naive
	VISTA	HMBD-002	Pembrolizumab + HMBD-002	NCT05082610 Phase I	Prior PD-(L)1 inhibitor
	TIM3	TSR-022	Nivolumab + TSR-022	NCT02817633 Phase I	Prior PD-(L)1 inhibitor
		RO7121661	PD1-TIM3 bispecific antibody	NCT03708328 Phase I	Prior PD-(L)1 inhibitor
	Siglec-15	NC318	Pembrolizumab + NC318	NCT04699123 Phase II	PD-(L)1 inhibitor naive; Prior PD-(L)1 inhibitor
	CD73	PT199	Anti-PD-1 mAb + PT199	NCT05431270 Phase I	Prior PD-(L)1 inhibitor
		LY3475070	Pembrolizumab + LY3475070	NCT04148937 Phase I	Pretreated
		NZV930	Spartalizumab + NZV930	NCT03549000 Phase I	Pretreated
		Oleclumab	Durvalumab + oleclumab consolidation after CRT	NCT03822351 Phase II	ICI-naive
	NKG2A	Monalizumab	Durvalumab + monalizumab consolidation after CRT	NCT03822351 Phase II	ICI-naive

(continued on next page)

Table 1
(continued)

Target	Agent	Strategy	NCT Identifier/ Phase	Population
Stimulatory immune checkpoints				
OX40/CD134	BGB-A445	Tislelizumab + BGB-A445	NCT04215978 Phase I	Prior PD-(L)1 inhibitor
	INBRX-106	Pembrolizumab + INBRX-106	NCT04198766 Phase I	Pretreated
	PF-04518600	Avelumab + PF-04518600	NCT02554812 Phase I/II	Pretreated
	GSK3174998	Pembrolizumab + GSK3174998	NCT02528357 Phase I	Pretreated
	INCAGN01949	Nivolumab + INCAGN01949, Nivolumab + ipilimumab + INCAGN01949	NCT03241173 Phase I/II	Pretreated; Prior PD-(L)1 inhibitor
4-1BB/CD137	GEN1046	Pembrolizumab + GEN1046	NCT05117242 Phase II	Pretreated
	ADG106	Nivolumab + ADG106	NCT05236608 Phase Ib/II	Pretreated; Prior ICI
	INBRX-105	Pembrolizumab + INBRX-105	NCT03809624 Phase I	Pretreated; Treatment-naive
CD40	APX005M	Nivolumab + APX005M	NCT03123783 Phase I/II	ICI-naive; Prior PD-(L)1 inhibitor
	CDX-1140	Pembrolizumab + CDX-1140	NCT03329950 Phase I	Prior PD-(L)1 inhibitor
GITR	INCAGN01876	Nivolumab + INCAGN01876, Nivolumab + ipilimumab + INCAGN01876	NCT03126110 Phase I/II	Pretreated
Vaccines	GEN-009	Pembrolizumab + GEN-009	NCT03633110 Phase I/II	Receiving pembrolizumab and chemo in 1L
	RO7198457	Atezolizumab + RO7198457	NCT03289962 Phase I	ICI-naive; Prior ICI
	GRT-C901/2	Nivolumab + ipilimumab + GRT-C901/2	NCT03639714 Phase I/II	Pretreated; Prior PD-(L)1 inhibitor
	TG4010	Nivolumab + TG4010	NCT02823990 Phase II	ICI-naive

Category	Type	Agent	Combination	Trial/Phase	Population
Adoptive T-cell therapies	TIL	LN-145	Pembrolizumab + LN-145	NCT03645928 Phase II	ICI-naive; Prior ICI
		TIL	Nivolumab + TIL	NCT03215810 Phase I	PD-(L)1 inhibitor naive
	TCR	Letetresgene autoleucel	Pembrolizumab + letetresgene autoleucel	NCT03709706 Phase I/II	Prior PD-(L)1 inhibitor; expresses NY-ESO-1 and/or LAGE-1a
Oncolytics		VSV-IFNβ-NIS	Pembrolizumab + VSV-IFNβ-NIS	NCT03647163 Phase I/II	Pretreated; Prior PD-(L)1 inhibitor
		ADV/HSV-tk	Pembrolizumab + ADV/HSV-tk	NCT03004183 Phase II	ICI-naive
		BT-001	Pembrolizumab + BT-001	NCT04725331 Phase I/II	Pretreated
Cytokines and other signaling-based therapies	IL-2	NKTR-214	Nivolumab + NKTR-214	NCT02983045 Phase I/II	No prior IL-2
		THOR-707	Anti-PD-1 mAb + THOR-707	NCT04009681 Phase I/II	Pretreated
		ALKS 4230	Pembrolizumab + ALKS 4230	NCT02799095 Phase I/II	Pretreated
	IL-1β	Canakinumab	Pembrolizumab + canakinumab vs canakinumab vs pembrolizumab as neoadjuvant therapy	NCT03968419 Phase II	No therapy in past 3 yrs
	IL-15	COH06	Atezolizumab + COH06	NCT05334329 Phase I	Prior PD-(L)1 inhibitor
		NIZ985	Spartalizumab + NIZ985	NCT04261439 Phase I	Prior PD-(L)1 inhibitor
	STING	TAK-676	Pembrolizumab + TAK-676	NCT04420884 Phase I	PD-(L)1 inhibitor naive; Prior PD-(L)1 inhibitor
		TAK-500	Pembrolizumab + TAK-500	NCT05070247 Phase I	Pretreated

(continued on next page)

Table 1
(continued)

Target	Agent	Strategy	NCT Identifier/ Phase	Population
Microbiome-based FMT	FMT	Pembrolizumab + FMT	NCT04951583 Phase II	PD-(L)1 inhibitor naive
Bacterial consortium	BMC128	Nivolumab + BMC128	NCT05354102 Phase I	Prior PD-(L)1 inhibitor
	MET-4	Anti-PD-1 mAb + MET-4	NCT03686202 Phase I	PD-(L)1 inhibitor naive; Prior PD-(L)1 inhibitor
E coli Nissle	SYNB1891	Atezolizumab + SYNB1891	NCT04167137 Phase I	Pretreated
Lactococcus lactis	GEN-001	Avelumab + GEN-001	NCT04601402 Phase I	Prior PD-(L)1 inhibitor
E gallinarum	MRx0518	Pembrolizumab + MRx0518	NCT03637803 Phase I	Prior PD-(L)1 inhibitor

Abbreviations: 1L, first-line; 2L, second-line; ATR, ataxia telangiectasia and Rad3-related protein kinase; AXL, AXL tyrosine kinase; cabo, cabozantinib; CRT, chemoradiotherapy; durva, durvalumab; *E. coli* Nissle, *Escherichia coli* Nissle; *E. gallinarum, Enterococcus gallinarum*; FMT, fecal microbiota transplantation; GITR, Glucocorticoid-induced TNFR-related protein; i, inhibitor; ICI, immune checkpoint inhibitor; IL-15, Interleukin-15; IL-1β, Interleukin-1β; IL-2, Interleukin-2; KRAS, Kirsten rat sarcoma viral oncogene homolog; LAG-3, Lymphocyte activation gene-3; MEK, mitogen-activated protein kinase 1; MET, MET protooncogene tyrosine kinase; NCT, National Clinical Trial; NKG2A, natural killer group protein A; non-sq, non-squamous; NSCLC, non-small cell lung cancer; NY-ESO-1, New York esophageal squamous cell carcinoma 1; PARP, poly ADP ribose polymerase; PD-(L)1, programmed death receptor (ligand) 1; pembro, pembrolizumab; PI3K, phosphatidylinositol-3-kinase; SCLC, small cell lung cancer; SLFN11, Schlafen Family Member 11 gene; sq, squamous; STING, stimulator of interferon genes; TCR, T-cell receptor; TIGIT, T-cell immunoreceptor with immunoglobulin and ITIM domains; TIL, tumor-infiltrating lymphocytes; TIM3, transmembrane immunoglobulin and mucin domain 3; TKI, tyrosine kinase inhibitor; VISTA, V-domain immunoglobulin suppressor of T-cell activation; yrs, years.

promotes local hypoxia and an immunosuppressive environment; combining anti-angiogenic agents with immunotherapy may help to reverse the immunosuppressive state by improving perfusion and allowing the infiltration of immune cells.[20] In NSCLC, patients treated with atezolizumab plus bevacizumab plus chemotherapy had longer median PFS and median OS compared with those treated with bevacizumab plus chemotherapy (8.3 months vs 6.8 months, 95% CI 0.52–0.74, $P < 0.001$; 19.2 months vs 14.7 months, 95% CI 0.64–0.96, $P = 0.02$).[21] Several anti-angiogenic monoclonal antibodies (mAbs) and multi-kinase inhibitors that include vascular endothelial growth factor receptor (VEGFR) as a target are currently being tested in combination with PD-(L)1 inhibitors. Preliminary encouraging results of the lung cancer master protocol (Lung-MAP) study investigating ramucirumab plus pembrolizumab (RP) compared with investigator's choice (SOC) (among docetaxel/ramucirumab, docetaxel, gemcitabine, and pemetrexed) in patients pretreated with PD-(L)1 inhibitors and chemotherapy were presented at American Society of Clinical Oncology (ASCO) 2022: OS was significantly improved with RP compared with SOC (14.5 months (80% CI 13.9–16.1) vs 11.5 (80% CI 9.9–13.0 months)) without increased adverse events.[22] In a phase Ib/II trial of multi-targeted tyrosine kinase inhibitor (TKI) lenvatinib and pembrolizumab, 22 patients with NSCLC (52% pretreated with PD-(L)1 inhibitors) showed an ORR of 33% and median PFS of 5.9 months.[23] This combination will be further tested in phase III trials,[24] as will multi-targeted TKI sitravatinib plus nivolumab[25] (NCT03906071) given the high response rates seen in a phase II trial (though this combination also demonstrated a high discontinuation rate).[26] The results of the COSMIC-021 study, which evaluated multi-targeted TKI cabozantinib and atezolizumab in PD-(L)1-pretreated NSCLC patients were presented at ASCO 2020 and revealed ORR 27% and median PFS 4.2 months.[27] Phase II (NCT04310007) and phase III (NCT04471428) studies are ongoing.

Novel immunomodulatory targets–checkpoints beyond programmed death ligand 1

Several alternative immunomodulatory checkpoints other than PD-(L)1 inhibitors have been identified, and clinical trials of these agents as monotherapies and in combination with PD-(L)1 inhibitors are ongoing (**Table 1**).

Inhibitory immune checkpoints

TIGIT T-cell immunoreceptor with immunoglobulin and immunoreceptor tyrosine-based inhibitory motif (ITIM) domains TIGIT (T-cell immunoreceptor with immunoglobulin and ITIM domains) is expressed on CD4 and CD8 T cells, natural killer (NK) cells, and Tregs, and binds to ligands present on cancer cells of different tumor types.[28] TIGIT inhibition in conjunction with PD-1 inhibition has demonstrated anti-tumor activity in preclinical studies.[28] Tiragolumab, a mAb-targeting TIGIT, was evaluated in combination with atezolizumab in the phase II CITYSCAPE trial in PD-L1-positive NSCLC patients; increased ORR and PFS were shown in the combination arm versus atezolizumab alone, though this was mostly driven by the TPS $\geq$ 50% subset.[29] However, the randomized phase III SKYSCRAPER-01 trial (NCT04294810) evaluating tiragolumab and atezolizumab as first-line treatment of PD-L1-high NSCLC patients did not meet its co-primary endpoint of PFS,[30] and in the randomized phase III SKYSCRAPER-02 trial, the addition of tiragolumab to atezolizumab, carboplatin and etoposide in patients with extensive stage small cell lung cancer did not provide benefit over atezolizumab and chemotherapy alone.[31] Although it is not clear why the promising data from phase II trials were not borne out in large, randomized, well-balanced phase III studies, multiple ongoing trials are still being conducted. Another anti-TIGIT antibody, vibostolimab, showed limited efficacy in NSCLC patients whose disease had progressed on ICI, both alone and in combination with pembrolizumab (ORR 7% and 5%, respectively).[32] Despite these results, a co-formulation of the two drugs (MK-7684A) is currently being tested in the ICI-resistant setting, alone and in combination with docetaxel (NCT04725188).

LAG-3 Lymphocyte activation gene-3 Lymphocyte activation gene-3 (LAG-3) is expressed on several immune cells[33] and is upregulated in multiple cancers.[28] In NSCLC, elevated LAG-3 expression in T cells has been associated with shorter PFS in response to anti-PD-1 agents.[34] In a phase II-III randomized trial of melanoma patients, the combination of LAG-3 inhibitor relatlimab with nivolumab improved PFS to 10.1 months (95% CI 6.4–15.7) compared with 4.6 months (95% CI 3.4–5.6) with nivolumab alone,[35] prompting its Food and Drug Administration (FDA) approval for melanoma in March 2022. Various agents targeting LAG-3 are now being tested in clinical trials (see **Table 1**).Others
Several other compounds targeting co-inhibitory receptors include antibodies against VISTA (V-domain immunoglobulin suppressor of T-cell activation),[36] TIM3 (transmembrane immunoglobulin and mucin domain 3),[37] S15 (Siglec-15),[38] and adenosine/ CD73 and NKG2A (natural killer group protein A) (antibodies against CD73 and NKG2A tested in the locally advanced setting in the COAST trial,[39] and in *EGFR*-mutant NSCLC[40]).

Stimulatory immune checkpoints In contrast to agents which inhibit negative immune checkpoints such as PD-1 and CTLA-4, agonist antibodies that target co-stimulatory receptors hold measured promise for future treatment, though clearly there are greater complexities and risks present than for inhibitory targets.[41] Several agonists of the tumor necrosis factor receptor family (such as OX40/CD134, 4-1BB/ CD137, CD40, ICOS, and glucocorticoid-induced tumor necrosis factor receptor (TNFR)-related protein [GITR]) have been tested in both the monotherapy and combination settings, with preliminary reports demonstrating more promise as part of a combinatorial treatment strategy.[42–47] For example, the phase I study of utomulimab, a 4-1BB/CD137 agonist, in patients with advanced solid tumors (including three with lung cancer) demonstrated an ORR of 3.8%,[44] whereas the phase Ib study of utomulimab plus pembrolizumab demonstrated an ORR of 26%, with one complete response in a patient with small cell lung cancer (SCLC) and one partial response in a patient with NSCLC.[46]

Novel Immunomodulatory Modalities–Beyond Checkpoint Inhibitors

Vaccines
Vaccines stimulate antigen-specific immunity, and strategies developed for cancer include targeting either single or a set of preselected tumor-associated antigens (TAA) or using a patient's tumor tissue to create a personalized neoantigen vaccine (**Fig. 1**). Early work involving single-antigen targets such as melanoma-associated antigen 3 (MAGE-A3), transmembrane glycoprotein mucin 1 (MUC-1), and preferentially expressed antigen in melanoma (PRAME) demonstrated limited efficacy.[48–50] Vaccines targeting multiple TAA have been variable; one successful example was OSE02101, a neoepitope vaccine targeting 5 TAA, which demonstrated an OS benefit over chemotherapy in advanced NSCLC that had progressed on PD-(L)1 inhibitor.[51,52] Combinations with PD-1 blockade and chemotherapy are being tested (NCT04884282).

Personalized neoantigen approaches, like NEO-PV-01, may prove to be more promising. This personalized vaccine was produced by whole-exome and RNA sequencing of patients' tumors, followed by the selection of high-quality neoepitopes and peptide

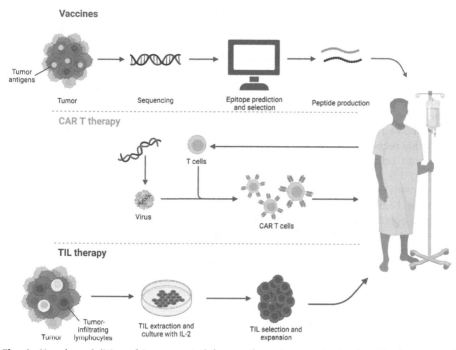

Fig. 1. Novel modalities of immunomodulatory therapies are depicted, with the steps of vaccine creation, CAR-T-cell production and TIL therapy shown in sequence. CAR, chimeric antigen receptor; IL-2, interleukin-2; TIL, tumor infiltrating lymphocytes. Figure created with BioRender.com.

production.[53] In a phase Ib trial of NEO-PV-01 in combination with PD-1 blockade in NSCLC, melanoma, and bladder cancer, 18 vaccinated patients showed ORR 39% in NSCLC and median PFS 8.5 months (95% CI 3.9 months to NE).[53] A subsequent phase Ib trial investigated the combination of NEO-PV-01 with pembrolizumab and chemotherapy in advanced non-squamous NSCLC and demonstrated ORR/clinical benefit rate (CBR) for the intention to treat group and vaccinated group were 34%/71% (95% CI 19.6–51.4/95% CI 54.1–84.6) and 69%/100% (95% CI 41.3–89.0/95% CI 79.4–100), respectively.[54] Despite these encouraging results and compelling scientific rationale, true efficacy remains elusive; an mRNA-based individualized neoantigen vaccine (RO7198457) in combination with atezolizumab in ICI-naive NSCLC patients showed an ORR of only 10%.[55] Many agents are currently in clinical trials alone or in combination with PD-1 blockade for patients with metastatic disease (NCT03633110, NCT02721043, NCT03289962, NCT03794128, NCT03639714) and for patients with resected disease in the adjuvant setting (NCT03633110, NCT04267237, NCT03313778). VB10.NEO is being tested in combination with bempegaldesleukin (pegylated IL-2) for advanced NSCLC without a complete response to PD-(L)1 inhibition (NCT03548467). In general, whereas there has been progress that offers more promise in personalized, neoantigen-specific vaccines, challenges remain with regard to cost, time investment, and neoantigen prediction models.

Adoptive T-cell therapies
Alternative methods to prime T cells include tumor-infiltrating lymphocyte (TIL) therapy, in which TILs are isolated from tumor, expanded and selected for antigen

recognition ex vivo, then reinfused into the lymphodepleted patient (see **Fig. 1**).[56] Advantages of TIL therapy include the ability to target multiple TAA due to the polyclonality of the T cells, as well as the ability to target truncal neoantigens clonally expressed by tumor cells.[57] In practice, TIL therapy may be limited by the intricate T-cell homing process, which is not solely antigen-dependent[58] and by several complex mechanisms including T-cell exhaustion.[57] One recent example of the application of this method in NSCLC was a phase I trial in which ICI-naive advanced NSCLC patients were treated with nivolumab, and then upon progression, treated with TIL infusion followed by maintenance nivolumab.[59] Twenty patients were enrolled and 16 ultimately received TIL following progression on nivolumab. Of 13 evaluable patients, 6 had an unconfirmed response, including two complete responses which were ongoing 1.5 years later. With regard to safety, two patients died before response assessment due to clinical decline before lymphodepletion, yielding a severe toxicity event of 12.5%, which met the pre-specified primary endpoint of ≤ 17%. Other adverse events (AEs) were primarily due to lymphodepletion and IL-2 administration. Interestingly, this study enrolled multiple patients with driver oncogenes that classically respond less briskly to immunotherapies, including two patients with classical *EGFR* Exon 19 deletions and two patients with *EML4-ALK* translocations. Preliminary results from a phase II study of TIL monotherapy in ICI-pretreated advanced NSCLC demonstrated an ORR of 21.4% in the full analysis set (6/28) and 25.0% in efficacy evaluable patients (6/24), one with a complete response ongoing at 20 months[60] with anticipated AE profile related to lymphodepletion and IL-2. This study is ongoing (NCT04614103).

This strategy may eventually be applied to driver oncogene subsets in NSCLC. Recently, Leidner and colleagues[61] described the treatment of a patient with *KRAS* G12D-mutant pancreatic cancer with an infusion of T cells genetically engineered to express T-cell receptors (TCRs) targeting mutant *KRAS* G12D. The patient formerly had been treated with TILs and high-dose IL-2 as described above, but progression was observed within 6 months. She was subsequently treated with autologous peripheral T cells that had been transduced to express HLA-C*08:02–restricted TCRs targeting mutant KRAS G12D, and experienced a partial response with tumor shrinkage of 72% at 6 months following cell transfer. This novel therapy may represent an alternative option for patients with oncogene-driven NSCLC whose disease progresses on standard therapy.

Chimeric antigen receptor T-cell therapy (CAR-T), in contrast to so-called endogenous T-cell recognition used by TILs, uses engineered synthetic receptors to target specific cancer cell antigens (see **Fig. 1**).[62] This methodology has enjoyed great success in B-cell hematologic malignancies, due to universal expression of target antigen CD19,[63,64] but has met challenges in its application to thoracic malignancies, given the heterogeneity of TAA expression.[65] The ideal target for CAR-T-cell therapy is exclusively expressed or overexpressed on tumor tissue, with very little expression in normal cells.[62] Potential targets in testing include epidermal growth factor receptor (EGFR), MSLN, MUC-1, PSCA, carcinoembryonic antigen (CEA), PD-L1, ROR-1, and human epidermal growth factor receptor 2 (HER-2),[62,66] though ongoing challenges remain with safety and with efficacy.[67] On-target but off-tumor effects have the potential to trigger severely toxic reactions,[67] and challenges with CAR-T cell infiltration into solid tumor tissue may mitigate anti-tumor potency.[66]

Oncolytic

Oncolytic virus therapy uses native or genetically modified viruses that selectively replicate within tumor cells, killing them via direct lysis, as well as simultaneously prompting systemic anti-tumor immune activation.[68] The majority of studies have used intratumoral delivery, which theoretically delivers more drugs without dilution and viral clearance seen intravenously.[28] This vehicle for anti-tumor activity depends on a complex balance in the body, in which a certain degree of viral infection must ensue, despite the potential for neutralizing antiviral responses which might limit their efficacy.[68] Many of the oncolytic viruses used clinically either have a natural tropism for aberrantly expressed markers on the cancer cell surface or are engineered to directly target such markers.[68] Clinical trials testing the use of oncolytic viruses have uncommonly included lung cancer patients, for whom intratumoral injection may be challenging (6% in one review[69]), and in aggregate have generally reported low response rates.[69] Combination strategies with chemotherapy and PD-1 checkpoint inhibitors may be promising[69] and are currently under study in lung cancer (NCT03004183, NCT00861627, NCT04725331). Modest activity was seen in KEYNOTE-200, which tested intravenously delivered coxsackievirus A21 in combination with pembrolizumab in advanced NSCLC, with an ORR of 23% in ICI-naive NSCLC patients and ORR of 33% in ICI-naive, *EGFR/ALK*-wild type NSCLC patients.[70]

Cytokines and other signaling-based therapies

Therapies based on cytokine signaling cascades have been shown to induce long-term remission in a small subset of patients with other cancers; in advanced melanoma patients, high-dose IL-2 produced 16% ORR, but in complete responders, the duration of response lasted several years.[71,72] Efforts to translate promising results to NSCLC have been disappointing overall. Bempegaldesleukin (NKTR-214), a pegylated recombinant IL-2 prodrug, demonstrated activation of CD8+ T cells and NK cells but did not produce any objective responses among 28 patients with advanced solid tumors.[73] In combination with nivolumab in PD-(L)1-naive patients, NKTR-214 induced a response in three of five patients; one patient had stable disease and one patient had progressive disease.[74] The activity of NKTR-214 in NSCLC is currently being explored in combination with the VB10.NEO vaccine (NCT03548467); a combination with pembrolizumab with or without chemotherapy (NCT03138889) has now been terminated. Another pegylated recombinant IL-2 molecule, THOR-707, is currently being investigated as monotherapy and in combination with pembrolizumab in the phase I/II HAMMER study.[75]

Transforming growth factor beta (TGF-β) has been identified as a potential target as a very influential immunomodulator. In early pre-malignant conditions, TGF-β promotes anti-tumor activity by enforcing regulation of the cell cycle, apoptosis, and cell differentiation, but once tumorigenesis occurs, cancer cells take advantage of TGF-β signaling cascades, transforming this cytokine into an oncogenic factor.[76,77] Of significant interest has been the opportunity to reverse the immunosuppressive environment promoted by TGF-β[77–79] as a way to enhance responsiveness to checkpoint inhibitors. Inhibition of TGF-β has been attempted through a multitude of mechanisms, including small molecule inhibitors, mAbs, ligand traps, and antisense oligonucleotides.[80] One of the most promising agents, bintrafusp alpha, a bifunctional fusion protein, which blocks TGF-β and PD-L1, showed promising results in a phase I trial of 80 ICI-naive NSCLC patients with an ORR of 21.3% overall, with higher response rates in PD-L1-positive (36.0%) and PD-L1 high (85.7%) patients.[81] Unfortunately, a subsequent phase III trial of bintrafusp alpha versus pembrolizumab in first-line treatment of high PD-L1 NSCLC patients was halted early for futility.[82]

Other attempts to use cytokine therapy in NSCLC have thus far met challenges. Early interest in the role of IL-1β was generated by a study investigating the use of canakinumab (anti-IL-1β mAb) for atherosclerosis; a post hoc analysis showed that patients treated with cankinumab were significantly less likely to die of lung cancer than patients in the placebo group.[83] The study authors posited that canakinumab may have slowed the progression and invasiveness of potentially pre-existing lung cancers, based on preclinical work demonstrating that IL-1 β can promote tumor invasiveness.[83] However, the phase III CANOPY-2 trial did not show an OS advantage of canakinumab and docetaxel compared with docetaxel alone in patients who had progressed on chemoimmunotherapy.[84] CANOPY-1 (evaluating canakinumab in the first line in combination with chemoimmunotherapy), CANOPY-A (evaluating canakinumab in the adjuvant setting), and CANOPY-N (evaluating canakinumab with pembrolizumab in the neoadjuvant setting) are ongoing. The pegylated recombinant IL-10 pegilodecakin did not demonstrate benefit as monotherapy or in combination with ICI in first-line or second-line treatment of NSCLC.[85] Preliminary results from a study of N803, a novel IL-15 complexed protein plus ICI in patients who had disease progression on the same ICI showed CR 0%, partial responses (PR) 8%,[86] and a study of single-agent NIZ985 showed no responses and significant toxicity,[87] though other IL-15-directed agents showed more promise. In a phase Ib study of ALT-803 with nivolumab in ICI-naive or pretreated NSCLC patients, this therapy was safely administered and induced partial response in 29% (6/21) patients.[88]

The cytosolic DNA sensor cyclic-GMP-AMP synthase (cGAS)- stimulator of interferon genes (STING) pathway has the central function of sensing central cytosolic double-stranded DNA, facilitating the innate immune response against infections, inflammation, and cancer.[89] STING agonists have thus generated interest as a way to restore responsiveness to ICI in preclinical models.[90] One of the most promising agents identified pre-clinically was 5,6-dimethylxanthenone-4-acetic acid (DMXAA) (ASA404),[91] and in a randomized phase II clinical trial, DMXAA in addition to chemotherapy in untreated NSCLC demonstrated no new safety signals as well as improved ORR and survival.[92] However, these results were not borne out in a larger phase III randomized trial of chemotherapy with or without DMXAA in advanced NSCLC.[93] A combination with ICI was explored in a phase I study of MK-1454 plus pembrolizumab in lymphomas or solid tumors, though results for NSCLC have not yet been published.[94] This and other studies (NCT04420884, NCT04879849, NCT05070247) of STING agonists as monotherapy or in combination with ICI are ongoing.

Microbiome-based

Interestingly, there has been a burgeoning interest in studying the effects of the human microbiome on the systemic immune response.[95] Alterations to the gut microbiome composition by antibiotics were found to attenuate response to ICI in cancer patients,[96] and supplementation with common bacterial flora restored the ability of PD-1 blockade to recruit T lymphocytes into mouse tumor beds.[97] Therapeutic strategies under investigation include fecal microbiota transplant (FMT), administration of defined bacterial strains and dietary changes.[98] FMT in combination with ICI for lung cancer patients is now under study in several trials (NCT05502913, NCT04951583, NCT05008861, NCT04521075, NCT04924374, NCT03819296), though the safety of this methodology remains a concern given FMT may unwittingly transfer parasites or multi-drug-resistant organisms in addition to the intended microbiota.[98] Specific bacterial isolates have been implicated in modulating the activity of checkpoint inhibitors, including *Bifidobacterium* spp.[99] and *Bacteroides* spp.,[100] and clinical trials of single-strain isolates in combination with immunotherapy are underway.[7] EDP1503, an orally deliverable strain of *Bifidobacterium animalis lactis*, was combined with pembrolizumab in phase I/II study of patients with solid tumors; this led to two PR in NSCLC patients (an ORR of 14% across tumor types).[101] A randomized phase I trial of metastatic renal cell carcinoma patients treated with nivolumab and ipilimumab with or without *Clostridium butyricum* demonstrated significantly longer PFS in the bacterial supplementation group (12.7 months vs 2.5 months, 95% CI 0.05–0.47, $P = 0.001$).[102] Lastly, dietary changes may influence the composition of gut microbiota and subsequent responses to immunomodulatory therapies.[98] A recent meta-analysis found that the use of probiotics in ICI-treated patients was associated with significantly higher ORR, PFS, and OS.[103] However, the use of probiotics remains controversial, with some clinical and preclinical studies suggesting worse outcomes in this setting. An observational study of melanoma patients treated with ICI showed that patients with adequate dietary fiber *without* probiotic supplementation had longer PFS, a finding recapitulated in murine models.[104] One prospective clinical trial is examining the effect of a fasting-mimicking diet on response and survival to chemo-immunotherapy in NSCLC (NCT03700437).

ANTIBODY-DRUG CONJUGATES

ADCs, a novel therapeutic comprised of an antibody moiety and a cytotoxic payload attached by a unique linker, have the potential to deliver highly potent treatment in a targeted manner. Advances in technology have now led to the impressive efficacy of ADCs in advanced cancers, leading to several approvals for various indications, including now in lung cancer. Despite substantial progress that has been made, the use of ADCs has still met various challenges, including toxicity profiles, unclear biomarker selection, and little information surrounding resistance.

Mechanism of Action of Antibody-Drug Conjugates

ADCs are comprised of three components: the antibody moiety, linker, and cytotoxic payload. The composition of each unique ADC affects the drug's delivery, potency, and toxicity. In this section, we review each individual part of the molecule and considerations that must be accounted for in designing the entire molecule (**Fig. 2**).

Antibody and target selection

The ideal target for a newly-designed ADC should demonstrate high expression on tumor and no or low expression on healthy cells,[105] should have minimal secretion in circulation and instead be displayed on the cell surface to be available for antibody binding,[106] and should, via internalization, facilitate ADC transportation into the cell.[107] However, there is generally still some expression of ADC targets across tissue types, including in normal tissues, which can subsequently affect binding affinity and toxicity profile.[108,109] In addition, cells neighboring those targeted by the ADC may also be killed by the so-called bystander effect, particularly if the payload is membrane-permeable.[110] Targets with high rates of turnover may result in more efficient drug delivery and, by extension, efficacy.[111] Interestingly, there is evidence that targets that are functionally oncogenic can facilitate ADC activity when compared with targets that are present on cell surface without functional significance.[105] The ideal antibody for incorporation into an ADC should have high target specificity[112] and affinity,[113] low immunogenicity (usually humanized or fully human immunoglobulins), and low cross-reactivity.[114] Differences in the immunoglobulin classes can affect the solubility and half-life of mAbs; Immunoglobulin G1 (IgG1) is the subclass most frequently used for ADC architecture to optimize these factors.[115,116]

Linker

Far from an inert component of the ADC, the linker that connects the antibody moiety to the cytotoxic payload must display specific properties to ensure the success of the

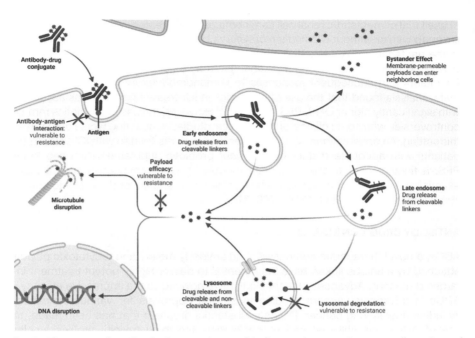

Fig. 2. The steps of antibody-drug conjugate binding and processing, as well as sites of payload action, are depicted. Steps particularly vulnerable to the development of resistance are labeled in red text accompanied by red "x." Figure created with BioRender.com.

overall molecule, and the recent advances in linker technology may have contributed substantially to the successes of the ADC class.[115] The linker must be stabilized to avoid premature release of the payload, which would result in unacceptable toxicity to the off-target tissue, and must maintain the payload in an inactive state while bound to the antibody.[117] Optimization of the linker chemistry must also allow the release of the payload once internalized.[118] Linkers are divided into two major classes, cleavable and non-cleavable, each with its own set of advantages. Cleavable linkers release the cytotoxic payload in response to environmental factors associated with tumors (eg, acidic conditions); imperfect designs show that available linkers display variable stability.[119] Non-cleavable linkers are more stable in plasma but rely on intracellular transport and degradation of the entire ADC to allow the release of the payload, which may affect cell permeability and subsequent clearance.[119] New data have indicated that the linker stability may also relate to target and payload selection as well as tumor microenvironment.[120–122]

Payload
Early work demonstrated that only a small fraction of traditional chemotherapy drugs penetrated tumor tissue when conjugated to antibodies[123,124]; subsequent experimentation with highly potent cytotoxic drugs such as auristatins, calicheamicins, topoisomerase inhibitors, and pyrrolobenzodiazepines indicated that these powerful payloads were critical for the efficacy of the overall molecule.[115,125] The drug-to-antibody ratio (DAR) represents the average number of payload moieties attached to each antibody; in general, ADCs with high DARs are expected to be more potent, though differences in clearance may actually render them more similar to lower-DAR ADCs.[126,127]

In vivo, ADCs represent a complex machinery with an intricate interplay of all the component molecules. Although the generally accepted model involves the binding of the antibody to the antigen, internalization into the cell, and payload release (see **Fig. 2**), the in vivo effect may be much more complicated when taking into account the pharmacokinetic variability of each component, incomplete penetration into tumor tissue, engagement of antibody-dependent cellular cytotoxicity (ADCC) or antibody-dependent cellular phagocytosis (ADCP), and the degree of "bystander effect" present via diffusion of lipophilic payloads across cell membranes, among other factors.[115]

Experience of Antibody-Drug Conjugates in Lung Cancer

ADCs have thus far been tested in patients with pretreated cancers, and due to their potent but targeted mechanism of action, have, in certain cases, been able to demonstrate impressive activity in treatment-refractory cancers.[115] However, activity in lung cancer specifically has been variable. **Table 2** lists promising ADCs undergoing further study in lung cancer; a selection is reviewed in more detail below.

Trophoblast cell-surface antigen-2

Trophoblast cell-surface antigen (TROP-2) is highly expressed in both NSCLC and SCLC. Two ADCs targeting TROP-2 have been tested in lung cancer patients regardless of TROP-2 expression in their tumors.

Sacituzumab govitecan (SG, IMMU-132) is composed of a humanized mAb sacituzumab and the payload SN-38, a topoisomerase I inhibitor, by a cleavable linker.[108] In the phase I/II dose-escalation and dose-expansion basket trial of 495 patients, which included 54 patients with heavily-pretreated metastatic NSCLC treated at doses of 8 and 10 mg/kg, there were confirmed PRs in 9 of 47 evaluable patients (19%) and stable disease (SD) in 23 patients (49%).[128] The median duration of response for responders was 6.0 months (95% CI, 4.8–8.3 months). Grade $\geq$ 3 events that occurred in $\geq$ 5% of patients were neutropenia (28%), leukopenia (9%), pneumonia (9%), diarrhea (7%), nausea (7%), and fatigue (6%). Given the vast majority of tumor specimens stained moderately or strongly by immunohistochemistry, it was not possible to correlate the response with TROP-2 expression. In the SCLC cohort, 53 pretreated patients were treated at 8 and 10 mg/kg. Seven of 50 evaluable patients demonstrated confirmed PR (14%), with a median duration of response of 5.7 months (95% CI, 3.6–19.9 months), and 21 of 50 patients had SD as the best response (42%). Grades 3 and 4 events were similar to those observed in the NSCLC cohort (neutropenia, 34%; diarrhea, 9%; fatigue, 13%; anemia 6%; hypoxia 4%). In the phase III randomized ASCENT trial, patients with advanced breast cancer that had progressed on at least two prior therapies received SG or physician's choice of standard chemotherapy. Patients in the SG cohort had significantly longer PFS (4.8 months, 95% CI 4.1–5.8 vs 1.7 months, 95% CI 1.5–2.5, $P < 0.0001$) and OS (11.8 months, 95% CI 10.5–13.8 vs 6.9 months, 95% CI 5.9–7.6, $P < 0.0001$) than patients in the standard chemotherapy arm. Based on these results, the FDA granted regular approval to SG for patients with unresectable or metastatic breast cancer that has progressed on at least two prior therapies in April 2021.

Datopotamab deruxtecan (Dato-DXd, DS-1062a) is a humanized mAb attached to deruxtecan by a cleavable linker. In the phase I TROPION-PanTumor01 study, patients with advanced solid tumors were treated with Dato-DXd. The NSCLC cohort included 180 patients from dose-escalation and dose-expansion phases treated at 4, 6, and 8 mg/kg.[129] ORR was similar among cohorts with 24% at 4 and 8 mg/kg, and 26% at 6 mg/kg. Grade $\geq$ 3 treatment-emergent AEs were seen in 47% of

Table 2
Selected clinical trials of antibody-drug conjugates under investigation in lung cancer

Target	ADC	Strategy	NCT Identifier/Phase	Population	Primary Endpoint
TROP-2	Sacituzumab govitecan (SG)	SG vs docetaxel (EVOKE-01)	NCT05089734 Phase III	Progressed on platinum doublet + PD-(L)1 inhibitor	OS
		SG ± chemo ± PD-(L)1 inhibitor (EVOKE-02)	NCT05186974 Phase II	Treatment-naive	ORR
		SG monotherapy (TROPiCS-03)	NCT03964727 Phase II	Progressed on platinum doublet + PD-(L)1 inhibitor	ORR
		SG + atezolizumab (Morpheus Lung)	NCT03337698 Phase I/II	Treatment-naive; Progressed on platinum doublet + PD-(L)1 inhibitor	ORR
		SG + berzosertib	NCT04826341 Phase I/II	SCLC progressed on platinum doublet	MTD, ORR
	Datopotamab deruxtecan (Dato-DXd)	Dato-DXd + pembrolizumab ± chemo (TROPION-Lung07)	NCT05555732 Phase III	Treatment-naive	PFS, OS
		Dato-DXd + pembro vs pembro (TROPION-Lung08)	NCT05215340 Phase III	Treatment-naive	PFS, OS
		Dato-DXd + pembrolizumab ± chemo (TROPION-Lung02)	NCT04526691 Phase I	Treatment-naive; ICI-naive; Pretreated	Safety
		Dato-DXd vs docetaxel (TROPION-Lung01)	NCT04656652 Phase III	Pretreated	PFS, OS
		Dato-DXd + osimertinib	NCT03944772 Phase II	Progressed on osimertinib	ORR
	SKB264	SKB264 monotherapy	NCT04152499 Phase I/II	Pretreated	MTD, ORR
HER2	Ado-Trastuzumab emtansine (TDM-1)	TDM-1 monotherapy	NCT02675829 Phase II	HER2-mutant or -amplified	ORR
		TDM-1 + osimertinib	-	HER2 bypass track resistance in EGFR-mutant pts	Safety, ORR
		TDM-1 monotherapy	NCT04591431 Phase II	Pretreated, HER2-mutant or -amplified	ORR
		TDM-1 monotherapy	NCT02465060 Phase II	Pretreated, HER2-amplified	ORR
	Trastuzumab deruxtecan (TDX-d)	TDX-d 6.4 mg/kg vs TDX-d 5.4 mg/kg (DESTINY-LUNG02)	NCT04644237 Phase II	Pretreated, HER2-mutant	ORR

Target	Agent	Trial/Combination	NCT Number, Phase	Patient population	Endpoint
		TDX-d vs platinum chemo + PD-(L)1 inhibitor	NCT05048797 Phase III	Treatment-naive, *HER2* mutant	PFS
		TDX-d + pembrolizumab	NCT04042701 Phase I	PD-(L)1 inhibitor naive, *HER2*-mutant or -amplified	Safety, ORR
		TDX-d + durvalumab + chemo (DESTINY-LUNG03)	NCT04686305 Phase I	Treatment-naive or pretreated, *HER2*-amplified	Safety
		TDX-d monotherapy (DESTINY-LUNG05)	NCT05246514 Phase II	Pretreated, *HER2*-mutant	ORR
		T-DXd + durvalumab (HUDSON)	NCT03334617 Phase II	Progression on PD-(L)1 inhibitor	ORR
	MRG002	MRG002 monotherapy	NCT05141786 Phase II	Pretreated, *HER2*-mutant	ORR
	GQ1001	GQ1001 monotherapy	NCT04450732 Phase I	Pretreated, *HER2*-amplified	Safety, MTD
	A166	A166 monotherapy	NCT03602079 Phase I/II	Pretreated, *HER2*-amplified	Safety, MTD
HER3	Patritumab deruxtecan (HER3-DXd)	HER3-DXd 5.6 mg/kg vs HER3-DXd up-titration (HERTHENA-Lung01)	NCT04619004 Phase II	Progressed on platinum doublet and osimertinib, *EGFR*-mutant	ORR
		HER3-DXd + osimertinib	NCT04676477 Phase I	Progression on osimertinib or treatment-naive, *EGFR*-mutant	Safety, ORR
		HER3-DXd vs chemotherapy (HERTHENA-Lung02)	NCT05338970 Phase III	Progression on EGFR TKI, *EGFR*-mutant	PFS
		HER3-DXd monotherapy	NCT03260491 Phase I	Pretreated, *EGFR*-mutant or –wild-type	Safety, ORR
MET	Telisotuzumab vedotin (Teliso-V)	Teliso-V monotherapy	NCT03539536 Phase II	Pretreated, c-Met+	Safety, ORR
		Teliso-V vs docetaxel	NCT04928846 Phase III	Pretreated, c-Met+	PFS, OS
		Teliso-V monotherapy	NCT05513703 Phase II	Treatment-naive, c-Met+	ORR
		Teliso-V + nivolumab	NCT02099058 Phase I	Pretreated	Safety, RP2D
		Teliso-V + osimertinib	NCT02099058 Phase I	Progressed on osimertinib, *EGFR*-mutant	Safety, RP2D
	REGN5093-M114	REGN5093-M114 monotherapy	NCT04982224 Phase I/II	Pretreated, c-Met+	Safety, ORR

(continued on next page)

Table 2
(continued)

Target	ADC	Strategy	NCT Identifier/ Phase	Population	Primary Endpoint
CEACAM5	Tusamitamab ravtansine	Tusamitamab ravtansine monotherapy	NCT05245071 Phase II	Pretreated, negative or moderate CEACAM5 and high CEA	ORR
		Tusamitamab ravtansine + pembrolizumab ± chemo	NCT04524689 Phase II	Treatment-naive, CEACAM5 ≥ 2+	Safety
		Tusamitamab ravtansine vs docetaxel	NCT04154956 Phase III	Pretreated, CEACAM5 ≥ 2+	PFS, OS
		Tusamitamab ravtansine + ramucirumab	NCT04394624 Phase II	Pretreated, CEACAM5 ≥ 2+	Safety, ORR
B7-H3	DS-7300a	DS-7300a monotherapy	NCT05280470 Phase II	Pretreated SCLC	ORR
	MCG018	MCG018 ± retifanlimab	NCT03729596 Phase I/II	Pretreated NSCLC	Safety
PTK7	Cofetuzumab pelidotin	Cofetuzumab pelidotin monotherapy	NCT04189614 Phase I	Pretreated, PTK7+	ORR
MUC1/EGFR	M1231	M1231 monotherapy	NCT04695847 Phase I	Pretreated, EGFR+ and MUC1+	Safety, ORR
Folate Receptor Alpha	MORAb-202	MORAb-202 monotherapy	NCT05577715 Phase II	Pretreated	Safety, ORR
	PRO1184	PRO1184 monotherapy	NCT05579366 Phase I/II	Pretreated	Safety
	AMT-151	AMT-151 monotherapy	NCT05498597 Phase I	Pretreated	Safety, MTD
AXL	BA3011	BA3011 ± PD-(L)1 inhibitor	NCT04681131 Phase II	Pretreated	Safety, ORR
NaPi2b	XMT-1592	XMT-1592 monotherapy	NCT04396340 Phase I/II	Pretreated	MTD
	XMT-1536	XMT-1536 monotherapy	NCT03319628 Phase I/II	Pretreated	Safety, ORR

Target	Drug name	Description	NCT / Phase	Population	Endpoint
EGFR	MRG003	MRG003 monotherapy	NCT04838548 Phase II	Pretreated, EGFR+	ORR
5T4	ASN004	ASN004 monotherapy	NCT04410224 Phase I	Pretreated	MTD
ROR2	BA3021	BA3021 ± PD-(L)1 inhibitor	NCT03504488 Phase I/II	Pretreated	Safety, ORR
Tissue Factor	XB002	XB002 ± nivolumab	NCT04925284 Phase I	Pretreated	MTD, ORR
CD71	CX-2029	CX-2029 monotherapy	NCT03543813 Phase I/II	Pretreated	Safety
CD30	Brentuximab vedotin	Brentuximab vedotin monotherapy	NCT03007030 Phase II	CD30+ mesothelioma	DCR

Abbreviations: 5T4, Trophoblast glycoprotein; ADC, antibody-drug conjugate; AXL, AXL tyrosine kinase; B7-H3, B7 homolog 3 protein; CEA, carcinoembryonic antigen; CEACAM5, Carcinoembryonic antigen-related cell adhesion molecule 5; chemo, chemotherapy; c-Met, tyrosine-protein kinase Met; DCR, disease control rate; EGFR, epidermal growth factor receptor; HER2, human epidermal growth factor receptor 2; HER3, receptor tyrosine-protein kinase erbB-3; ICI, immune checkpoint inhibitor; MET, MET proto-oncogene tyrosine kinase; MTD, maximum tolerated dose; MUC1, mucin 1, cell-surface associated; NaPi2b, sodium-dependent phosphate transport protein 2B; NCT, National Clinical Trial; NSCLC, non-small cell lung cancer; ORR, objective response rate; OS, overall survival; pembro, pembrolizumab; PFS, progression-free survival; PTK7, protein tyrosine kinase 7; ROR2, Tyrosine-protein kinase transmembrane receptor ROR2; SCLC, small cell lung cancer; TROP-2, Trophoblast cell-surface antigen 2.

patients, though neutropenia and diarrhea were infrequent. Drug-related interstitial lung disease occurred in 11% (19 patients) with three grade 5 events at the 8 mg/kg dose. Dato-DXd is now being explored at the 6 mg/kg dose in the phase III TROPION-Lung01 study versus docetaxel in metastatic NSCLC without actionable mutations[130] and in combination with PD-(L)1 inhibitors in phase Ib trials (NCT04526691, NCT04612751).

Human epidermal growth factor receptor 2

Human epidermal growth factor receptor 2 (HER2) plays a critical role in oncogenesis in several cancer types[131] and can be altered in NSCLC through protein overexpression, gene amplification, or gene mutation. HER2 mutations are present in NSCLC in about 1% to 5% cases[132,133] and define a subset of patients who might particularly benefit from HER2-directed ADCs, as activating mutations have been shown to increase HER2 receptor internalization.[134]

Ado-trastuzumab emtansine (T-DM1) is composed of anti-HER2 mAb trastuzumab linked to the microtubule inhibitor emtansine (DM1) by a non-cleavable linker. In a phase II basket trial of T-DM1, 18 patients with HER2-mutant NSCLC, 50% of whom had had prior HER2-directed TKI or mAb, demonstrated ORR 44% (95% CI, 22%–69%) with median PFS 5 months (95% CI, 3–9 months).[135] Treatment-related AEs were mainly grade 1 or 2, and infusion reactions occurred in 28% of patients. A Japanese phase II trial of T-DM1 in 22 NSCLC patients with exon 20 insertion mutations demonstrated ORR 38.1% (90% confidence interval, 23.0–55.9%) with median PFS 2.8 months (95% CI, 1.4–4.4 months); thrombocytopenia was the only notable grade ≥ 3 event in more than one patient (4, 18.2%).[136] Results of testing T-DM1 in NSCLC patients with HER2 overexpression have been less promising: one phase II trial in patients with an immunohistochemistry (IHC) score of 3+, an IHC score of 2+ and positive fluorescence in situ (FISH), or exon 20 mutation was terminated early due to limited efficacy,[137] and another in patients with IHC 2–3+ showed zero responses in the 2+ cohort and four PR in the 3+ cohort.[138]

Recently, there has been great enthusiasm for trastuzumab deruxtecan (T-DXd), an ADC constructed with the same anti-HER2 mAb but conjugated instead to a topoisomerase inhibitor by a cleavable linker. The higher DAR, membrane-permeable payload, and cleavable linker combine to produce an overall more potent molecule.[139] In the DESTINY-Lung01 study of 6.4 mg/kg of T-DXd in 91 patients with HER2-mutant NSCLC, objective responses were observed in 55% of patients (95% CI, 44–65) and the median PFS was 8.2 months (95% CI, 6.0–11.9).[140] The toxicity profile was notable for 26% of patients who developed interstitial lung disease (ILD), which resulted in two treatment-related deaths. At ESMO 2022, interim results of the DESTINY-Lung02 phase II trial of T-DXd 5.4 mg/kg compared with 6.4 mg/kg in HER2-mutant NSCLC were presented. In the pre-specified early cohort, confirmed ORR was 53.8% (95% CI 39.5–67.8) to the lower dose and 42.9% (95% CI 24.5–62.8) to the higher dose, and the lower dose resulted in fewer instances of ILD.[141] Given the impressive efficacy in a heavily-pretreated population, in August 2022, T-DXd received accelerated approval by the FDA for use in HER2-mutant NSCLC at the 5.4 mg/kg dose.

Human epidermal growth factor receptor-3

HER3, a member of the HER family of protein receptors, is expressed in approximately 80% of NSCLC tumors[142,143] and has been associated with poorer outcomes.[143]

Patritumab deruxtecan (HER3-DXd) is an ADC with the same payload as in T-DXd and Dato-DXd, conjugated to a fully human HER3 mAb by a cleavable linker. In a phase I study of patients with advanced EGFR-mutant NSCLC, whose disease had progressed on prior EGFR TKI, 57 patients received the recommended dose for expansion of 5.6 mg/kg and confirmed ORR was 39% (95% CI, 26.0–52.4), disease control rate (DCR) 72%, and mPFS 8.2 months.[144] Of note, responses were observed in tumors with a wide range of resistance mechanisms, and across all HER3 expression levels. Grade ≥ 3 treatment-related AEs occurred in 64% of patients, and the most common were thrombocytopenia and neutropenia. Treatment-related ILD occurred in 5% of patients. Further studies are ongoing, including the HERTHENA-Lung01 study, which is evaluating HER3-DXd at 5.6 mg/kg versus dose up-titration in patients with *EGFR*-mutant NSCLC, HERTHENA-Lung02, which will study HER3-DXd versus chemotherapy after disease progression on EGFR TKI, and a phase I study of combination therapy with osimertinib (NCT04676477).

MET proto-oncogene

Ligand binding to MET, a receptor tyrosine kinase encoded by the mesenchymal to epithelial transition gene (*MET*), results in the activation of downstream signaling pathways which promote cell proliferation and survival. Alterations in *MET* comprise an important subset of oncogene-driven NSCLC, including MET exon 14 skipping mutations which occur in 3% to 4% of NSCLC patients,[145] and *MET* amplification, which occurs in 1% to 6% of NSCLC patients.[146-148] *MET* amplification is also an important mechanism of resistance for patients with oncogene-driven NSCLC whose disease progresses on targeted therapy.[149]

Telisotuzumab vedotin (Teliso-V) is an ADC comprised of anti c-MET mAb ABT-700 conjugated to cytotoxic monomethyl auristatin E (MMAE) via a cleavable linker. In a first-in-human study of 16 patients with c-Met positive, heavily-pretreated NSCLC, three patients had a PR (19%) and DCR was 56%; median PFS was 5.7 months (95% CI, 1.2 –15.4 months).[150] The patients who exhibited response were all *KRAS* and *EGFR* wild type. With regard to safety, given multiple dose-limiting toxicities (DLTs) in two patients in the 3 and 3.3 mg/kg dose level groups, though the maximum-tolerated dose (MTD) was not formally identified, 2.7 mg/kg was selected for expansion. Grade 3 or 4 AEs attributed to the drug were seen in 12.8% of the dose-escalation cohort and 33.3% of dose expansion cohort; the most common grade ≥ 3 treatment-related adverse events (TRAEs) were fatigue, hypoalbuminemia, anemia, and neutropenia. A subsequent study which evaluated every 2- or 3-week dosing enrolled 52 NSCLC patients.[151] Of 40 patients whose tumors were c-Met positive, ORR was 23% with median PFS 5.2 months (95% CI 1.7–6.4 months); 65% of patients reported grade ≥ 3 TRAEs, including 68% receiving the therapy every 2 weeks and 63% every 3 weeks. Unfortunately, the phase II study of Teliso-V in patients with c-MET positive squamous cell carcinoma was terminated early for lack of efficacy (ORR 9%, 95% CI 0%–20%) in addition to concerns about safety (three grade 5 events, two pneumonitis, and one bronchopulmonary hemorrhage).[152] Teliso-V in combination with erlotinib was also studied in *EGFR*-mutant c-MET positive NSCLC following progression on EGFR TKI.[153] An ORR of 34.5% (17.9%–54.3%) was achieved with a median PFS not reached at 4-month follow-up. The most frequent grade ≥ 3 TEAEs were pulmonary embolism (14%), peripheral neuropathy (7%), and diarrhea (7%). Further studies are ongoing (NCT03539536, NCT04928846, NCT05513703).

Carcinoembryonic antigen (CEA)-related cell adhesion molecule 5

Carcinoembryonic antigen (CEA)-related cell adhesion molecule 5 (CEACAM5) is expressed weakly in normal tissues but highly expressed in several tumor types, including lung,[154] and may facilitate tumor invasion and metastasis.[155]

Tusamitamab ravtansine (SAR408701) is an ADC that combines a humanized mAb with the cytotoxic payload maytansinoid (DM4) via a cleavable linker. Based on promising preclinical models,[156] a first-in-human study was conducted[157] with a dose expansion cohort in non-squamous NSCLC patients;[158] 92 patients were treated in two cohorts, moderate expressers (28 patients) and high expressers (64 patients). In the moderate expresser cohort, ORR was 7.1%, and in the high expresser cohort, ORR was 20.3% (95% confidence interval 12.27%–31.71%) and 42.2% had stable disease. Grade $\geq$3 TEAEs occurred in 47.8% of patients and were assessed as drug-related in 15.2%. Notable toxicities included keratopathy/keratitis in 38.0% and peripheral neuropathy in 26.1%. A phase III trial comparing tusamitamab ravtansine with docetaxel in NSCLC patients pretreated with chemo and ICI whose tumors express CEACAM5 in at least 50% of tumor cells is ongoing (NCT04154956), as well as phase II trials of tusamitamab ravtansine in combination with ramucirumab (NCT04394624) and with pembrolizumab with or without platinum-based chemotherapy (NCT04524689).

Others in development
Table 2 lists several other targets currently under investigation in lung cancer. Of note, Delta-like protein 3 (DLL3), which is expressed in high-grade neuroendocrine cancers and may contribute to neuroendocrine tumorigenesis,[159] has been an attractive target in neuroendocrine lung cancer. Unfortunately, trials with DLL3-targeting ADCs Rovalpituzumab tesirine (Rova-T) and SC-002 yielded disappointing results in terms of both efficacy and toxicity, and both of these agents are no longer in development.[160–163] Other halted therapies include glembatumumab vedotin, an ADC targeting glycoprotein NMB,[164] and anetumab ravtansine, an ADC targeting mesothelin.[165]

Resistance to Antibody-Drug Conjugates

The complexity of the ADC molecule reveals several vulnerable sites for the development of resistance, though a full understanding of these mechanisms is still somewhat limited. Drago and colleagues[115] suggest that the major steps at which resistance can occur include antibody-antigen interaction, ADC internalization and processing, and payload activity (see **Fig. 2**). The antibody–antigen interaction may be compromised by the downregulation of antigen, loss of antigen expression, mutations in the antigen, or the presence of competing ligands for the antigen.[166] The ADC internalization process has several steps which may be sites of resistance, including altered trafficking to lysosomes, lysosomal degradation hindered by reduced proteolytic or acidification function, and the overexpression of drug efflux transporters.[166] With regard to payload efficacy, there may be dysregulation in the apoptotic pathway or upregulation of ATP-binding cassette proteins which hinder payload activity.[115,166] One recent study investigating resistance to sacituzumab govitecan in triple-negative breast cancer through RNA and whole-exome sequencing of pre-treatment and post-treatment specimens identified mutations in *TOP1* (encoding the payload target topoisomerase 1) and *TACSTD2* (encoding TROP2) as important acquired resistance mechanisms.[167]

In identifying strategies to overcome resistance to ADCs, the precise mechanism that is impaired must be recognized. If lysosomal proteolysis and acidification are compromised, ensuring the cleavability of the linker could be a rational strategy.[108] If drug efflux pump upregulation is identified as a culprit, the selection of a cytotoxic payload that is a poor efflux substrate could mitigate resistance.[166] It is clear that there is still much to be learned regarding response and resistance to these novel therapies as they are integrated more commonly into the clinic.

DISCUSSION OF FUTURE DIRECTIONS

There are many strategies in development to augment the efficacy of ADCs. These include the use of bispecific antibodies to target two different antigens or two distinct epitopes of the same antigens,[108] combination treatment with kinase inhibitors or other mAb such as ICI or anti-VEGF therapies,[108,115,168] the conjugation of cytotoxic payloads to PD-1 antibodies,[108] the use of targeted agents or ICI as a payload agent,[115] and the integration of molecular-based imaging to confirm in vivo target expression and drug delivery.[166] As investigations into underlying mechanisms of ADC efficacy continue, promising therapeutic strategies will gain further clarity.

SUMMARY

The immune checkpoint inhibitor therapy has revolutionized the treatment of lung cancer over the past several years, and the field is now on the precipice of a marked expansion of innovative strategies to address primary and acquired resistance to ICIs. Strategies under study include the combination of ICI with alternative agents to augment efficacy, novel immune-mediated therapeutics, and the growing use of ADCs, a powerful vehicle to deliver potent cytotoxic therapy in a more targeted manner. As these strategies are tested further in clinical trials, we anticipate that more effective therapies for patients with lung cancer are integrated into regular clinical practice.

CLINICS CARE POINTS

- Patients with acquired resistance may benefit from combination therapies intended to restore sensitivity to immune modulation, whereas those with primary resistance to PD-(L)1 inhibitors might require alternative novel modalities entirely

- Several novel combinations with PD-(L)1 inhibitors are under investigation, and though there have been some promising results, none have yet been approved

- Immunomodulatory therapies such as vaccination, adoptive T-cell therapies, oncolytic viruses, cytokines, and microbiome-based therapies are novel strategies to address lung cancers unresponsive to traditional chemo- or immunotherapies

- ADCs are a potent new class of agents that combine the advantages of targeted therapies and cytotoxic therapy and hold great promise as potentially efficacious agents for heavily-pretreated patients

---

DISCLOSURE OF FUNDING

There was no funding received for this work.

CONFLICTS OF INTEREST

A.J. Cooper has received consulting honoraria from MJH Life Sciences. R.S. Heist reports Consulting: Abbvie, Astrazeneca, Claim Therapeutics, Daichii Sankyo, EMD Serono, Lilly, Novartis, Regeneron, Sanofi Research funding to institution not to self: Abbvie, United States, Agios, United States, Corvus, Daichii Sankyo, Erasca, Exelixis, United States, Lilly, United States, Mirati, Novartis, Switzerland, Turning Point.

REFERENCES

1. Gandhi L, Rodriguez-Abreu D, Gadgeel S, et al. Pembrolizumab plus chemotherapy in metastatic non-small-cell lung cancer. N Engl J Med 2018;378(22): 2078–92.
2. Paz-Ares L, Luft A, Vicente D, et al. Pembrolizumab plus chemotherapy for squamous non-small-cell lung cancer. N Engl J Med 2018;379(21):2040–51.
3. Reck M, Rodriguez-Abreu D, Robinson AG, et al. Pembrolizumab versus chemotherapy for PD-L1-positive non-small-cell lung cancer. N Engl J Med 2016;375(19):1823–33.
4. Mok TSK, Wu Y-L, Kudaba I, et al. Pembrolizumab versus chemotherapy for previously untreated, PD-L1-expressing, locally advanced or metastatic non-small-cell lung cancer (KEYNOTE-042): a randomised, open label, controlled, phase 3 trial. Lancet 2019;393(10183):1819–30.
5. Paz-Ares L, Dvorkin M, Chen Y, et al. Durvalumab plus platinum–etoposide versus platinum–etoposide in first-line treatment of extensive-stage small-cell lung cancer (CASPIAN): a randomised, controlled, open-label, phase 3 trial. Lancet 2019;394(10212):1929–39.
6. Horn L, Mansfield AS, Szczesna A, et al. First-line atezolizumab plus chemotherapy in extensive-stage small-cell lung cancer. N Engl J Med 2018; 379(23):2220–9.
7. Passaro A, Brahmer J, Antonia S, et al. Managing resistance to immune checkpoint inhibitors in lung cancer: treatment and novel strategies. J Clin Oncol 2022;40(6):598–610.
8. Sharma P, Hu-Lieskovan S, Wargo JA, et al. Primary, adaptive, and acquired resistance to cancer immunotherapy. Cell 2017;168(4):707–23.
9. Tang T, Huang X, Zhang G, et al. Advantages of targeting the tumor immune microenvironment over blocking immune checkpoint in cancer immunotherapy. Signal Transduct Targeted Ther 2021;6(1):72.
10. Binnewies M, Roberts EW, Kersten K, et al. Understanding the tumor immune microenvironment (TIME) for effective therapy. Nat Med 2018;24(5):541–50.
11. Devaud C, John LB, Westwood JA, et al. Immune modulation of the tumor microenvironment for enhancing cancer immunotherapy. OncoImmunology 2013; 2(8):e25961.
12. Gandara D, Reck M, Moro-Sibilot D, et al. Fast progression in non-small cell lung cancer: results from the randomized phase III OAK study evaluating second-line atezolizumab versus docetaxel. J Immunother Cancer 2021;9(3):e001882. https://doi.org/10.1136/jitc-2020-001882.
13. National Comprehensive Cancer Network Non-Small Cell Lung Cancer Guidelines. 2022;3.2022.
14. Stewart RA, Pilie PG, Yap TA. Development of PARP and immune-checkpoint inhibitor combinations. Cancer Res 2018;78(24):6717–25.
15. Clarke JM, Patel JD, Robert F, et al. Veliparib and nivolumab in combination with platinum doublet chemotherapy in patients with metastatic or advanced non-small cell lung cancer: a phase 1 dose escalation study. Lung Cancer 2021; 161:180–8.
16. Ramalingam SS, Thara E, Awad MM, et al. JASPER: Phase 2 trial of first-line niraparib plus pembrolizumab in patients with advanced non–small cell lung cancer. Cancer 2021;128(1):65–74.

17. Besse B, Awad M, Forde P, et al. OA07.08 HUDSON: an open-label, multi-drug, biomarker-directed, phase II platform study in patients with NSCLC, who Progressed on Anti-PD(L)1 Therapy. J Thorac Oncol 2021;16(3):S118–9.

18. Kwok M, Davies N, Agathanggelou A, et al. ATR inhibition induces synthetic lethality and overcomes chemoresistance in TP53- or ATM-defective chronic lymphocytic leukemia cells. Blood 2016;127(5):582–95.

19. Reaper PM, Griffiths MR, Long JM, et al. Selective killing of ATM- or p53-deficient cancer cells through inhibition of ATR. Nat Chem Biol 2011;7(7): 428–30.

20. Chen W, Shen L, Jiang J, et al. Antiangiogenic therapy reverses the immunosuppressive breast cancer microenvironment. Biomark Res 2021;9(1):59.

21. Socinski MA, Jotte RM, Cappuzzo F, et al. Atezolizumab for first-line treatment of metastatic nonsquamous NSCLC. N Engl J Med 2018;378(24):2288–301.

22. Reckamp KL, Redman MW, Dragnev KH, et al. Phase II randomized study of ramucirumab and pembrolizumab versus standard of care in advanced non-small-cell lung cancer previously treated with immunotherapy-lung-MAP S1800A. J Clin Oncol 2022;40(21):2295–306.

23. Taylor MH, Lee CH, Makker V, et al. Phase IB/II Trial of lenvatinib plus pembrolizumab in patients with advanced renal cell carcinoma, endometrial cancer, and other selected advanced solid tumors. J Clin Oncol 2020;38(11):1154–63.

24. Taylor MH, Schmidt EV, Dutcus C, et al. The LEAP program: lenvatinib plus pembrolizumab for the treatment of advanced solid tumors. Future Oncol 2021; 17(6):637–48.

25. Percent IJ, Reynolds CH, Konduri K, et al. Phase III trial of sitravatinib plus nivolumab vs. docetaxel for treatment of NSCLC after platinum-based chemotherapy and immunotherapy (SAPPHIRE). J Clin Oncol 2020;38(15_suppl): TPS9635.

26. Leal TA, Spira AI, Blakely C, et al. Stage 2 enrollment complete: Sitravatinib in combination with nivolumab in NSCLC patients progressing on prior checkpoint inhibitor therapy. Ann Oncol 2018;29:viii400–1.

27. Neal JW, Lim FL, Felip E, et al. Cabozantinib in combination with atezolizumab in non-small cell lung cancer (NSCLC) patients previously treated with an immune checkpoint inhibitor: Results from cohort 7 of the COSMIC-021 study. J Clin Oncol 2020;38(15_suppl):9610.

28. Sanborn RE, Schneiders FL, Senan S, et al. Beyond checkpoint inhibitors: enhancing antitumor immune response in lung cancer. Am Soc Clin Oncol Educ Book 2022;42:1–14.

29. Rodriguez-Abreu D, Johnson ML, Hussein MA, et al. Primary analysis of a randomized, double-blind, phase II study of the anti-TIGIT antibody tiragolumab (tira) plus atezolizumab (atezo) versus placebo plus atezo as first-line (1L) treatment in patients with PD-L1-selected NSCLC (CITYSCAPE). J Clin Oncol 2020; 38(15_suppl):9503.

30. Roche News Release. Roche reports interim results for phase III SKYSCRAPER-01 study in PD-L1-high metastatic non-small cell lung cancer. 2022. Available at: https://bitly/37EbDJX. Accessed September 15, 2022.

31. Rudin CM, Liu SV, Lu S, et al. SKYSCRAPER-02: Primary results of a phase III, randomized, double-blind, placebo-controlled study of atezolizumab (atezo) + carboplatin + etoposide (CE) with or without tiragolumab (tira) in patients (pts) with untreated extensive-stage small cell lung cancer (ES-SCLC). J Clin Oncol 2022;40(17_suppl):LBA8507.

32. Ahn M, Niu J, Kim D, et al. 1400P - Vibostolimab, an anti-TIGIT antibody, as monotherapy and in combination with pembrolizumab in anti-PD-1/PD-L1-refractory NSCLC. Ann Oncol 2020;31:S754–840.

33. Shi AP, Tang XY, Xiong YL, et al. Immune checkpoint LAG3 and Its Ligand FGL1 in Cancer. Front Immunol 2021;12:785091.

34. Datar I, Sanmamed MF, Wang J, et al. Expression analysis and significance of PD-1, LAG-3, and TIM-3 in human non-small cell lung cancer using spatially resolved and multiparametric single-cell analysis. Clin Cancer Res 2019; 25(15):4663–73.

35. Tawbi HA, Schadendorf D, Lipson EJ, et al. Relatlimab and nivolumab versus nivolumab in untreated advanced melanoma. N Engl J Med 2022;386(1):24–34.

36. Radhakrishnan V, Banavali S, Gupta S, et al. Excellent CBR and prolonged PFS in non-squamous NSCLC with oral CA-170, an inhibitor of VISTA and PD-L1. Ann Oncol 2019;30.

37. Curigliano G, Gelderblom H, Mach N, et al. Abstract CT183: Phase (Ph) I/II study of MBG453± spartalizumab (PDR001) in patients (pts) with advanced malignancies. Cancer Res 2019;79(13_Supplement):CT183.

38. Tolcher A, Hamid O, Weber J, et al. Single agent anti-tumor activity in PD-1 re-fractory NSCLC: phase 1 data from the first-in-human trial of NC318, a Siglec-15-targeted antibody. SITC 2019. Abstract 032.

39. Herbst RS, Majem M, Barlesi F, et al. COAST: an open-label, phase II, multidrug platform study of durvalumab alone or in combination with oleclumab or mona-lizumab in patients with unresectable, stage III non-small-cell lung cancer. J Clin Oncol 2022;40(29):3383–93.

40. Bendell JC, LoRusso P, Overman MJ, et al. Safety and efficacy of the anti-CD73 monoclonal antibody (mAb) oleclumab ± durvalumab in patients (pts) with advanced colorectal cancer (CRC), pancreatic ductal adenocarcinoma (PDAC), or EGFR-mutant non-small cell lung cancer (EGFRm NSCLC). J Clin Oncol 2021;39(15_suppl):9047.

41. Mayes PA, Hance KW, Hoos A. The promise and challenges of immune agonist antibody development in cancer. Nat Rev Drug Discov 2018;17(7):509–27.

42. Grilley-Olson JE, Curti BD, Smith DC, et al. SEA-CD40, a non-fucosylated CD40 agonist: Interim results from a phase 1 study in advanced solid tumors. J Clin Oncol 2018;36(15_suppl):3093.

43. Zappasodi R, Sirard C, Li Y, et al. Rational design of anti-GITR-based combina-tion immunotherapy. Nat Med 2019;25(5):759–66.

44. Segal NH, He AR, Doi T, et al. Phase I Study of Single-Agent Utomilumab (PF-05082566), a 4-1BB/CD137 Agonist, in Patients with Advanced Cancer. Clin Cancer Res 2018;24(8):1816–23.

45. Chiappori A, THompson J, Eskens F, et al. P860 Results from a combination of OX40 (PF-04518600) and 4–1BB (utomilumab) agonistic antibodies in mela-noma and non-small cell lung cancer in a phase 1 dose expansion cohort. Jour-nal for ImmunoTherapy of Cancer 2020;8.

46. Tolcher AW, Sznol M, Hu-Lieskovan S, et al. Phase Ib Study of Utomilumab (PF-05082566), a 4-1BB/CD137 Agonist, in Combination with Pembrolizumab (MK-3475) in Patients with Advanced Solid Tumors. Clin Cancer Res 2017;23(18): 5349–57.

47. Geva R, Voskoboynik M, Dobrenkov K, et al. First-in-human phase 1 study of MK-1248, an anti-glucocorticoid-induced tumor necrosis factor receptor agonist monoclonal antibody, as monotherapy or with pembrolizumab in patients with advanced solid tumors. Cancer 2020;126(22):4926–35.

48. Vansteenkiste JF, Cho BC, Vanakesa T, et al. Efficacy of the MAGE-A3 cancer immunotherapeutic as adjuvant therapy in patients with resected MAGE-A3-positive non-small-cell lung cancer (MAGRIT): a randomised, double-blind, placebo-controlled, phase 3 trial. Lancet Oncol 2016;17(6):822–35.

49. Butts C, Socinski MA, Mitchell PL, et al. Tecemotide (L-BLP25) versus placebo after chemoradiotherapy for stage III non-small-cell lung cancer (START): a randomised, double-blind, phase 3 trial. Lancet Oncol 2014;15(1):59–68.

50. Pujol JL, De Pas T, Rittmeyer A, et al. Safety and immunogenicity of the PRAME cancer immunotherapeutic in patients with resected non-small cell lung cancer: a phase I dose escalation Study. J Thorac Oncol 2016;11(12):2208–17.

51. Giaccone G, Felip E, Cobo M, et al. 1260MO Activity of OSE-2101 in HLA-A2+ non-small cell lung cancer (NSCLC) patients after failure to immune checkpoint inhibitors (ICI): Step 1 results of phase III ATALANTE-1 randomised trial. Ann Oncol 2020;31:S814–5.

52. Besse B, Campelo RG, Cobo Dols M, et al. LBA47 Activity of OSE-2101 in HLA-A2+ non-small cell lung cancer (NSCLC) patients after failure to immune checkpoint inhibitors (IO): Final results of phase III Atalante-1 randomised trial. Ann Oncol 2021;32(suppl_5):S1283–346. https://doi.org/10.1016/annonc/annonc741.

53. Ott PA, Hu-Lieskovan S, Chmielowski B, et al. A phase Ib trial of personalized neoantigen therapy plus anti-PD-1 in patients with advanced melanoma, non-small cell lung cancer, or bladder cancer. Cell 2020;183(2):347–362 e324.

54. Awad MM, Govindan R, Balogh KN, et al. Personalized neoantigen vaccine NEO-PV-01 with chemotherapy and anti-PD-1 as first-line treatment for non-squamous non-small cell lung cancer. Cancer Cell 2022;40(9):1010–1026 e1011.

55. Lopez J., Camidge D., Iafolla M.A.J., et al., CT301 - A phase Ib study to evaluate RO7198457, an individualized Neoantigen Specific immunoTherapy (iNeST), in combination with atezolizumab in patients with locally advanced or metastatic solid tumors. 2020. Articles, Abstracts, and Reports. 3949. Available at: https://digitalcommons.psjhealth.org/publications/3949.

56. Rosenberg SA, Restifo NP. Adoptive cell transfer as personalized immunotherapy for human cancer. Science 2015;348(6230):62–8.

57. Kast F, Klein C, Umana P, et al. Advances in identification and selection of personalized neoantigen/T-cell pairs for autologous adoptive T cell therapies. OncoImmunology 2021;10(1):1869389.

58. Sackstein R, Schatton T, Barthel SR. T-lymphocyte homing: an underappreciated yet critical hurdle for successful cancer immunotherapy. Lab Invest 2017;97(6):669–97.

59. Creelan BC, Wang C, Teer JK, et al. Tumor-infiltrating lymphocyte treatment for anti-PD-1-resistant metastatic lung cancer: a phase 1 trial. Nat Med 2021;27(8):1410–8.

60. Schoenfeld A, Lee S, Paz-Ares L, et al. 458 First phase 2 results of autologous tumor-infiltrating lymphocyte (TIL; LN-145) monotherapy in patients with advanced, immune checkpoint inhibitor-treated, non-small cell lung cancer (NSCLC). Journal for ImmunoTherapy of Cancer 2021;9(Suppl 2):A486–7.

61. Leidner R, Sanjuan Silva N, Huang H, et al. Neoantigen T-Cell receptor gene therapy in pancreatic cancer. N Engl J Med 2022;386(22):2112–9.

62. Kiesgen S, Chicaybam L, Chintala NK, et al. Chimeric antigen receptor (CAR) T-Cell therapy for thoracic malignancies. J Thorac Oncol 2018;13(1):16–26.

63. Sadelain M, Riviere I, Riddell S. Therapeutic T cell engineering. Nature 2017;545(7655):423–31.

64. Maude SL, Frey N, Shaw PA, et al. Chimeric antigen receptor T cells for sustained remissions in leukemia. N Engl J Med 2014;371(16):1507–17.

65. Jamal-Hanjani M, Quezada SA, Larkin J, et al. Translational implications of tumor heterogeneity. Clin Cancer Res 2015;21(6):1258–66.

66. Zhong S, Cui Y, Liu Q, et al. CAR-T cell therapy for lung cancer: a promising but challenging future. J Thorac Dis 2020;12(8):4516–21.

67. Fuca G, Reppel L, Landoni E, et al. Enhancing chimeric antigen receptor T-Cell efficacy in solid tumors. Clin Cancer Res 2020;26(11):2444–51.

68. Kaufman HL, Kohlhapp FJ, Zloza A. Oncolytic viruses: a new class of immunotherapy drugs. Nat Rev Drug Discov 2015;14(9):642–62.

69. Macedo N., Miller D.M., Haq R., et al., Clinical landscape of oncolytic virus research in 2020, J Immunother Cancer, 8 (2), 2020, e001486. https://doi.org/10.1136/jitc-2020-001486.

70. Rudin CM, Pandha HS, Gupta S, et al. Phase Ib KEYNOTE-200: A study of an intravenously delivered oncolytic virus, coxsackievirus A21 in combination with pembrolizumab in advanced NSCLC and bladder cancer patients. Ann Oncol 2018;29.

71. Atkins MB, Lotze MT, Dutcher JP, et al. High-dose recombinant interleukin 2 therapy for patients with metastatic melanoma: analysis of 270 patients treated between 1985 and 1993. J Clin Oncol 1999;17(7):2105–16.

72. Atkins MB, Kunkel L, Sznol M, Rosenberg SA. High-dose recombinant interleukin-2 therapy in patients with metastatic melanoma: long-term survival update. Cancer J Sci Am 2000;6(Suppl 1):S11–4.

73. Bentebibel SE, Hurwitz ME, Bernatchez C, et al. A first-in-human study and biomarker analysis of NKTR-214, a novel IL2Rbetagamma-biased cytokine, in patients with advanced or metastatic solid tumors. Cancer Discov 2019;9(6):711–21.

74. Diab A, Tannir NM, Bentebibel SE, et al. Bempegaldesleukin (NKTR-214) plus nivolumab in patients with advanced solid tumors: phase I dose-escalation study of safety, efficacy, and immune activation (PIVOT-02). Cancer Discov 2020;10(8):1158–73.

75. Janku F, Abdul-Karim R, Azad A, et al. Abstract LB041: THOR-707 (SAR444245), a novel not-alpha IL-2 as monotherapy and in combination with pembrolizumab in advanced/metastatic solid tumors: Interim results from HAMMER, an open-label, multicenter phase 1/2 Study. Cancer Res 2021;81(13_Supplement):LB041.

76. Kubiczkova L, Sedlarikova L, Hajek R, et al. TGF-beta - an excellent servant but a bad master. J Transl Med 2012;10:183.

77. Ciardiello D, Elez E, Tabernero J, et al. Clinical development of therapies targeting TGFβ: current knowledge and future perspectives. Ann Oncol 2020;31(10):1336–49.

78. Gao Y, Souza-Fonseca-Guimaraes F, Bald T, et al. Tumor immunoevasion by the conversion of effector NK cells into type 1 innate lymphoid cells. Nat Immunol 2017;18(9):1004–15.

79. Derynck R, Turley SJ, Akhurst RJ. TGFbeta biology in cancer progression and immunotherapy. Nat Rev Clin Oncol 2021;18(1):9–34.

80. Kim BG, Malek E, Choi SH, et al. Novel therapies emerging in oncology to target the TGF-beta pathway. J Hematol Oncol 2021;14(1):55.

81. Paz-Ares L, Kim TM, Vicente D, et al. Bintrafusp Alfa, a Bifunctional Fusion Protein Targeting TGF-beta and PD-L1, in Second-Line Treatment of Patients With

NSCLC: Results From an Expansion Cohort of a Phase 1 Trial. J Thorac Oncol 2020;15(7):1210–22.

82. Merck Press Release. Merck KGaA, Darmstadt, Germany Announces Update on the INTR@PID Clinical Program Including Lung 037 Study. 2021. Available at: https://wwwemdgroupcom/en/news/bintrafusp-alfa-037-update-20-01-2021html. Accessed September 15, 2022.

83. Ridker PM, MacFadyen JG, Thuren T, et al. Effect of interleukin-1β inhibition with canakinumab on incident lung cancer in patients with atherosclerosis: exploratory results from a randomised, double-blind, placebo-controlled trial. Lancet 2017;390(10105):1833–42.

84. Novartis Press Release. Novartis provides update on Phase III CANOPY-A study evaluating canakinumab as adjuvant treatment in non-small cell lung cancer. 2022. Available at: https://wwwnovartiscom/news/media-releases/novartis-provides-update-phase-iii-canopy-study-evaluating-canakinumab-adjuvant-treatment-non-small-cell-lung-cancer. Accessed September 15, 2022.

85. Spigel D, Jotte R, Nemunaitis J, et al. Randomized Phase 2 Studies of Checkpoint Inhibitors Alone or in Combination With Pegilodecakin in Patients With Metastatic NSCLC (CYPRESS 1 and CYPRESS 2). J Thorac Oncol 2021;16(2):327–33.

86. Wrangle JM, Awad MM, Badin FB, et al. Preliminary data from QUILT 3.055: A phase 2 multi-cohort study of N803 (IL-15 superagonist) in combination with checkpoint inhibitors (CPI). J Clin Oncol 2021;39(15_suppl):2596.

87. Conlon K, Watson DC, Waldmann TA, et al. Phase I study of single agent NIZ985, a recombinant heterodimeric IL-15 agonist, in adult patients with metastatic or unresectable solid tumors. J Immunother Cancer 2021;9(11).

88. Wrangle JM, Velcheti V, Patel MR, et al. ALT-803, an IL-15 superagonist, in combination with nivolumab in patients with metastatic non-small cell lung cancer: a non-randomised, open-label, phase 1b trial. Lancet Oncol 2018;19(5):694–704.

89. Jiang M, Chen P, Wang L, et al. cGAS-STING, an important pathway in cancer immunotherapy. J Hematol Oncol 2020;13(1):81.

90. Flood BA, Higgs EF, Li S, et al. STING pathway agonism as a cancer therapeutic. Immunol Rev 2019;290(1):24–38.

91. Amouzegar A., Chelvanambi M., Filderman J.N., et al., STING agonists as cancer therapeutics, *Cancers*, 13 (11), 2021, 2695.

92. McKeage MJ, Von Pawel J, Reck M, et al. Randomised phase II study of ASA404 combined with carboplatin and paclitaxel in previously untreated advanced non-small cell lung cancer. Br J Cancer 2008;99(12):2006–12.

93. Lara PN Jr, Douillard JY, Nakagawa K, et al. Randomized phase III placebo-controlled trial of carboplatin and paclitaxel with or without the vascular disrupting agent vadimezan (ASA404) in advanced non-small-cell lung cancer. J Clin Oncol 2011;29(22):2965–71.

94. Harrington K.J., Brody J., Ingham M., et al., Preliminary results of the first-in-human (FIH) study of MK-1454, an agonist of stimulator of interferon genes (STING), as monotherapy or in combination with pembrolizumab (pembro) in patients with advanced solid tumors or lymphomas, *Ann Oncol*, 29, 2018, viii712.

95. Zitvogel L, Ma Y, Raoult D, et al. The microbiome in cancer immunotherapy: diagnostic tools and therapeutic strategies. Science 2018;359(6382):1366–70.

96. Derosa L, Hellmann MD, Spaziano M, et al. Negative association of antibiotics on clinical activity of immune checkpoint inhibitors in patients with advanced renal cell and non-small-cell lung cancer. Ann Oncol 2018;29(6):1437–44.

97. Routy B, Le Chatelier E, Derosa L, et al. Gut microbiome influences efficacy of PD-1-based immunotherapy against epithelial tumors. Science 2018; 359(6371):91–7.

98. Soto Chervin C, Gajewski TF. Microbiome-based interventions: therapeutic strategies in cancer immunotherapy. Immunooncol Technol 2020;8:12–20.

99. Sivan A, Corrales L, Hubert N, et al. Commensal Bifidobacterium promotes antitumor immunity and facilitates anti-PD-L1 efficacy. Science 2015;350(6264): 1084–9.

100. Vetizou M, Pitt JM, Daillere R, et al. Anticancer immunotherapy by CTLA-4 blockade relies on the gut microbiota. Science 2015;350(6264):1079–84.

101. McHale D, Francisco-Anderson L, Sandy P, et al. P-325 Oral delivery of a single microbial strain, EDP1503, induces anti-tumor responses via gut-mediated activation of both innate and adaptive immunity. Ann Oncol 2020;31.

102. Dizman N, Meza L, Bergerot P, et al. Nivolumab plus ipilimumab with or without live bacterial supplementation in metastatic renal cell carcinoma: a randomized phase 1 trial. Nat Med 2022;28(4):704–12.

103. Zhang L, Jin Q, Chai D, et al. The correlation between probiotic use and outcomes of cancer patients treated with immune checkpoint inhibitors. Front Pharmacol 2022;13:937874.

104. Spencer CN, McQuade JL, Gopalakrishnan V, et al. Dietary fiber and probiotics influence the gut microbiome and melanoma immunotherapy response. Science 2021;374(6575):1632–40.

105. Damelin M, Zhong W, Myers J, et al. Evolving Strategies for Target Selection for Antibody-Drug Conjugates. Pharm Res (N Y) 2015;32(11):3494–507.

106. Tipton TR, Roghanian A, Oldham RJ, et al. Antigenic modulation limits the effector cell mechanisms employed by type I anti-CD20 monoclonal antibodies. Blood 2015;125(12):1901–9.

107. Donaghy H. Effects of antibody, drug and linker on the preclinical and clinical toxicities of antibody-drug conjugates. mAbs 2016;8(4):659–71.

108. Reuss JE, Gosa L, Liu SV. Antibody drug conjugates in lung cancer: state of the current therapeutic landscape and future developments. Clin Lung Cancer 2021;22(6):483–99.

109. Ritchie M, Tchistiakova L, Scott N. Implications of receptor-mediated endocytosis and intracellular trafficking dynamics in the development of antibody drug conjugates. mAbs 2013;5(1):13–21.

110. Staudacher AH, Brown MP. Antibody drug conjugates and bystander killing: is antigen-dependent internalisation required? Br J Cancer 2017;117(12): 1736–42.

111. de Goeij BE, Satijn D, Freitag CM, et al. High turnover of tissue factor enables efficient intracellular delivery of antibody-drug conjugates. Mol Cancer Ther 2015;14(5):1130–40.

112. Peters C, Brown S. Antibody-drug conjugates as novel anti-cancer chemotherapeutics. Biosci Rep 2015;35(4).

113. Khongorzul P, Ling CJ, Khan FU, et al. Antibody-Drug Conjugates: A Comprehensive Review. Mol Cancer Res 2020;18(1):3–19.

114. Hughes JP, Rees S, Kalindjian SB, et al. Principles of early drug discovery. Br J Pharmacol 2011;162(6):1239–49.

115. Drago JZ, Modi S, Chandarlapaty S. Unlocking the potential of antibody-drug conjugates for cancer therapy. Nat Rev Clin Oncol 2021;18(6):327–44.

116. Goulet DR, Atkins WM. Considerations for the design of antibody-based therapeutics. J Pharm Sci 2020;109(1):74–103.

117. Alley SC, Benjamin DR, Jeffrey SC, et al. Contribution of linker stability to the activities of anticancer immunoconjugates. Bioconjug Chem 2008;19(3):759–65.
118. Nagayama A, Ellisen LW, Chabner B, et al. Antibody-drug conjugates for the treatment of solid tumors: clinical experience and latest developments. Target Oncol 2017;12(6):719–39.
119. Jain N, Smith SW, Ghone S, et al. Current ADC linker chemistry. Pharm Res (N Y) 2015;32(11):3526–40.
120. Tsuchikama K, An Z. Antibody-drug conjugates: recent advances in conjugation and linker chemistries. Protein Cell 2018;9(1):33–46.
121. Goldenberg DM, Cardillo TM, Govindan SV, et al. Trop-2 is a novel target for solid cancer therapy with sacituzumab govitecan (IMMU-132), an antibody-drug conjugate (ADC). Oncotarget 2015;6(26):22496–512.
122. Polson AG, Calemine-Fenaux J, Chan P, et al. Antibody-drug conjugates for the treatment of non-Hodgkin's lymphoma: target and linker-drug selection. Cancer Res 2009;69(6):2358–64.
123. Teicher BA, Chari RV. Antibody conjugate therapeutics: challenges and potential. Clin Cancer Res 2011;17(20):6389–97.
124. Beck A, Goetsch L, Dumontet C, et al. Strategies and challenges for the next generation of antibody-drug conjugates. Nat Rev Drug Discov 2017;16(5):315–37.
125. McCombs JR, Owen SC. Antibody drug conjugates: design and selection of linker, payload and conjugation chemistry. AAPS J 2015;17(2):339–51.
126. Sun X, Ponte JF, Yoder NC, et al. Effects of drug-antibody ratio on pharmacokinetics, biodistribution, efficacy, and tolerability of antibody-maytansinoid conjugates. Bioconjug Chem 2017;28(5):1371–81.
127. Hamblett KJ, Senter PD, Chace DF, et al. Effects of drug loading on the antitumor activity of a monoclonal antibody drug conjugate. Clin Cancer Res 2004;10(20):7063–70.
128. Heist RS, Guarino MJ, Masters G, et al. Therapy of Advanced Non-Small-Cell Lung Cancer With an SN-38-Anti-Trop-2 Drug Conjugate, Sacituzumab Govitecan. J Clin Oncol 2017;35(24):2790–7.
129. Garon E, Johnson M, Lisberg A, et al. MA03.02 TROPION-PanTumor01: Updated Results From the NSCLC Cohort of the Phase 1 Study of Datopotamab Deruxtecan in Solid Tumors. J Thorac Oncol 2021;16(10):S892–3.
130. Yoh K, Goto Y, Thomas M, et al. A randomized, phase 3 study of datopotamab deruxtecan (Dato-DXd; DS-1062) versus docetaxel in previously treated advanced or metastatic non-small cell lung cancer (NSCLC) without actionable genomic alterations (TROPION-Lung01). J Clin Oncol 2021;39(15_suppl):TPS9127.
131. Subramanian J, Katta A, Masood A, et al. Emergence of ERBB2 Mutation as a Biomarker and an Actionable Target in Solid Cancers. Oncol 2019;24(12):e1303–14.
132. Mazières J, Peters S, Lepage B, et al. Lung Cancer that harbors an HER2 mutation: epidemiologic characteristics and therapeutic perspectives. J Clin Oncol 2013;31(16):1997–2003.
133. Arcila ME, Chaft JE, Nafa K, et al. Prevalence, clinicopathologic associations, and molecular spectrum of ERBB2 (HER2) tyrosine kinase mutations in lung adenocarcinomas. Clin Cancer Res 2012;18(18):4910–8.
134. Li BT, Michelini F, Misale S, et al. HER2-mediated internalization of cytotoxic agents in ERBB2 amplified or mutant lung cancers. Cancer Discov 2020;10(5):674–87.

135. Li BT, Shen R, Buonocore D, et al. Ado-trastuzumab emtansine for patients with HER2-mutant lung cancers: results from a phase II basket trial. J Clin Oncol 2018;36(24):2532–7.
136. Iwama E, Zenke Y, Sugawara S, et al. Trastuzumab emtansine for patients with non-small cell lung cancer positive for human epidermal growth factor receptor 2 exon-20 insertion mutations. Eur J Cancer 2022;162:99–106.
137. Hotta K, Aoe K, Kozuki T, et al. A phase II study of trastuzumab emtansine in HER2-positive non-small cell lung cancer. J Thorac Oncol 2018;13(2):273–9.
138. Peters S, Stahel R, Bubendorf L, et al. Trastuzumab emtansine (T-DM1) in patients with previously treated HER2-overexpressing metastatic non-small cell lung cancer: efficacy, safety, and biomarkers. Clin Cancer Res 2019;25(1):64–72.
139. Modi S, Saura C, Yamashita T, et al. Trastuzumab deruxtecan in previously treated HER2-positive breast cancer. N Engl J Med 2020;382(7):610–21.
140. Li BT, Smit EF, Goto Y, et al. Trastuzumab deruxtecan in HER2-mutant non-small-cell lung cancer. N Engl J Med 2022;386(3):241–51.
141. Goto K, Sang-We K, Kubo T, et al. LBA55 - Trastuzumab deruxtecan (T-DXd) in patients (Pts) with HER2-mutant metastatic non-small cell lung cancer (NSCLC): Interim results from the phase 2 DESTINY-Lung02 trial. Ann Oncol 2022;33:S808–69.
142. Li Q, Zhang R, Yan H, et al. Prognostic significance of HER3 in patients with malignant solid tumors. Oncotarget 2017;8(40):67140–51.
143. Scharpenseel H, Hanssen A, Loges S, et al. EGFR and HER3 expression in circulating tumor cells and tumor tissue from non-small cell lung cancer patients. Sci Rep 2019;9(1):7406.
144. Janne PA, Baik C, Su WC, et al. Efficacy and safety of patritumab deruxtecan (HER3-DXd) in EGFR inhibitor-resistant, EGFR-mutated non-small cell lung cancer. Cancer Discov 2022;12(1):74–89.
145. Awad MM, Oxnard GR, Jackman DM, et al. MET exon 14 mutations in non-small-cell lung cancer are associated with advanced age and stage-dependent MET genomic amplification and c-Met overexpression. J Clin Oncol 2016;34(7):721–30.
146. Onozato R, Kosaka T, Kuwano H, et al. Activation of MET by gene amplification or by splice mutations deleting the juxtamembrane domain in primary resected lung cancers. J Thorac Oncol 2009;4(1):5–11.
147. Okuda K, Sasaki H, Yukiue H, et al. Met gene copy number predicts the prognosis for completely resected non-small cell lung cancer. Cancer Sci 2008;99(11):2280–5.
148. Cappuzzo F, Marchetti A, Skokan M, et al. Increased MET gene copy number negatively affects survival of surgically resected non-small-cell lung cancer patients. J Clin Oncol 2009;27(10):1667–74.
149. Cooper AJ, Sequist LV, Lin JJ. Third-generation EGFR and ALK inhibitors: mechanisms of resistance and management. Nat Rev Clin Oncol 2022;19(8):499–514.
150. Strickler JH, Weekes CD, Nemunaitis J, et al. First-in-human phase I, Dose-escalation and -expansion study of telisotuzumab vedotin, an antibody-drug conjugate targeting c-Met, in patients with advanced solid tumors. J Clin Oncol 2018;36(33):3298–306.
151. Camidge DR, Morgensztern D, Heist RS, et al. Phase I Study of 2- or 3-week dosing of telisotuzumab vedotin, an antibody–drug conjugate targeting c-Met,

monotherapy in patients with advanced non–small cell lung carcinoma. Clin Cancer Res 2021;27(21):5781–92.

152. Waqar SN, Redman MW, Arnold SM, et al. A Phase II Study of Telisotuzumab Vedotin in Patients With c-MET-positive Stage IV or Recurrent Squamous Cell Lung Cancer (LUNG-MAP Sub-study S1400K, NCT03574753). Clin Lung Cancer 2021;22(3):170–7.

153. Camidge DR, Barlesi F, Goldman JW, et al. Results of the phase 1b study of ABBV-399 (telisotuzumab vedotin; teliso-v) in combination with erlotinib in patients with c-Met+ non-small cell lung cancer by EGFR mutation status. J Clin Oncol 2019;37(15_suppl):3011.

154. Hammarstrom S. The carcinoembryonic antigen (CEA) family: structures, suggested functions and expression in normal and malignant tissues. Semin Cancer Biol 1999;9(2):67–81.

155. Tong G, Xu W, Zhang G, et al. The role of tissue and serum carcinoembryonic antigen in stages I to III of colorectal cancer-A retrospective cohort study. Cancer Med 2018;7(11):5327–38.

156. Decary S, Berne PF, Nicolazzi C, et al. Preclinical Activity of SAR408701: a novel Anti-CEACAM5-maytansinoid Antibody-drug Conjugate for the Treatment of CEACAM5-positive Epithelial Tumors. Clin Cancer Res 2020;26(24):6589–99.

157. Gazzah A, Bedard PL, Hierro C, et al. Safety, pharmacokinetics, and antitumor activity of the anti-CEACAM5-DM4 antibody-drug conjugate tusamitamab ravtansine (SAR408701) in patients with advanced solid tumors: first-in-human dose-escalation study. Ann Oncol 2022;33(4):416–25.

158. Gazzah A, Ricordel C, Cousin S, et al. Efficacy and safety of the antibody-drug conjugate (ADC) SAR408701 in patients (pts) with non-squamous non-small cell lung cancer (NSQ NSCLC) expressing carcinoembryonic antigen-related cell adhesion molecule 5 (CEACAM5). J Clin Oncol 2020;38(15_suppl):9505.

159. Saunders LR, Bankovich AJ, Anderson WC, et al. A DLL3-targeted antibody-drug conjugate eradicates high-grade pulmonary neuroendocrine tumor-initiating cells in vivo. Sci Transl Med 2015;7(302):302ra136.

160. Rudin CM, Pietanza MC, Bauer TM, et al. Rovalpituzumab tesirine, a DLL3-targeted antibody-drug conjugate, in recurrent small-cell lung cancer: a first-in-human, first-in-class, open-label, phase 1 study. Lancet Oncol 2017;18(1):42–51.

161. Morgensztern D, Besse B, Greillier L, et al. Efficacy and safety of rovalpituzumab tesirine in third-line and beyond patients with DLL3-expressing, relapsed/refractory small-cell lung cancer: results from the phase II TRINITY study. Clin Cancer Res 2019;25(23):6958–66.

162. Blackhall F, Jao K, Greillier L, et al. Efficacy and safety of rovalpituzumab tesirine compared with topotecan as second-line therapy in DLL3-High SCLC: results from the phase 3 TAHOE study. J Thorac Oncol 2021;16(9):1547–58.

163. Morgensztern D, Johnson M, Rudin CM, et al. SC-002 in patients with relapsed or refractory small cell lung cancer and large cell neuroendocrine carcinoma: Phase 1 study. Lung Cancer 2020;145:126–31.

164. Khan SA, Sun Z, Dahlberg S, et al. Efficacy and Safety of Glembatumumab Vedotin in Patients With Advanced or Metastatic Squamous Cell Carcinoma of the Lung (PrECOG 0504). JTO Clin Res Rep 2021;2(5):100166.

165. Kindler HL, Novello S, Fennell D, et al. OA 02.01 randomized phase II study of anetumab ravtansine or vinorelbine in patients with metastatic pleural mesothelioma. J Thorac Oncol 2017;12(11):S1746.

166. Hafeez U., Parakh S., Gan H.K., et al., Antibody-drug conjugates for cancer therapy, *Molecules*, 25 (20), 2020, 4764.
167. Coates JT, Sun S, Leshchiner I, et al. Parallel genomic alterations of antigen and payload targets mediate polyclonal acquired clinical resistance to sacituzumab govitecan in triple-negative breast cancer. Cancer Discov 2021;11(10):2436–45.
168. Nicolo E, Giugliano F, Ascione L, et al. Combining antibody-drug conjugates with immunotherapy in solid tumors: current landscape and future perspectives. Cancer Treat Rev 2022;106:102395.